MW00452769

Pediatric Anesthesia:
A Guide for the Non-Pediatric
Anesthesia Provider
Part I

Edited by

Bharathi Gourkanti

Irwin Gratz

Grace Dippo
Department of Anesthesiology,
Cooper Medical School of Rowan University,
Cooper University Health Care,
Camden, NJ
USA

Nathalie Peiris
Department of Anesthesiology and Perioperative Medicine,
Nemours Children's Health,
Delaware Valley,
Wilmington, DE
USA

&

Dinesh K. Choudhry
Department of Anesthesiology,
Shriners Hospitals for Children,
Philadelphia, PA
USA

Pediatric Anesthesia: A Guide for the Non-Pediatric Anesthesia Provider

Part I

Editors: Bharathi Gourkanti, Irwin Gratz and Grace Dippo

ISBN (Online): 978-981-5036-27-5

ISBN (Print): 978-981-5036-28-2

ISBN (Paperback): 978-981-5036-29-9

© 2022, Bentham Books imprint.

Published by Bentham Science Publishers Pte. Ltd. Sharjah. All Rights Reserved.

BENTHAM SCIENCE PUBLISHERS LTD.
End User License Agreement (for non-institutional, personal use)

This is an agreement between you and Bentham Science Publishers Ltd. Please read this License Agreement carefully before using the ebook/echapter/ejournal (**"Work"**). Your use of the Work constitutes your agreement to the terms and conditions set forth in this License Agreement. If you do not agree to these terms and conditions then you should not use the Work.

Bentham Science Publishers agrees to grant you a non-exclusive, non-transferable limited license to use the Work subject to and in accordance with the following terms and conditions. This License Agreement is for non-library, personal use only. For a library / institutional / multi user license in respect of the Work, please contact: permission@benthamscience.net.

Usage Rules:

1. All rights reserved: The Work is the subject of copyright and Bentham Science Publishers either owns the Work (and the copyright in it) or is licensed to distribute the Work. You shall not copy, reproduce, modify, remove, delete, augment, add to, publish, transmit, sell, resell, create derivative works from, or in any way exploit the Work or make the Work available for others to do any of the same, in any form or by any means, in whole or in part, in each case without the prior written permission of Bentham Science Publishers, unless stated otherwise in this License Agreement.
2. You may download a copy of the Work on one occasion to one personal computer (including tablet, laptop, desktop, or other such devices). You may make one back-up copy of the Work to avoid losing it.
3. The unauthorised use or distribution of copyrighted or other proprietary content is illegal and could subject you to liability for substantial money damages. You will be liable for any damage resulting from your misuse of the Work or any violation of this License Agreement, including any infringement by you of copyrights or proprietary rights.

Disclaimer:

Bentham Science Publishers does not guarantee that the information in the Work is error-free, or warrant that it will meet your requirements or that access to the Work will be uninterrupted or error-free. The Work is provided "as is" without warranty of any kind, either express or implied or statutory, including, without limitation, implied warranties of merchantability and fitness for a particular purpose. The entire risk as to the results and performance of the Work is assumed by you. No responsibility is assumed by Bentham Science Publishers, its staff, editors and/or authors for any injury and/or damage to persons or property as a matter of products liability, negligence or otherwise, or from any use or operation of any methods, products instruction, advertisements or ideas contained in the Work.

Limitation of Liability:

In no event will Bentham Science Publishers, its staff, editors and/or authors, be liable for any damages, including, without limitation, special, incidental and/or consequential damages and/or damages for lost data and/or profits arising out of (whether directly or indirectly) the use or inability to use the Work. The entire liability of Bentham Science Publishers shall be limited to the amount actually paid by you for the Work.

General:

1. Any dispute or claim arising out of or in connection with this License Agreement or the Work (including non-contractual disputes or claims) will be governed by and construed in accordance with the laws of Singapore. Each party agrees that the courts of the state of Singapore shall have exclusive jurisdiction to settle any dispute or claim arising out of or in connection with this License Agreement or the Work (including non-contractual disputes or claims).
2. Your rights under this License Agreement will automatically terminate without notice and without the

need for a court order if at any point you breach any terms of this License Agreement. In no event will any delay or failure by Bentham Science Publishers in enforcing your compliance with this License Agreement constitute a waiver of any of its rights.

3. You acknowledge that you have read this License Agreement, and agree to be bound by its terms and conditions. To the extent that any other terms and conditions presented on any website of Bentham Science Publishers conflict with, or are inconsistent with, the terms and conditions set out in this License Agreement, you acknowledge that the terms and conditions set out in this License Agreement shall prevail.

Bentham Science Publishers Pte. Ltd.
80 Robinson Road #02-00
Singapore 068898
Singapore
Email: subscriptions@benthamscience.net

CONTENTS

PREFACE

I have been practicing the art and science of anesthesia for almost three decades, and for the past 23 years as a pediatric anesthesiologist. It is my strong belief that providing anesthesia for children is not just a job; it is a privilege. Parents trust anesthesia providers with their child's life, which they value more than their own lives. Guarding a child's life, taking charge of their care, and handing them back safely to their family is a great honor and an immense responsibility. When I was approached to edit a textbook on pediatric anesthesia, I did not wish to produce a formal or standard text, but to make it more informative, clinically oriented, practical, and user-friendly.

WHO THIS BOOK IS WRITTEN FOR

Though this is written for general anesthesia providers who occasionally are required to provide pediatric anesthesia, many others who provide pediatric anesthesia, sedation, pain control, resuscitation, or emergency care may also benefit. This book is an excellent starting point for providers in training, and a handy clinical reference for those who are many years into clinical practice. Our goal is to provide a source with the most critical and clinically relevant information that can be easily referenced by a busy practitioner in the middle of the night.

WHO CONTRIBUTED TO THIS BOOK

Every member of the anesthesia care team has a unique perspective and an abundance of knowledge to share. Our editors and contributors include board-certified pediatric anesthesiologists, general anesthesiologists who occasionally treat children, pediatric anesthesia fellows in training, anesthesia residents, and certified registered nurse anesthetists. Our collective knowledge and teamwork have given this text its unique and approachable voice.

WHAT IS IN THIS BOOK

Our goal in this book was to present the scientific data as it relates to current clinical practice in an approachable and easily understood fashion. The information presented ranges from basic topics that will be useful for residents and nurses preparing for their exams, to a comprehensive analysis of the current controversies and common practices in pediatric anesthesia. We summarize the information into tables, figures, and illustrations where possible for easy reference. We review the key differences in a pediatric patient's anatomy, physiology, and pharmacology for those providers accustomed to treating adults, and outline how to modify anesthetic techniques accordingly. We highlight topics critical to the safe perioperative care of infants and children. A thorough discussion of the management of common pediatric comorbidities is included, and commonly encountered anesthetic complications and their treatments are presented.

THANKS

I am extremely grateful to all the contributors for bringing their invaluable knowledge, various points of view, and unique expertise to this book.

I thank my co-editors Dr. Irwin Gratz, Dr. Grace Dippo, Dr. Nathalie Peiris and Dr. Dinesh K.

Choudhry, for their knowledge, competence, patience, and scrupulous attention to detail to make this manuscript more meaningful.

My warmest thanks to Hira Aftab, Manager-Publications, and our Project Coordinator whose unrelenting support has helped make this project possible.

Finally, I would like to thank Bentham Science for providing the opportunity to create this body of work.

SUMMARY

In summary, we designed this book for all those who routinely or occasionally provide pediatric anesthesia with theoretical, clinical, and practical knowledge, and a readily available quick reference.

We sincerely hope this book will be of help to you in providing the safe practice of pediatric anesthesia.

Bharathi Gourkanti
Associate Professor of Clinical Anesthesiology,
Department of Anesthesiology,
Cooper Medical School of Rowan University,
Cooper University Health Care,
Camden, NJ,
USA

List of Contributors

Abraham G. Oommen	Department of Anesthesiology and Perioperative Medicine, Nemours A.I. duPont Hospital for Children, Sidney Kimmel Medical College at Thomas Jefferson University, Wilmington, DE, USA
Andrea Gomez-Morad	Department of Anesthesiology, Boston Children's Hospital, Boston, MA, USA
Arvind Chandrankantan	Department of Anesthesiology, Texas Children's Hospital, Houston, TX, USA
Aysha Hasan	Department of Anesthesiology, St. Christopher's Hospital for Children, Philadelphia, PA, USA
Bharathi Gourkanti	Department of Anesthesiology, Cooper Medical School of Rowan University, Cooper University Health Care, Camden, NJ, USA
Dinesh K. Choudhry	Department of Anesthesiology, Shriners Hospital for Children, Philadelphia, PA, USA
Fatimah Habib	Department of Anesthesiology, Cooper Medical School of Rowan University, Cooper University Health Care, Camden, NJ, USA
Grace Dippo	Department of Anesthesiology, Cooper Medical School of Rowan University, Cooper University Health Care, Camden, NJ, USA
Ian Brotman	Department of Anesthesiology, Cooper Medical School of Rowan University, Cooper University Health Care, Camden, NJ, USA
Kathleen Kwiatt	Department of Anesthesiology, Cooper Medical School of Rowan University, Cooper University Health Care, Camden, NJ, USA
Malgorzata Lutwin-Kawalec	Department of Anesthesia and Perioperative Medicine, Nemours Children's Health, Wilmington, DE, USA
Manish Purohit	Department of Anesthesiology and Perioperative Medicine, Nemours A.I. duPont Hospital for Children, Sidney Kimmel Medical College at Thomas Jefferson University, Wilmington, DE, USA
Mark A. Dobish	Department of Anesthesiology, MedStar Georgetown University Hospital, Washington D.C., USA
Marlo DiDonna	Department of Anesthesiology, Cooper Medical School of Rowan University, Cooper University Health Care, Camden, NJ, USA
Mary Theroux	Department of Anesthesiology and Perioperative Medicine, Nemours A.I. duPont Hospital for Children, Sidney Kimmel Medical College at Thomas Jefferson University, Wilmington, DE, USA
Melissa Lester	Department of Anesthesiology, Cooper Medical School of Rowan University, Cooper University Health Care, Camden, NJ, USA
Michael R. Schwartz	Department of Anesthesiology, Cooper Medical School of Rowan University, Cooper University Health Care, Camden, NJ, USA
Nathalie Peiris	Department of Anesthesiology and Perioperative Medicine, Nemours Children's Health, Delaware Valley, Wilmington, DE, USA

Pravin Taneja   Department of Anesthesiology, St. Christopher's Hospital for Children, Philadelphia, PA, USA

Rachel Koehler   Department of Anesthesiology, Cooper Medical School of Rowan University, Cooper University Health Care, Camden, NJ, USA

Rosemary De La Cruz   Department of Anesthesiology, Cooper Medical School of Rowan University, Cooper University Health Care, Camden, NJ, USA

Sabina DiCindio   Department of Anesthesiology and Perioperative Medicine, Nemours A.I. duPont Hospital for Children, Sidney Kimmel Medical College at Thomas Jefferson University, Wilmington, DE, USA

Shaharyar Ahmad   Department of Anesthesiology, Cooper Medical School of Rowan University, Cooper University Health Care, Camden, NJ, USA

Sheaba Varghese   Department of Anesthesia and Perioperative Medicine, Nemours Children's Health, Delaware Valley, Wilmington, DE, USA

Sindhu Samba   Department of Anesthesiology, Cooper Medical School of Rowan University, Cooper University Health Care, Camden, NJ, USA

Yue Monica Li   Department of Anesthesiology, Cooper Medical School of Rowan University, Cooper University Health Care, Camden, NJ, USA

CHAPTER 1

Anatomy and Physiology

Rachel Koehler[1], Pravin Taneja[2] and Nathalie Peiris[3]

[1] *Department of Anesthesiology, Cooper Medical School of Rowan University, Cooper University Health Care, Camden, NJ, USA*

[2] *Department of Anesthesiology, St. Christopher's Hospital for Children, Philadelphia, PA, USA*

[3] *Department of Anesthesiology and Perioperative Medicine, Nemours Children's Health, Delaware Valley, Wilmington, DE, USA*

Abstract: Knowing the anatomical differences between the pediatric patient and the adult patient are important for perioperative anesthetic care. This chapter will describe the head, neck, and airway anatomical differences in pediatric patients and their perioperative implications. In addition, this chapter will explore the physiology of different organ systems in the pediatric patient and the perioperative considerations for the anesthesia provider.

Keywords: Anatomy and physiology, Pediatric airway anatomy, Pediatric cardiovascular physiology, Pediatric endocrine physiology, Pediatric hematology physiology, Pediatric renal and hepatic physiology, Pediatric respiratory physiology, Temperature regulation.

AIRWAY

The pediatric airway is unique compared to the adult airway. These differences at times can cause dire consequences when not in care of experienced hands [1]. See (Fig. **1**) below for comparison.

Infants have a larger head size compared to their body causing difficulties with proper positioning. A shoulder roll is helpful to raise the shoulders to better align the oral, pharyngeal, and tracheal axises for a more optimized view [2]. The first thing a provider will notice is that the tongue of the infant is larger compared to the size of the oral cavity. This makes obstruction (particularly when doing a mask induction) more likely to occur and the anesthesia provider should be prepared to manage an obstructed airway. In addition, it makes it more difficult to

* **Corresponding author Bharathi Gourkanti:** Department of Anesthesiology, Cooper Medical School of Rowan University, Cooper University Health Care, Camden, NJ, United States; E-mail: gourkantibharathi@cooperhealth.edu

Bharathi Gourkanti, Irwin Gratz, Grace Dippo, Nathalie Peiris and Dinesh K. Choudhry (Eds.)
All rights reserved-© 2022 Bentham Science Publishers

"sweep" it out of the way to obtain a view of the vocal cords. The epiglottis in children is narrow, omega-shaped, floppy, and long which makes it challenging to directly lift in order to obtain a good view of the vocal cords. The larynx is closer to the head (at the level of C3-4 *versus* C4-5) and appears to be more anterior compared to adults [3]. This produces a more acute angle between the different airway axises, making visualization more difficult. The anterior attachment of the vocal cords of an infant is also angled more caudally compared to an adult (which are attached perpendicular to the trachea) which may cause difficulty with guiding the endotracheal tube through the glottic opening. Due to these anatomic differences, a Miller blade is typically used over a Macintosh blade because it allows for better control and lift of the epiglottis and it is also able to move the large tongue out of the way [3 - 5]. The anesthesia provider managing the airway should also know that the narrowest part of the pediatric airway is the cricoid cartilage, in comparison to adults where it is the glottic opening. This is important because the endotracheal tube may pass through the glottic opening but encounter resistance in the subglottic region. It is thought that the differences in the subglottic region of the airway become similar to adults by the age of 10 [6].

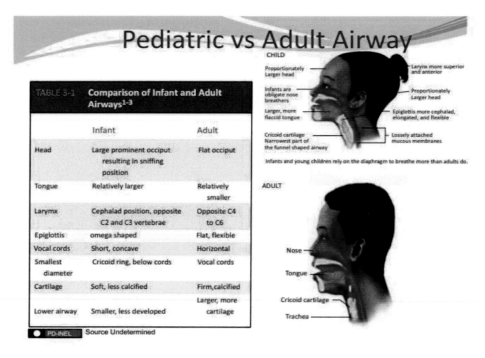

Fig. (1). Comparison of the pediatric and adult airways.

This reported "funnel shaped" airway has led to the debate between using cuffed *versus* uncuffed endotracheal tubes in pediatric patients. The cricoid ring is the only complete ring of cartilage in the airway and thus, does not have any distensibility. The concern with cuffed endotracheal tubes is that the balloon will be overfilled, leading to mucosal ischemia, fibrosis, and edema to the surrounding anatomy causing inflammation and reduced airway diameter upon extubation. This would lead to post-extubation complications such as croup or subglottic stenosis. This is particularly concerning for the youngest population, where any decrease in airway diameter would increase airway resistance significantly. The benefits of an uncuffed endotracheal tube are the removal of the risk of the cuff causing mucosal trauma, and a larger internal diameter of the endotracheal tube which allows for easier suctioning and lower airway resistance [7]. However, drawbacks of an uncuffed endotracheal tube include increased risk of multiple tube exchanges due to inability to adequately ventilate secondary to an air leak. An adequate fit is when a leak occurs at an airway pressure of 15-25 cm of H_2O pressure [8]. Multiple tube exchanges could lead to increased risk of trauma due to multiple airway manipulation attempts in addition to increasing operating room contamination due to leak of volatile anesthetics.

A Cochrane Review from 2017 which looked at the benefit of using a cuffed *versus* uncuffed endotracheal tube for general anesthesia in pediatric patients under 8 years old was not able to draw definite conclusions [9]. However, a meta-analysis done a year later did find that cuffed endotracheal tubes showed no difference in duration of intubation, reintubation occurrence, accidental extubation rate, croup occurrence and racemic epinephrine use during the intubation process and no increased rate of croup post-extubation [10].

Respiratory Physiology

The respiratory center in a neonate is not fully developed at birth. Neonates have an impaired response to hypoxia and hypercarbia. Preterm infants will typically have the paradoxical reaction of decreased respiratory rate and apnea in response to hypoxia and hypercapnia. An increased ventilatory drive does not occur in full term infants until after the first week of life. High concentration of inspired oxygen in a neonate also leads to depressed respiratory drive and complications such as retinopathy of prematurity and bronchopulmonary dysplasia due to the inability to break down oxygen free radicals. However, a low concentration of oxygen has been found to stimulate a neonate's respiratory drive [11]. In addition, the medications used commonly in the anesthesia world can dull the response to hypercapnia and hypoxia [12]. Due to the combination of general anesthesia and a neonate's immature response to hypoxia and hypercapnia, life-threatening apneas can occur in neonates - particularly in premature ones. This risk is typically highest in the first 12 hours postoperatively. This is why it is recommended to keep premature infants (those under 60 weeks post conceptual age) for overnight monitoring of postoperative apnea [6].

Infants are obligate nasal breathers. This is due to immature coordination between breathing and swallowing mechanisms. The ability to switch to oral breathing does not occur until 3-5 months [6]. Thus, it is important to remember to ensure nasal passages are clear because the infant may not have the ability to switch to oral breathing when its nasal passages are obstructed. One can do this by gentle nasal suctioning with a soft suction prior to induction and extubation.

The main purpose of the lungs is to oxygenate the blood and to ventilate carbon dioxide from the body [13, 14]. The pulmonary system overall is incomplete when a baby is first born and matures over a child's development [15]. The lungs of an infant have less alveoli compared to adults. They also do not have the interconnections between them or as much elastic tissue around the alveoli which help prevent atelectasis [16 - 18]. Infants have defined tidal volumes which cannot change during inspiration due to their chest anatomy. The intercostal muscles are poorly developed and the ribs of pediatric patients are horizontally placed and result in significantly more chest wall compliance compared to adults. This increased chest wall compliance results in the infant relying solely on the diaphragm for inspiration - thus increasing the work of breathing for the infant. In addition, the diaphragm in the infant and neonate has proportionally less type 1 muscle fibers compared to an adult - which makes the younger population more prone to respiratory failure due to fatigue. Pediatric patients also have lower functional residual capacity (FRC) and smaller lung volumes compared to adults. This leads to a higher closing volume than FRC, which results in the premature closure of small airways. Pediatric patients compensate for this through different respiratory mechanics such as increased respiratory rate, quick expiratory times, and laryngeal adduction [3, 19 - 22]. However, under general anesthesia, these mechanics are ablated. During anesthesia, a provider should provide at least 5 cm H_2O of PEEP in an attempt to avoid atelectasis and conserve FRC [23]. The ratio of their minute ventilation to their FRC is much higher than it is in an adult. They also have a much higher oxygen consumption rate at 7 mL/kg/min compared to an adult which is roughly 3 mL/kg/min [8]. All of these factors combined make an infant more susceptible to desaturation during induction of anesthesia at a much faster rate [11].

Inhalational induction is usually used for children *versus* intravenous induction due to difficulty getting an IV in an awake patient and the rate of induction is often quicker in this patient population. Lerman *et al.* found that blood-gas partition coefficients were about 18% less than those in adults with a p-value of

<0.005. The fast rising rate of alveolar anesthetic partial pressure is due to multiple factors. Infants have an increased cardiac output per kg and have greater perfusion of vascular organs. As mentioned previously, they have a greater ratio of minute ventilation to their FRC and thus have a greater alveolar ventilation [24, 25].

Cardiac Physiology

The main role of the heart is to deliver oxygenated blood from the lungs to the various organs and tissues throughout the body. There are a multitude of structures, signals, and steps involved in the formation of the heart and vascular system. This process starts during the third week of gestation and is completed around the seventh week [26]. A provider should be aware that when something goes awry in one of these steps this could lead to a congenital heart defect. The incidence of congenital heart disease in the United States is roughly 1%, which is around 40,000 births per year [27, 28].

Fetal circulation, neonatal circulation, and adult circulation vary greatly from one another and every child must transition through each of these. During gestation (Fig. **2**), oxygenated blood comes from the placenta *via* the umbilical vein. Half the oxygenated blood goes to the liver and supplies oxygen while the other half bypasses the liver *via* the ductus venosus and travels *via* the inferior vena cava to the right atrium. The oxygenated blood goes through the right atrium to the left atrium *via* the patent foramen ovale, down to the left ventricle and pumps oxygenated blood through the aorta, brain and upper half of the body. Deoxygenated blood comes from two sources; the inferior vena cava (bringing the deoxygenated blood from the lower half of the body) and the superior vena cava (bringing deoxygenated blood from the upper half of the body). This deoxygenated blood passes from the right atrium to the right ventricle and up to the pulmonary artery. However, pulmonary vascular resistance is high, causing blood to flow through the ductus arteriosus which connects the pulmonary artery to the descending aorta. Thus, deoxygenated blood bypasses the lungs, travels through the descending aorta (some supplying the lower half of the body with blood) to the umbilical artery back to the placenta for reoxygenation. Thus, the fetal circulation is said to run in parallel (with the left ventricle supplying oxygenated blood to the brain and upper half of body while the right ventricle supplying blood with less oxygen to the placenta and lower half of the body) [11].

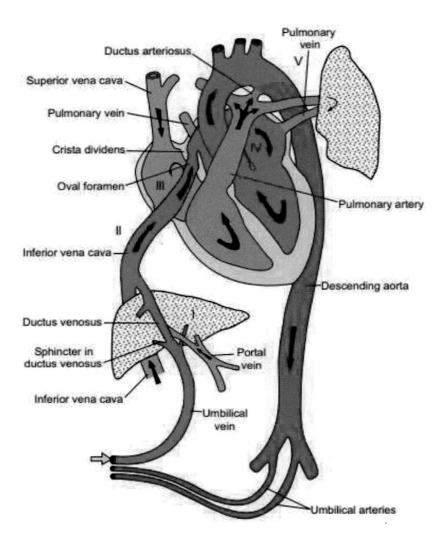

Fig. (2). Fetal circulation.

Once a baby is born, their circulation must transition from fetal life to neonatal life (Fig. **3**). When a baby takes their first breath this causes the pulmonary arterial pressure to dramatically decrease. After the placenta is separated from the baby this causes the systemic vascular resistance to increase. This leads to change in flow and helps to increase pulmonary artery blood flow and return of oxygenated blood to the left atrium. Ductus venosus narrows and decreases right atrium pressure. The increase in left atrium pressure compared to right atrium pressure results in functional closure of the patent foramen ovale. The rise in partial pressure of oxygen and decrease in prostaglandin production due to placenta removal causes constriction of the ductus arteriosus. This functionally closes in 24-48 hours and permanently closes after 4-8 weeks [11].

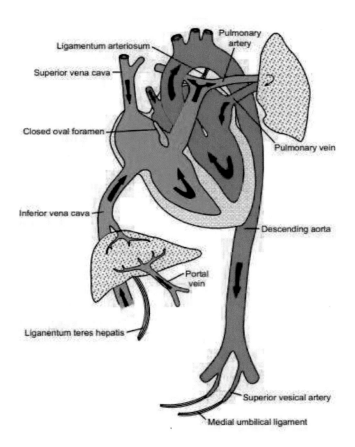

Fig. (3). Neonatal circulation.

The transitional period is very vulnerable and changes during the perioperative period could cause increase in pulmonary vascular resistance and reversal to fetal circulation. Factors that one must be mindful of include hypoxia, hypercarbia, hypothermia or acidosis in a neonate. These conditions can cause increased pulmonary vascular resistance and lead to right to left shunting through the ductus arteriosus. One way to monitor for this intraoperatively would be to place two pulse oximeters on a neonatal patient - one preductal such as the right hand and one post-ductal such as a lower extremity. An increase in 3% of oxygen saturation in a pre-ductal pulse oximeter compared to a post-ductal pulse oximeter indicates a right to left shunt [11]. Persistent fetal circulation and right to left shunting leads to decreased perfusion to systemic circulation resulting in peripheral tissue ischemia and a prolonged time for anesthesia induction *via* inhalational induction.

The newborn heart has less actin and myosin proteins and is less compliant than the adult heart. When a newborn heart has an increase of volume within their ventricles, it does not respond as well based on the well-known Frank-Starling curve due to the rigidity present. The main way an infant increases their cardiac output is through their heart rate which is why children are known to be heart rate dependent. See Table **1** below for normal hemodynamic values.

Table 1. Average hemodynamic values [29 - 32].

	Newborn	1 mo - 1 yo	1 yo - 5 yo	5 yo - 12 yo	≥ 13 yo (adult values)
BP	60/30	90-110/45-65	95-115/45-65	100-120/50-80	<120/<80
MAP	40	60-80	62-82	67-93	≥ 65
HR	100-165	100-140	80-130	65-115	60-100

Renal Physiology

Renal function in a pediatric patient is not fully formed at birth. This is due to low renal perfusion pressure and immature glomerular and tubular function [33]. The kidneys play an important role with fluid, pH, electrolyte balance, and drug metabolism and excretion. Anesthesia providers should be aware that the pediatric population can experience decreased creatinine clearance, compromised electrolyte balance, and issues maintaining proper concentration of urine [34]. The newborn's glomerular filtration rate (GFR) is low at around 40 ml/min/1.73 m^2 and does not reach adult range until around two years of age [35]. Due to this immaturity of renal clearance, metabolism of many common drugs used during anesthesia is slowed which can lead to prolonged duration of action of medications. These drugs include antibiotics, narcotics, and neuromuscular blocking drugs. Thus, one could consider a pediatric patient as if he or she is similar to an adult patient with renal failure (in particular to antibiotic dosing and in conjunction with a pediatric pharmacist)-with longer intervals between redosing. In extremely premature patients, one can also consider using medications that completely bypass renal metabolism when possible such as cisatracurium for neuromuscular blockade. Since renal blood flow and GFR values are decreased in the pediatric population, fluids should not be carelessly given [36, 37]. Administration of fluids should be given in a volume-controlled device such as on an infusion pump or Buretrol.

Electrolyte disturbances occur due to decreased absorption in the renal tubules. This puts pediatric patients at risk for electrolyte derangements such as hyponatremia, hypoglycemia, and metabolic acidosis. Thus, if a pediatric child comes to the operating room with maintenance fluids or TPN, it is prudent to continue those fluids to avoid electrolyte disturbances.

Hematologic Physiology

Blood within our body is mainly made up of red blood cells, white blood cells, platelets, plasma, and proteins. The hematological system has a multitude of functions including delivering oxygen to different tissues, fighting infections, and hemostasis. The bone marrow is the main site of hematopoiesis at birth. When the infant is experiencing some type of stress, extramedullary enters can be seen in the liver, lymph nodes, spleen, and paravertebral regions [38, 39]. A clinician has to be mindful of the values of each cell line and how they differ from adults. Platelet counts in neonates are roughly the same as adults [40]. The average lymphocyte count is also within the range of adults [41]. A newborn is born with an average hemoglobin of 16.8 g/dL due to the production of fetal hemoglobin and adult hemoglobin A [6]. After a child is born, hemoglobin values start to fall due to decrease in fetal hemoglobin and slow increase of erythropoietin levels. This nadir is reached around 8-12 weeks of age and decreases to a hemoglobin level of 9.5-11 g/dL [42, 43]. Preterm infants have a quicker reduction and lower nadir values of hemoglobin compared to term infants [44]. This phenomenon is physiologic and occurs for a few reasons. In healthy adults, red blood cells have an average lifespan of 120 days. This timeline is cut in half in infants, where they will only last for 60-70 days. Preterm infants' red blood cells have an even shorter life span of 35-50 days. Preterm infants are also at a disadvantage because the majority of iron transfer from the mother occurs late in the last trimester [45, 46]. While the baby is *in utero* the oxygen saturation is around 50%. The oxygen saturation dramatically increases to 95% once the baby is born and takes their first breath. This causes a downregulation of erythropoietin which is the hormone that stimulates the production of red blood cells. During a child's development the hemoglobin concentration gradually increases and reaches adult values at the age of adolescence [47]. Typical treatment of anemia is to limit blood draws or give blood transfusions [48].

Premature babies also may have an increased risk of bleeding due to decreased synthesis of vitamin K dependent coagulation factors and thrombocytopenia due to association with concerning neonatal pathologies such as retinopathy of prematurity, intraventricular hemorrhage, and sepsis [49]. One treatment that helps prevent intraventricular hemorrhage is vitamin K injection which is given prophylactically to babies when they are first born [50]. If a premature patient is scheduled for surgery, it is prudent to check a platelet count and coagulation levels in order to have the pertinent blood products available.

Gastrointestinal Physiology

The gastrointestinal and hepatic systems carry out many functions, including breaking down foods, processing and absorbing nutrients, metabolizing drugs, glucose control, and removal of waste [51, 52]. The gastrointestinal system is not fully formed at birth and intestinal motility is stimulated by enteral feeds. Breast milk has been shown to decrease common ailments a preterm infant may encounter such as necrotizing enterocolitis, retinopathy of prematurity, and sepsis [53 - 55]. Lactose is the main carbohydrate found in a baby's diet and it is a disaccharide containing glucose and galactose.

Around 10% of healthy infants can experience hypoglycemia, and this rate can go even higher in premature, small for gestational age, intrauterine growth restriction, or babies of diabetic mothers. There are multiple processes behind this including decreased glycogen storage, increased energy demands, insufficient muscle mass which would provide amino acids for gluconeogenesis, and low-fat stores which would be used to make ketones [56 - 60]. The American Academy of Pediatrics defines hypoglycemia as < 47 mg/dL [61]. There are many signs and symptoms of hypoglycemia including diaphoresis, irritability, pallor, hunger, tachycardia, vomiting, apnea, hypotonia, seizures, and coma which could lead to death [62]. However, under general anesthesia, these symptoms are often masked. Oftentimes, due to the increased catecholamine release from stresses of surgery, pediatric patients may not require as much glucose supplementation. If an anesthesia provider is suspicious about hypoglycemia, one should immediately obtain a point-of-care glucose level which is quick and easy. Treatment is with intravenous dextrose [6].

The liver is the primary source of drug metabolism in the body. Functional hepatic metabolism does not reach adult levels until 1 year of age. This is due to immaturity of liver enzymes, reduction of hepatic proteins (such as albumin) and low hepatic perfusion pressure (which results in less drug delivery to the liver) [6]. All of these factors result in decreased drug metabolism and caution should be taken in the administration of medications that are highly protein bound (such as certain antibiotics, antiepileptics), or rely on perfusion-limited hepatic clearance (such as propofol or narcotics) in order to avoid toxicity. Another consideration would be to bypass hepatic metabolism altogether by using medications such as cisatracurium for neuromuscular blockade and remifentanil for opioids. More about pharmacodynamics will be discussed in the pharmacology chapter.

Temperature Physiology

Humans are normothermic and maintain an internal body temperature at ~37 degrees Celsius plus or minus 0.2 degrees Celsius [63]. Temperature is sensed by myelinated A-delta and unmyelinated C nerve fibers and travels along the spinothalamic tracts in the anterior spinal cord to convey information to the hypothalamus [64 - 66]. The hypothalamus is the primary regulator of internal body temperature. If body temperature is perceived to be above threshold, sweating and vasodilation will occur. Conversely, if body temperature is perceived to be below threshold, vasoconstriction, and shivering will occur [67].

The administration of general anesthesia changes this normal thermoregulation. Volatile anesthetics, propofol and narcotics such as morphine have vasodilatory effects and inhibit hypothalamic thermoregulation by decreasing the shivering threshold and increasing the sweating threshold as seen in Fig. (**4**) below.

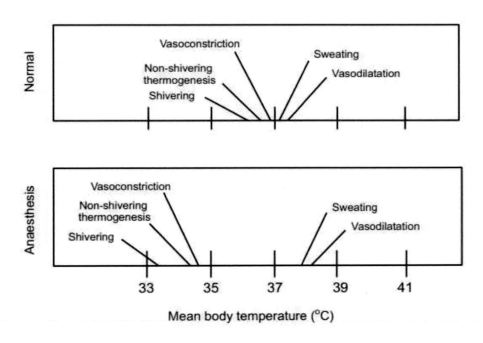

Fig. (4). Comparison of changes in thermogenesis under anesthesia.

There are 3 phases of hypothermia under general anesthesia: rapid decline, slow decline, and steady state. The first phase involves redistribution of heat from the core to the periphery. This causes a 1-2 degree Celsius drop in temperature. The slow decline is when heat loss is greater than heat production. Once the heat loss and production are equal, the patient is said to be in a steady state [68].

There are four modes of heat loss that occur under general anesthesia in the operating room as seen in Fig. (5). Radiation is the transfer of heat to the surrounding air *via* photons. This is the primary mode of heat loss during the redistribution of heat from the core to the periphery.

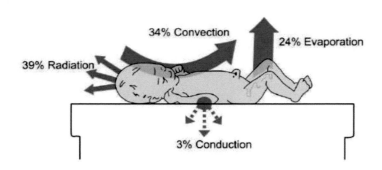

Fig. (5). Different modes and percentages of heat loss in babies.

Convection is the transfer of heat due to air movement which occurs due to the cool laminar air flow in the operating room. Evaporation is when heat loss occurs when water turns into a gas. In the operating room, this occurs due to exposed skin, respiratory exchange and surgical wound exposure. Conduction is the transfer of heat between two objects directly in contact with each other - such as the patient on the operating room table [63, 69].

Heat loss is greater in pediatric patients compared to adults due to their increased body surface areas relative to their total body volume, nominal amount of subcutaneous fat, and thin skin [63, 70, 71]. In addition, the younger the patient is, the more inefficient heat generation is. For the first 3 months of life, neonatal patients do not have the ability to shiver and rely instead on non-shivering thermogenesis (*via* brown fat metabolism, which does not develop until 26-30 weeks of gestation) for their primary source of heat generation. Non-shivering thermogenesis is inhibited by volatile anesthetics and thus leads to decreased ability of the neonate to thermoregulate.

Regulation of core body temperature is important to maintain optimal organ and enzymatic function. Hypothermia occurs when the temperature goes below 36 degrees Celsius. Hypothermia during surgery is well known to cause increased rates of surgical site infection, poor wound healing, platelet dysfunction, coagulopathy, increased rate of blood transfusion, increased myocardial events, decreased rate of drug metabolism, delayed awakening, and increased length of hospital stay [63, 70]. Conversely, hyperthermia (body temperature > 38 degrees Celsius) can cause tachycardia, vasodilation, and neurological injury. However, the biggest concern when encountering hyperthermia in a pediatric patient in the operating room is malignant hyperthermia, which can be deadly if not detected and treated in a timely manner.

Temperature monitoring should be performed for all anesthetics in order to prevent and treat derangements in body temperature. There are multiple different areas one can measure temperature. A provider can measure the core or peripheral, the core temperature being the most accurate. The core temperature can be measured *via* nasopharyngeal, distal esophageal, pulmonary arterial catheter or tympanic membrane. Near core temperatures can be measured *via* rectum or bladder. Skin temperature probes are the most common temperature probe used however, measure peripheral temperature which may be a 2-4 degree Celsius difference from core temperature. Each of these modalities have their limitations [63]. The easiest way to measure core temperature in a pediatric patient typically is nasopharyngeal or distal esophageal - taking care to avoid causing trauma with placement.

There are multiple methods an anesthesia provider can use to warm a pediatric patient. The first way to prevent initial heat loss is by warming the operating room to 75-80 degrees Fahrenheit prior to the patient's arrival to decrease radiation and convective losses. If a neonatal patient needs to be transported to and from the operating room, one can ensure that the patient has a hat on, wrapped in warm blankets, and transported in a warming incubator or on a warming mattress. Once in the operating room, one can warm the patient prior to inducing anesthesia by forced air blankets and radiant heat lamps [70, 72]. This will increase the heat content of the body overall [73]. Unless a pediatric patient is receiving large volumes of fluids or blood products a fluid warmer adds little value for treating hypothermia [63]. Also, keep in mind pediatric patients may need a higher temperature compared to adults within the operating room to maintain normothermia [74]. Humidifying the breathing circuit minimizes heat loss *via* evaporation. This can be done actively by evaporative or ultrasonic humidifiers or passively by heat and moisture exchanger (HME). HMEs have commonly been referred to as "artificial noses" [75, 76]. HMEs can humidify the circuit up to 50% which preserves normal cilia function, prevents bronchospasm, and maintains normothermia in the pediatric population. This is due to higher minute ventilation observed in children which is why this is a more effective means of heat conversation compared to adults [77 - 80]. The patient can be kept warm during the operation by use of forced air blankets while continued temperature monitoring will ensure that the patient does not overheat.

CONCLUSION

Children are not just miniature adults, but differ significantly in the anatomy and physiology of the cardiovascular, respiratory, neurologic, renal, and hepatic organ systems. Also, infants and neonates respond quite differently to various medications due to differences in pharmacokinetics and pharmacodynamics. The understanding of these differences in the developmental phase is essential to providing safe anesthetic care and a complication-free perioperative course.

CONSENT FOR PUBLICATION

Not applicable.

CONFLICT OF INTEREST

The author declares no conflict of interest, financial or otherwise.

ACKNOWLEDGEMENT

The authors thank Eureka Science for the medical illustrations seen throughout the chapter.

REFERENCES

[1]   Auroy Y, Ecoffey C, Messiah A, Rouvier B. Relationship between complications of pediatric anesthesia and volume of pediatric anesthetics. Anesth Analg 1997; 84(1): 234-5.
[http://dx.doi.org/10.1213/00000539-199701000-00060] [PMID: 8989044]

[2]   Jones R, Stewart J. An alternative to a shoulder roll for infants. Anaesthesia 2012; 67(4): 424.
[http://dx.doi.org/10.1111/j.1365-2044.2012.07085.x] [PMID: 22409794]

[3]   Huang AS, Hajduk J, Rim C, Coffield S, Jagannathan N. Focused review on management of the difficult paediatric airway. Indian J Anaesth 2019; 63(6): 428-36.
[http://dx.doi.org/10.4103/ija.IJA_250_19] [PMID: 31263293]

[4]   Miller RA. A new laryngoscope for intubation of infants. Anesthesiology 1946; 7: 205.
[http://dx.doi.org/10.1097/00000542-194603000-00014] [PMID: 21023368]

[5]   Passi Y, Sathyamoorthy M, Lerman J, Heard C, Marino M. Comparison of the laryngoscopy views with the size 1 Miller and Macintosh laryngoscope blades lifting the epiglottis or the base of the tongue in infants and children <2 yr of age. Br J Anaesth 2014; 113(5): 869-74.
[http://dx.doi.org/10.1093/bja/aeu228] [PMID: 25062740]

[6]   Coté CJ, Lerman J, Anderson BJ. A practice of anesthesia for infants and children. 6th ed., Philadelphia, PA: Elsevier 2019.

[7]   Litman RS, Maxwell LG. Cuffed *versus* uncuffed endotracheal tubes in pediatric anesthesia: the debate should finally end. Anesthesiology 2013; 118(3): 500-1.
[http://dx.doi.org/10.1097/ALN.0b013e318282cc8f] [PMID: 23314108]

[8]   McNiece WL, Dierdorf SF. The pediatric airway. Semin Pediatr Surg 2004; 13(3): 152-65.
[http://dx.doi.org/10.1053/j.sempedsurg.2004.04.008] [PMID: 15272423]

[9]   De Orange FA, Andrade RG, Lemos A, Borges PS, Figueiroa JN, Kovatsis PG. Cuffed *versus* uncuffed endotracheal tubes for general anaesthesia in children aged eight years and under. Cochrane Database Syst Rev 2017; 11: CD011954.
[http://dx.doi.org/10.1002/14651858.CD011954.pub2] [PMID: 29149469]

[10]   Chen L, Zhang J, Pan G, Li X, Shi T, He W. Cuffed *versus* Uncuffed Endotracheal Tubes in Pediatrics: A Meta-analysis. Open Med (Wars) 2018; 13: 366-73.
[http://dx.doi.org/10.1515/med-2018-0055] [PMID: 30211319]

[11]   Saikia D, Mahanta B. Cardiovascular and respiratory physiology in children. Indian J Anaesth 2019; 63(9): 690-7.
[http://dx.doi.org/10.4103/ija.IJA_490_19] [PMID: 31571681]

[12]   Kurth CD, Spitzer AR, Broennle AM, Downes JJ. Postoperative apnea in preterm infants. Anesthesiology 1987; 66(4): 483-8.
[http://dx.doi.org/10.1097/00000542-198704000-00006] [PMID: 3565813]

[13]   Davis RP, Mychaliska GB. Neonatal pulmonary physiology. Semin Pediatr Surg 2013; 22(4): 179-84.
[http://dx.doi.org/10.1053/j.sempedsurg.2013.10.005] [PMID: 24331091]

[14]   Neumann RP, von Ungern-Sternberg BS. The neonatal lung--physiology and ventilation. Paediatr Anaesth 2014; 24(1): 10-21.
[http://dx.doi.org/10.1111/pan.12280] [PMID: 24152199]

[15]   Carroll JL, Agarwal A. Development of ventilatory control in infants. Paediatr Respir Rev 2010; 11(4): 199-207.
[http://dx.doi.org/10.1016/j.prrv.2010.06.002] [PMID: 21109177]

[16]   Langston C, Kida K, Reed M, Thurlbeck WM. Human lung growth in late gestation and in the neonate. Am Rev Respir Dis 1984; 129(4): 607-13.
[PMID: 6538770]

[17]   Hislop A, Reid L. Development of the acinus in the human lung. Thorax 1974; 29(1): 90-4.
[http://dx.doi.org/10.1136/thx.29.1.90] [PMID: 4825556]

[18]   Mansell A, Bryan C, Levison H. Airway closure in children. J Appl Physiol 1972; 33(6): 711-4.
[http://dx.doi.org/10.1152/jappl.1972.33.6.711] [PMID: 4643846]

[19]   Keens TG, Bryan AC, Levison H, Ianuzzo CD. Developmental pattern of muscle fiber types in human ventilatory muscles. J Appl Physiol 1978; 44(6): 909-13.
[http://dx.doi.org/10.1152/jappl.1978.44.6.909] [PMID: 149779]

[20]   Hutten GJ, van Eykern LA, Latzin P, Thamrin C, van Aalderen WM, Frey U. Respiratory muscle activity related to flow and lung volume in preterm infants compared with term infants. Pediatr Res 2010; 68(4): 339-43.
[http://dx.doi.org/10.1203/PDR.0b013e3181eeeaf4] [PMID: 20606599]

[21]   Harding R. Function of the larynx in the fetus and newborn. Annu Rev Physiol 1984; 46: 645-59.
[http://dx.doi.org/10.1146/annurev.ph.46.030184.003241] [PMID: 6370121]

[22]   Kosch PC, Stark AR. Dynamic maintenance of end-expiratory lung volume in full-term infants. J Appl Physiol 1984; 57(4): 1126-33.
[http://dx.doi.org/10.1152/jappl.1984.57.4.1126] [PMID: 6501029]

[23]   von Ungern-Sternberg BS, Hammer J, Schibler A, Frei FJ, Erb TO. Decrease of functional residual capacity and ventilation homogeneity after neuromuscular blockade in anesthetized young infants and preschool children. Anesthesiology 2006; 105(4): 670-5.
[http://dx.doi.org/10.1097/00000542-200610000-00010] [PMID: 17006063]

[24]   Lerman J, Gregory GA, Willis MM, Eger EI II. Age and solubility of volatile anesthetics in blood.

Anesthesiology 1984; 61(2): 139-43.
[http://dx.doi.org/10.1097/00000542-198408000-00005] [PMID: 6465597]

[25] Salanitre E, Rackow H. The pulmonary exchange of nitrous oxide and halothane in infants and children. Anesthesiology 1969; 30(4): 388-94.
[http://dx.doi.org/10.1097/00000542-196904000-00006] [PMID: 5773948]

[26] Tan CMJ, Lewandowski AJ. The Transitional Heart: From Early Embryonic and Fetal Development to Neonatal Life. Fetal Diagn Ther 2020; 47(5): 373-86.
[http://dx.doi.org/10.1159/000501906] [PMID: 31533099]

[27] Hoffman JI, Kaplan S. The incidence of congenital heart disease. J Am Coll Cardiol 2002; 39(12): 1890-900.
[http://dx.doi.org/10.1016/S0735-1097(02)01886-7] [PMID: 12084585]

[28] Reller MD, Strickland MJ, Riehle-Colarusso T, Mahle WT, Correa A. Prevalence of congenital heart defects in metropolitan Atlanta, 1998-2005. J Pediatr 2008; 153(6): 807-13.
[http://dx.doi.org/10.1016/j.jpeds.2008.05.059] [PMID: 18657826]

[29] Atchabahian A, Gupta R. The anesthesia guide. New York: McGraw-Hill Medical 2013.

[30] Hines MH. Neonatal cardiovascular physiology. Semin Pediatr Surg 2013; 22(4): 174-8.
[http://dx.doi.org/10.1053/j.sempedsurg.2013.10.004] [PMID: 24331090]

[31] Neuhauser HK, Thamm M, Ellert U, Hense HW, Rosario AS. Blood pressure percentiles by age and height from nonoverweight children and adolescents in Germany. Pediatrics 2011; 127(4): e978-88.
[http://dx.doi.org/10.1542/peds.2010-1290] [PMID: 21382947]

[32] Flynn JT, Kaelber DC, Baker-Smith CM, *et al.* Clinical Practice Guideline for Screening and Management of High Blood Pressure in Children and Adolescents. Pediatrics 2017; 140(3): e20171904.
[http://dx.doi.org/10.1542/peds.2017-1904]

[33] Maheshwari M, Sanwatsarkar S, Katakwar M. Pharmacology related to paediatric anaesthesia. Indian J Anaesth 2019; 63(9): 698-706.
[http://dx.doi.org/10.4103/ija.IJA_487_19] [PMID: 31571682]

[34] Sulemanji M, Vakili K. Neonatal renal physiology. Semin Pediatr Surg 2013; 22(4): 195-8.
[http://dx.doi.org/10.1053/j.sempedsurg.2013.10.008] [PMID: 24331094]

[35] Schwartz GJ, Brion LP, Spitzer A. The use of plasma creatinine concentration for estimating glomerular filtration rate in infants, children, and adolescents. Pediatr Clin North Am 1987; 34(3): 571-90.
[http://dx.doi.org/10.1016/S0031-3955(16)36251-4] [PMID: 3588043]

[36] Elmas AT, Tabel Y, Elmas ON. Reference intervals of serum cystatin C for determining cystatin C-based glomerular filtration rates in preterm neonates. J Matern Fetal Neonatal Med 2013; 26(15): 1474-8.
[http://dx.doi.org/10.3109/14767058.2013.789844] [PMID: 23528044]

[37] Treiber M, Pecovnik-Balon B, Gorenjak M. Cystatin C *versus* creatinine as a marker of glomerular filtration rate in the newborn. Wien Klin Wochenschr 2006; 118 (Suppl. 2): 66-70.
[http://dx.doi.org/10.1007/s00508-006-0555-8] [PMID: 16817048]

[38] Diaz-Miron J, Miller J, Vogel AM. Neonatal hematology. Semin Pediatr Surg 2013; 22(4): 199-204.
[http://dx.doi.org/10.1053/j.sempedsurg.2013.10.009] [PMID: 24331095]

[39] Sohawon D, Lau KK, Lau T, Bowden DK. Extra-medullary haematopoiesis: a pictorial review of its typical and atypical locations. J Med Imaging Radiat Oncol 2012; 56(5): 538-44.
[http://dx.doi.org/10.1111/j.1754-9485.2012.02397.x] [PMID: 23043573]

[40] Sell EJ, Corrigan JJ Jr. Platelet counts, fibrinogen concentrations, and factor V and factor VIII levels in healthy infants according to gestational age. J Pediatr 1973; 82(6): 1028-32.

[http://dx.doi.org/10.1016/S0022-3476(73)80436-6] [PMID: 4702894]

[41]   Henry E, Christensen RD. Reference Intervals in Neonatal Hematology. Clin Perinatol 2015; 42(3): 483-97.
[http://dx.doi.org/10.1016/j.clp.2015.04.005] [PMID: 26250912]

[42]   Matoth Y, Zaizov R, Varsano I. Postnatal changes in some red cell parameters. Acta Paediatr Scand 1971; 60(3): 317-23.
[http://dx.doi.org/10.1111/j.1651-2227.1971.tb06663.x] [PMID: 5579856]

[43]   Aher S, Malwatkar K, Kadam S. Neonatal anemia. Semin Fetal Neonatal Med 2008; 13(4): 239-47.
[http://dx.doi.org/10.1016/j.siny.2008.02.009] [PMID: 18411074]

[44]   Lundström U, Siimes MA. Red blood cell values in low-birth-weight infants: ages at which values become equivalent to those of term infants. J Pediatr 1980; 96(6): 1040-2.
[http://dx.doi.org/10.1016/S0022-3476(80)80636-6] [PMID: 7373464]

[45]   Juul S. Erythropoiesis and the approach to anemia in premature infants. J Matern Fetal Neonatal Med 2012; 25 (Suppl. 5): 97-9.
[http://dx.doi.org/10.3109/14767058.2012.715467] [PMID: 23025780]

[46]   Bard H, Widness JA. The life span of erythrocytes transfused to preterm infants. Pediatr Res 1997; 42(1): 9-11.
[http://dx.doi.org/10.1203/00006450-199707000-00002] [PMID: 9212030]

[47]   Jorgensen JM, Crespo-Bellido M, Dewey KG. Variation in hemoglobin across the life cycle and between males and females. Ann N Y Acad Sci 2019; 08;1450(1): 105-25.
[http://dx.doi.org/10.1111/nyas.14096]

[48]   Strauss RG. Anaemia of prematurity: pathophysiology and treatment. Blood Rev 2010; 24(6): 221-5.
[http://dx.doi.org/10.1016/j.blre.2010.08.001] [PMID: 20817366]

[49]   Christensen RD, Baer VL, Gordon PV, *et al.* Reference ranges for lymphocyte counts of neonates: associations between abnormal counts and outcomes. Pediatrics 2012; 129(5): e1165-72.
[http://dx.doi.org/10.1542/peds.2011-2661] [PMID: 22508916]

[50]   Kuperman AA, Kenet G, Papadakis E, Brenner B. Intraventricular hemorrhage in preterm infants: coagulation perspectives. Semin Thromb Hemost 2011; 37(7): 730-6.
[http://dx.doi.org/10.1055/s-0031-1297163] [PMID: 22187395]

[51]   Lenfestey MW, Neu J. Gastrointestinal Development: Implications for Management of Preterm and Term Infants. Gastroenterol Clin North Am 2018; 12;47(4): 773-91.

[52]   Montgomery RK, Mulberg AE, Grand RJ. Development of the human gastrointestinal tract: twenty years of progress. Gastroenterology 1999; 116(3): 702-31.
[http://dx.doi.org/10.1016/S0016-5085(99)70193-9] [PMID: 10029630]

[53]   Meinzen-Derr J, Poindexter B, Wrage L, Morrow AL, Stoll B, Donovan EF. Role of human milk in extremely low birth weight infants' risk of necrotizing enterocolitis or death. J Perinatol 2009; 29(1): 57-62.
[http://dx.doi.org/10.1038/jp.2008.117] [PMID: 18716628]

[54]   Howie PW, Forsyth JS, Ogston SA, Clark A, Florey CD. Protective effect of breast feeding against infection. BMJ 1990; 300(6716): 11-6.
[http://dx.doi.org/10.1136/bmj.300.6716.11] [PMID: 2105113]

[55]   Heller CD, O'Shea M, Yao Q, *et al.* Human milk intake and retinopathy of prematurity in extremely low birth weight infants. Pediatrics 2007; 120(1): 1-9.
[http://dx.doi.org/10.1542/peds.2006-1465] [PMID: 17606555]

[56]   Gustafsson J. Neonatal energy substrate production. Indian J Med Res 2009; 130(5): 618-23.
[PMID: 20090117]

[57]   Heck LJ, Erenberg A. Serum glucose levels in term neonates during the first 48 hours of life. J Pediatr

1987; 110(1): 119-22.
[http://dx.doi.org/10.1016/S0022-3476(87)80303-7] [PMID: 3794870]

[58] Thompson-Branch A, Havranek T. Neonatal Hypoglycemia. Pediatr Rev 2017; 38(4): 147-57.
[http://dx.doi.org/10.1542/pir.2016-0063] [PMID: 28364046]

[59] Hawdon JM, Ward Platt MP, Aynsley-Green A. Patterns of metabolic adaptation for preterm and term infants in the first neonatal week 1992.
[http://dx.doi.org/10.1136/adc.67.4_Spec_No.357]

[60] Stanley CA, Rozance PJ, Thornton PS, *et al*. Re-evaluating "transitional neonatal hypoglycemia": mechanism and implications for management. J Pediatr 2015; 166(6): 1520-5.e1.
[http://dx.doi.org/10.1016/j.jpeds.2015.02.045] [PMID: 25819173]

[61] Lucas A, Morley R, Cole TJ. Adverse neurodevelopmental outcome of moderate neonatal hypoglycaemia. BMJ 1988; 297(6659): 1304-8.
[http://dx.doi.org/10.1136/bmj.297.6659.1304] [PMID: 2462455]

[62] Mitrakou A, Ryan C, Veneman T, *et al*. Hierarchy of glycemic thresholds for counterregulatory hormone secretion, symptoms, and cerebral dysfunction. Am J Physiol 1991; 260(1 Pt 1): E67-74.
[PMID: 1987794]

[63] Bissonnette B. Temperature monitoring in pediatric anesthesia. Int Anesthesiol Clin 1992; 30(3): 63-76.
[http://dx.doi.org/10.1097/00004311-199230030-00005] [PMID: 1516974]

[64] Pierau FK, Wurster RD. Primary afferent input from cutaneous thermoreceptors. Fed Proc 1981; 40(14): 2819-4.
[PMID: 7308494]

[65] Poulos DA. Central processing of cutaneous temperature information. Fed Proc 1981; 40(14): 2825-9.
[PMID: 6796435]

[66] Hellon RF. Neurophysiology of temperature regulation: problems and perspectives. Fed Proc 1981; 40(14): 2804-7.
[PMID: 7308492]

[67] Sessler DI. Temperature monitoring and perioperative thermoregulation. Anesthesiology 2008; 109(2): 318-38.
[http://dx.doi.org/10.1097/ALN.0b013e31817f6d76] [PMID: 18648241]

[68] Bindu B, Bindra A, Rath G. Temperature management under general anesthesia: Compulsion or option. J Anaesthesiol Clin Pharmacol 2017; 33(3): 306-16.
[http://dx.doi.org/10.4103/joacp.JOACP_334_16] [PMID: 29109627]

[69] Sessler DI. Perioperative heat balance. Anesthesiology 2000; 92(2): 578-96.
[http://dx.doi.org/10.1097/00000542-200002000-00042] [PMID: 10691247]

[70] Barash P. Clinical Anesthesia. 6th ed. Philadelphia: Wolters Kluwer/Lippincott Williams & Wilkins 2009. 282-, 284, 376-377.

[71] Litman R. Pediatric Anesthesia. 1st ed. Philadelphia, Penn.: Elsevier Mosby 2004; pp. 112-3.

[72] Sessler DI. Malignant hyperthermia. J Pediatr 1986; 109(1): 9-14.
[http://dx.doi.org/10.1016/S0022-3476(86)80563-7] [PMID: 3522838]

[73] Just B, Trévien V, Delva E, Lienhart A. Prevention of intraoperative hypothermia by preoperative skin-surface warming. Anesthesiology 1993; 79(2): 214-8.
[http://dx.doi.org/10.1097/00000542-199308000-00004] [PMID: 8251019]

[74] Bennett EJ, Patel KP, Grundy EM. Neonatal temperature and surgery. Anesthesiology 1977; 46(4): 303-4.
[http://dx.doi.org/10.1097/00000542-197704000-00016] [PMID: 842890]

[75]   Newton DEF. Proceedings: The effect of anaesthetic gas humidification on body temperature. Br J Anaesth 1975; 47(9): 1026.
[PMID: 1191469]

[76]   Chalon J, Markham JP, Ali MM, Ramanathan S, Turndorf H. The pall ultipor breathing circuit filter--an efficient heat and moisture exchanger. Anesth Analg 1984; 63(6): 566-70.
[http://dx.doi.org/10.1213/00000539-198406000-00003] [PMID: 6731877]

[77]   Chalon J, Loew DA, Malebranche J. Effects of dry anesthetic gases on tracheobronchial ciliated epithelium. Anesthesiology 1972; 37(3): 338-43.
[http://dx.doi.org/10.1097/00000542-197209000-00010] [PMID: 4115208]

[78]   Forbes AR. Temperature, humidity and mucus flow in the intubated trachea. Br J Anaesth 1974; 46(1): 29-34.
[http://dx.doi.org/10.1093/bja/46.1.29] [PMID: 4820930]

[79]   Bissonnette B, Sessler DI, LaFlamme P. Passive and active inspired gas humidification in infants and children. Anesthesiology 1989; 71(3): 350-4.
[http://dx.doi.org/10.1097/00000542-198909000-00006] [PMID: 2774261]

[80]   Bissonnette B, Sessler DI. Passive or active inspired gas humidification increases thermal steady-state temperatures in anesthetized infants. Anesth Analg 1989; 69(6): 783-7.
[http://dx.doi.org/10.1213/00000539-198912000-00017] [PMID: 2589661]

CHAPTER 2

Pediatric Pharmacology and Fluid Management

Shaharyar Ahmad[1] and Grace Dippo[1]

[1] *Department of Anesthesiology, Cooper Medical School of Rowan University, Cooper University Health Care, Camden, NJ, USA*

Abstract: Medication management and fluid resuscitation are the cornerstones of providing safe procedural sedation for any patient, pediatric or adult. Due to the immature organ systems, vastly different body sizes and compositions, unique pathologies, and altered metabolic pathways, knowledge of adult pharmacology and fluid management cannot be directly applied to the pediatric patient. This chapter describes the principles of pediatric pharmacology and their applications in various common healthy and diseased physiologic states. Drug administration, clinical effects, common pitfalls, and metabolism and elimination for the most important perioperative medications are discussed in detail. Knowledge of proper perioperative fluid administration in the healthy pediatric patient, as well as fluid resuscitation in shock states and common electrolyte disturbances common to pediatric patients, can easily be lifesaving. The assessment and treatment of these pathologic states are described in detail.

Keywords: Acetaminophen, Benzodiazepines, Circulating blood volumes, Context-sensitive half time, Dehydration in infants and children, Diuretics, Drug excretion, Drug metabolism, Fluid and electrolyte requirements in children, Fluid compartments, Genetic variations affecting pharmacokinetics, Intravenous anesthetics, Local anesthetics, Neuromuscular blocking drugs, Nitrous oxide, NSAIDs, Opioids, Parenteral fluids and electrolytes, Pharmacodynamics in children, Pharmacokinetics, Postoperative nausea and vomiting, Postoperative pulmonary edema, Sedatives, Shock states, Volatile anesthetics, Volume of distribution.

PHARMACOKINETICS

Pharmacokinetics is the study of how the body responds to drug administration, and encompasses drug absorption, distribution, and elimination. Common routes of drug administration include intravascular, submucosal, oral, transdermal, and

* **Corresponding author Bharathi Gourkanti:** Department of Anesthesiology, Cooper Medical School of Rowan University, Cooper University Health Care, Camden, NJ, USA; E-mail: gourkantibharathi@cooperhealth.edu

Bharathi Gourkanti, Irwin Gratz, Grace Dippo, Nathalie Peiris and Dinesh K. Choudhry (Eds.)
All rights reserved-© 2022 Bentham Science Publishers

intrathecal. Bioavailability is a measure of the amount of an administered dose that reaches the bloodstream. Thus, it represents the fraction of the dose that is absorbed and escapes first-pass elimination [1].

Zero order kinetics is dose-independent. In zero order kinetics, the elimination capacity is saturated so only a constant amount of drug is excreted over time. An example of this, even in infants, is how alcohol is metabolized at a constant rate by alcohol dehydrogenase regardless of the amount of alcohol consumed [2]. **First order kinetics is dose-dependent.** In first order kinetics, as drug concentration rises there is an increase in the rate of elimination until a point where the dose rate is equal to the clearance, a point called the steady-state. This process takes about 3-5 half lives in a continuous infusion. The purpose of a loading dose is to quickly get to the desired drug concentration needed to balance out the clearance. This would allow the desired drug effect to be obtained and maintained faster [5].

Context-sensitive Half Time

What happens when the infusion of the drug is stopped? The context-sensitive half time (CSHT) is the time it takes for the drug concentration to decrease by half after an infusion is stopped. This is a property unique to different drugs. The longer the infusion, the more tissues become saturated with a drug leading it to have a longer CSHT. Of note, the CSHT is only determined from computer simulation [6].

Remifentanil, for instance, is a methyl ester that is metabolized by plasma and nonspecific tissue esterases, has a short duration and undergoes rapid elimination. Because the drug does not accumulate, the CSHT remains relatively constant and the pharmacokinetics remain stable regardless of how long the drug is infused. Given that remifentanil is metabolized independently of renal and hepatic routes which can be immature in neonates, and that it is cleared faster in neonates than older individuals, remifentanil is a favorable analgesic for pediatric patients [7,8].

Half Life and Volume of Distribution

The elimination half life of a drug is the time it takes for half the drug to be metabolized (Table **1**). Elimination half life is directly related to the volume of distribution (Vd) and inversely related to clearance [3]. Because drugs distribute down a gradient from areas of high concentration to low concentration, Vd can be thought of as the volume of tissue that the drug is able to reach. For example, fentanyl is a very lipid soluble drug and has a large Vd. In contrast, glycopyrrolate is highly ionized, does not readily cross lipid membranes, and has a low Vd [28].

V_d = dose / concentration

Chloroquine, for instance, has a high clearance but still has a very long half life (up to 1-2 months) due to its large volume of distribution. The utility of half life for measuring drug elimination is limited in case of liver or kidney disease [4].

Table 1. Percent of drug removed based on number of half-lives past.

Number of Half Lives (t)	Percent of Drug Removed
1	50%
2	75%
3	88%
4	94%
5	97%

Percent of Drug Removed = $(1 - 0.5^t)$ x 100%)

Pediatric Pharmacokinetic Considerations

These properties of pharmacokinetics can be very different in the pediatric population. Absorption, plasma protein binding, metabolism, and excretion levels are decreased in children. The volume of distribution is increased [9]. The fetal circulation has notable differences compared to adults. Neonates have increased pulmonary vascular resistance, decreased systemic vascular resistance, and right-to-left shunting through a patent foramen ovale. There is also decreased cardiac compliance, and with a constant stroke volume, neonates are dependent on their heart rate to maintain cardiac output [10].

Administration, Absorption, and Distribution

Absorption is the way a drug moves from the administration site to the systemic circulation. In infants, there is a more rapid absorption from the inhalation and intramuscular routes, giving these drugs a faster onset. Due to delayed gastric emptying and immature intestinal motility, enteral absorption from orally administered medications can be slower in children [11]. **Distribution** is how a drug moves from the systemic circulation into the various body compartments. Pediatric drug distribution differs from that of adults because children have a higher fat content (22.4% at 12 months *vs.* 13% at 15 years). This means that lipophilic drugs have a larger Vd in children than adults [29].

Increased Total Body Water

There is a change in the total body water (TBW) with age. In neonates, TBW is

80% and after 1 year it is 60%, which remains the same through adulthood. This difference comes from a reduction in the extracellular fluid (ECF) (45% in a neonate to 26% in a 1-year old). The ECF continues to decline in childhood and into adulthood as the fat and muscle content increase. This is clinically significant because the higher relative ECF in the pediatric population contributes to the larger volume of distribution of all drugs [39].

Increased Permeability of the Blood-Brain Barrier

Neonates have a particular sensitivity to sedatives and hypnotics in comparison to adults, partly related to increased permeability from an immature BBB. The BBB consists of tight-junctions between endothelial cells of brain capillaries and serves as a barrier to large molecules to prevent them from freely entering the cerebral circulation from the systemic circulation [12].

Clearance, Metabolism, Excretion

Hepatic drug metabolism can be categorized into phase I reactions (oxidation, reduction, and hydrolysis) and phase II reactions (conjugation with various molecules such as sulfate, glycine, glucuronide). Newborns have a reduced or entirely absent content of microsomal enzymes and reduced cytochrome P450 activity, leading to slowed drug metabolism. There is also a reduction in the liver's ability to form glucuronide conjugates due to a reduction in the activity of glucuronyl transferase and uridine 5'-diphospho-glucose (UDPG) dehydrogenase which can cause unconjugated hyperbilirubinemia, especially in premature infants. In this particular population, the provider should be cautious with drugs that have a reduced clearance from immature hepatic function, such as morphine, acetaminophen, and dexmedetomidine.

The **renal system** is important in regulating the volume and composition of body fluids and the elimination of toxins. The maturation of renal function, as expressed by the glomerular filtration rate, approaches mature capacity at 2 years old [14].

PHARMACODYNAMICS

Our understanding of pharmacodynamics is not as complete as our understanding of pharmacokinetics [15]. Pharmacodynamics concerns the relationship between drug doses and their response. This response represents a continuum from desired effect to toxicity. This relationship, for most drugs, is not linear (Fig. **1**). As a drug is administered and its serum concentration rises, it reaches a point on its dose-response curve of a maximum effect called the Emax, after which there is not a significant increase in the drug's effect with rising drug concentration.

In the concentration-effect relationship as seen in Fig. (**1**), the point where 50% of the Emax is obtained is known as the EC50. Pharmacodynamics can be divided into two main topics: the transduction of signals caused by drugs and the evaluation of the drug effects [12, 15].

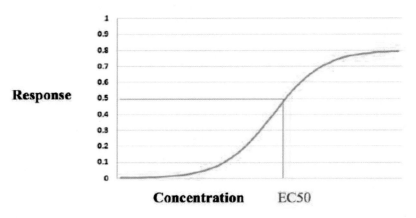

Fig. (1). Concentration Response Curve. Original figure design by Shaharyar Ahmad MD.

Signal Transduction

Drugs are in a constant state of binding to their receptors and dissociating from their receptors. Steady state is a condition where the rate of drug binding is equal to the rate of drug dissociating from receptors. Kd is the dissociation constant, which is a ratio of bound drug to free drug at equilibrium. The dissociation constant (Kd) is equal to the drug concentration when 50% of receptors are occupied and is indirectly proportional to how tight the drug binds the receptor [16].

Types of Agonists

Full agonists bind their receptors and achieve a maximal response with their drug concentration. **Partial agonists** only achieve a partial response regardless of being at high concentrations. **Inverse agonists** bind the receptor but cause an effect that is the opposite of what the original drug intended to cause. Receptors are constantly in a state of flux and altering their conformations. Agonists are thought to increase the amount of time that receptors stay in a particular conformation that facilitates the drug response. **Competitive antagonists** block other drugs from binding receptors by binding the receptors in their place. **Noncompetitive antagonists** irreversibly bind the receptor and cause it to change conformation, thus preventing the original drug from binding its receptor and causing an appropriate response.

Types of Receptors

The most common receptors are the **G-protein coupled receptors** with distinct subtypes, that have secondary messenger cascades mediated by cAMP and IP3/DAG, for instance that cause downstream biochemical effects. **Ligand-gated ion channels** conduct the flow of sodium, potassium, calcium, and chloride and regulate nerve conduction through changes in membrane polarization. **Voltage-gated ion channels** conduct nerve transduction through the transmission of action potentials.

Drug Effects

Potency is a measure of how drug activity produces a defined effect and efficacy measures the therapeutic effectiveness of the drug in humans [15]. Drugs with a concentration-response curve shifted to the left are more potent, and right-shifted curves represent drugs that are less potent.

The ED_{50} is the dose of a drug required to produce the desired effect in 50% of patients. LD_{50} is the dose of the drug lethal to 50% of patients. The **therapeutic index** is a ratio between the LD_{50} and ED_{50} and is descriptive of drug safety, such that safer drugs have a higher LD_{50} relative to the ED_{50}. For example, alfentanil has a high therapeutic index with LD_{50}/ED_{50} ratio of 1080 *versus* that of morphine and fentanyl with therapeutic indices of 70 and 227 respectively [30].

Drug-Drug Interactions

When two or more drugs are administered, their individual pharmacodynamics and pharmacokinetic properties can change to alter the intended drug effect. For instance, giving a CYP3A4 inhibitor such as St. John's Wort can prolong the metabolism of codeine [12, 15]. Table **2** below illustrates commonly encountered inhibitors and inducers of the CYP450 enzyme system.

Table 2. Common inhibitors and inducers of CYP450.

Inhibitors	Inducers
Mnemonic is 'SICKFACES.COM'	Mnemonic is 'CRAPS'
• Sodium valproate • Isoniazid • Cimetidine • Ketoconazole • Fluconazole • Alcohol • Chloramphenicol • Erythromycin • Sulfonylurea • Ciprofloxacin • Omeprazole • Metronidazole	• Carbamazepine • Rifampin • bArbiturates • Phenytoin • St. John's Wort

ANESTHETIC DRUGS & PHARMACOLOGY

Volatile Anesthetics are the most commonly used maintenance anesthetic in children. They are associated with minimal effects on cardiac physiology and are low-cost. Nitrous oxide is used as an adjuvant to other induction and maintenance anesthetics [39]. Potency and gas properties of nitrous oxide and the volatile anesthetics are found below in Table **3**.

Table 3. Properties of Volatile Anesthetics.

Property	Halothane	Isoflurane	Sevoflurane	Desflurane	Nitrous Oxide
Vapor Pressure (mm Hg)	244	240	185	664	39,000
Blood: gas partition coefficient	2.4	1.4	0.66	0.42	0.47
Fat: blood partition coefficient	51	45	48	27	2.3
MAC (adult) %	0.75	1.2	2.0	7	104
MAC (2 year old) %	0.97	1.6	2.6	8.7	Not known

Halothane

Though rarely used in the United States, halothane is still used in some countries. Halothane has a sweet, non-pungent odor, intermediate solubility, and high potency, and can be used for inhalational induction in the pediatric population. Halothane is also a negative inotrope and undergoes the most metabolism of any of the volatile anesthetics and should therefore be used with caution in patients with liver dysfunction [31].

Sevoflurane

Sevoflurane is the least pungent volatile anesthetic and is consequently associated with a lower incidence of coughing, laryngospasm, and breath holding compared to other volatile anesthetics. Sevoflurane has a low blood solubility, is a potent respiratory depressant, and maintains cardiovascular stability at up to 1 MAC in the pediatric population [39].

Desflurane

Due to its low blood solubility compared to the other volatile anesthetics, desflurane has the fastest induction and elimination. Desflurane is more pungent than sevoflurane and is used for maintenance of anesthesia [39].

Isoflurane

Isoflurane has increased blood solubility compared to the other fluorinated volatile anesthetics, so it has a slower onset of induction and elimination compared to desflurane and sevoflurane. Isoflurane is not as expensive as the other volatile anesthetics and is useful in long-duration cases. Like desflurane, isoflurane is also more pungent than sevoflurane [39].

Nitrous Oxide

Nitrous oxide can decrease the requirement of other volatile anesthetics. N_2O also provides the second gas effect, whereby it enhances the uptake of the "second gas." As nitrous oxide is rapidly taken up from the alveolus to the bloodstream, the other gas in the mixture (typically a volatile anesthetic) is drawn into the trachea to replace the lost volume, increasing the concentration of the second gas to drive enhanced uptake through an enhanced concentration gradient. Situations where N_2O can be dangerous include venous or air embolism, pneumothorax, intestinal obstruction, pneumocephalus, intraocular air bubbles, ear surgery, and pulmonary hypertension. N_2O can increase PONV risk [32].

Physiologic Properties of Volatile Anesthetics

The rate of rise of volatile anesthetic depends on a variety of factors such as the fraction of the inspired drug and minute ventilation. Uptake of these drugs depends on cardiac output, blood and tissue solubility, and the gradient between the alveolus and the pulmonary vasculature. The rate of rise of the fraction of drug inspired in the alveolus (FA) divided by the fraction of the inspired drug concentration (FI) called FA/FI is a useful ratio that can be compared among different volatile anesthetics. Steady state is defined as when FA = FI or FA/FI = 1. As cardiac output increases, as in neonates, the time needed for equilibration of

FA/FI takes longer than in conditions of low cardiac output, resulting in a slower induction compared to adults. The rate of increase of FA/FI also has an inverse relationship with drug solubility such that the **drugs with the fastest induction** are: nitrous oxide > desflurane > sevoflurane > isoflurane > halothane.

Mask induction is faster in children. Infants have a smaller functional residual capacity (FRC) and higher minute ventilation than adults, and higher blood flow to vessel-rich organs [32].

A **right-to-left shunt** will slow induction more for poorly-soluble volatile anesthetics than soluble anesthetics such as isIV anesthetic agents oflurane. In a right-to-left shunt, the volatile anesthetic in the left ventricle gets diluted with blood from the right ventricle, so there is less anesthetic included in the cardiac output to the brain. Because this prolongs the time to equilibrium when the partial pressure is equal in the brain and the alveolus, there is a **longer induction time**. In contrast, there is **no significant effect of a left-to-right shunt** on uptake of volatile anesthetics.

Premedication

The goal of premedication is to assist with anxiolysis, amnesia, and reduce the stress associated with surgery. The ideal drugs used for premedication have a rapid onset, few side effects, and do not prolong recovery time. Midazolam, ketamine, and clonidine are effective premedication agents and are suitable for various administration routes [35, 36, 39]. See Table **4** below for routes and dosing of these common premedications.

Table 4. Premedication Drug Dosing [35, 36, 39].

Drug	Midazolam	Ketamine	Clonidine
Dose	PO: 0.5-1 mg/kg (max 20mg) IV: 0.05-0.15 mg/kg IM: 0.1-0.2 mg/kg Rectal: 0.75-1.0 mg/kg Nasal: 0.1-0.2 mg/kg Sublingual: 0.2-0.3 mg/kg	PO: 3-5 mg/kg IM: 2-5 mg/kg Rectal: 5 mg/kg Nasal: 3 mg/kg	PO: 4 mcg/kg IM: 1-5 mcg/kg Rectal: 5 mcg/kg

Intravenous Anesthetic Agents

Commonly used IV anesthetic agents are described in detail below, and in brief for easy reference in Table **5**.

Table 5. IV anesthetic agents [21].

Drug	Receptor Site	Metabolism	Induction & Infusion Dose	Hemodynamic Effects	Systemic Effects
Propofol	Agonist ofbeta-subunit of GABA-A receptor	Hepatic glucuronidation	Induction dose 2.5-3.5 mg/kg *age>3y Infusion loading dose: 2.5-5 mg/kg, Infusion rate: 200- 300 mcg/kg/min	Reduce MAP, SVR, $CMRO_2$, CBF, antiepileptic	propofolinfusion syndrome, hypotension, apnea, pain oninjection, antiemetic, antiepileptic, spontaneous excitatory movements
Ketamine	NMDA noncompetitive antagonist	Hepatic demethylation to norketamine, renal excretion	Induction dose IV: 1-2 mg/kg IM: 5-10 mg/kg For sedation IV 0.25-0.5mg/kg	Increase MAP,CBF, $CMRO_2$, bronchodilation, increased ICP, IOP	hallucination, delirium, analgesia, preserved respiratorydrive, laryngospasm, increased secretions
Etomidate	Increases affinity of GABA at GABA-A receptor	Hepatic andplasma esterases	Induction dose 0.2-0.6 mg/kg	Minimalchanges in BP and CO, reduce CBF, $CMRO_2$, ICP	Inhibit 11-betahydroxylase, adrenalin sufficiency, myoclonus, pain on injection, nausea and vomiting
Dexmedetomidine	Selective Alpha-2 agonist	Hepatic glucuronidation, oxidation	Loading dose 1-2 mcg/kg Infusion dose 0.5-1 mcg/kg/hr (age <12mo) 0.5-1.5 mcg/kg/hr (age >12 mo)	Increase BP, reduce CO, bradycardia, reduce IOP	Respiratory depression, opioid sparing, analgesia, anxiolysis, reduce postoperative shivering
Thiopental	Potentiate GABA-A receptor and increase chloride influx	Hepatic metabolism	neonate 3-4 mg/kg infant 5-8 mg/kg age 1-12 yr 5-6 mg/kg age >12yr 3-5 mg/kg	Reduce CBF, $CMRO_2$, ICP, MAP, increase HR, reduce BP	contraindicated in porphyria, can cause shivering, sneezing, coughing, and bronchospasm

(Table 5) cont.....

Drug	Receptor Site	Metabolism	Induction & Infusion Dose	Hemodynamic Effects	Systemic Effects
Methohexital	Potentiate GABA-A receptor and increase chloride influx	Hepatic metabolism	Induction dose IV 1-2 mg/kg Rectal: 20-30 mg/kg	Reduce CBF, $CMRO_2$, ICP, increase HR, reduce BP	Similar to thiopental but 3x more potent
Pentobarbital	Potentiate GABA-A receptor and increase chloride influx	Hepatic metabolism	Aliquots of 1-3 mg/kg until max dose 100 mg/kg	Reduce CBF, $CMRO_2$, ICP	Similar to thiopental, nausea, vomiting, prolonged recovery period

Propofol

Propofol is an alkylphenyl derivative made as an emulsion of water with soybean oil, glycerol, and egg phosphatide. In a patient with an egg allergy, it is important to determine whether the patient is allergic to egg yolk or egg white. Patients with egg allergies are usually sensitive to egg whites, but the lecithin in propofol is derived from yolk [17]. Regarding propofol pharmacokinetics, infants have an increased volume of distribution and a decreased clearance but the propofol clearance approaches adult value by approximately 50 weeks postnatal age in a term neonate [16, 40]. Children have a lower sensitivity to propofol and may require higher doses for sedation than adults. The context sensitive half time (CSHT) is higher for children with propofol infusion. In one study, a four-hour infusion of propofol was found to have a CSHT of about 20 minutes in children aged 3 to 11 years compared to 6-9 minutes in adults. This means that the drug will remain longer in systemic circulation for children than adults.

The most clinically significant adverse effect with propofol is **propofol infusion syndrome** (PRIS) which occurs with continuous infusions of high-dose propofol > 4 mg/kg/hour over a period > 48 hours. PRIS is associated with bradycardia, metabolic acidosis, rhabdomyolysis, myoglobinuria, and death. The pathogenesis is thought to be due to propofol interfering with the metabolism of fatty acids or inhibition of coQ at complex II, cytochrome C, or complex IV in the electron transport chain in aerobic metabolism in the mitochondria [18, 19].

Ketamine

Ketamine is a cyclohexylamine derivative that is a noncompetitive antagonist at the central NMDA receptor and also affects the opioid receptor, muscarinic receptor, and the voltage-gated sodium and L-type calcium channels. Ketamine can be used as an effective preoperative medication and low-dose ketamine infusions (0.1-0.3 mg/kg/hr) can be used for analgesia and to decrease opioid requirements in the perioperative period [39].

Etomidate

Etomidate is a potent short-acting sedative-hypnotic GABA agonist, known for its hemodynamic stability with induction. Adrenal insufficiency can be observed even with a single induction dose. Etomidate can also cause bradycardia, and pre-treatment is indicated [39].

Clonidine

Clonidine is an alpha-2 agonist with sedative and analgesic properties. Used in some instances as a premedication (4 mcg/kg), clonidine was found to decrease the postoperative rates of nausea, vomiting, and shivering. A 2014 study found that a clonidine infusion at 1 mcg/hr decreased the requirements of fentanyl and midazolam intraoperatively in neonates undergoing mechanical ventilation. Clonidine has also been used to prolong the duration of caudal anesthesia [35, 36].

Dexmedetomidine

Dexmedetomidine is an alpha-2 agonist that is about 1000 times more selective for the alpha-2 receptor than clonidine. Its sedative effects are due to the reduction of neuronal activity in the locus coeruleus. Dexmedetomidine can also be used for anxiolysis and can provide analgesia with opioid-sparing effects.

Barbiturates

Barbiturates interact with alpha and beta subunits of the GABA-A receptor which leads to a chloride influx resulting in GABA induced postsynaptic inhibition [41]. Barbiturates undergo hepatic metabolism and renal elimination. Since neonates take up to 3 weeks to develop their phase 2 glucuronidation enzymes in the liver, they can have decreased metabolism of barbiturates leading to high serum blood levels. Therefore, barbiturates are less used than sedatives of other drug classes in this population. Barbiturates are also associated with cardiac depression and have largely been replaced by drugs in other classes [32].

IV Anesthetics

Neuromuscular Blockers

Commonly used neuromuscular blocking agents are described in detail below, and in brief for easy reference in Table **6**.

Table 6. Nondepolarizing Neuromuscular Blockers [39, 42].

NDNMB	Duration	ED95 Dose	Metabolism/ Excretion
Rocuronium	Intermediate, 20-30 minutes	3 mg/kg (Intubating dose 0.6 mg/kg, RSI dose 1.2 mg/kg)	Hepatic / Biliary and renal
Vecuronium	Intermediate, 20-30 minutes	0.05 mg/kg	Hepatic / Biliary and renal *active metabolite renally excreted
Pancuronium	Long, 60-90 minutes	0.07 mg/kg	Hepatic metabolism / renal elimination
Atracurium	Intermediate, 20-30 minutes	0.2 mg/kg	Hofmann elimination *Laudanosine active metabolite
Cisatracurium	Intermediate, 20-30 minutes	0.05 mg/kg	Hofmann elimination
Mivacurium	Short, 15-20 minutes	0.07 mg/kg	Plasma cholinesterase

Succinylcholine

Succinylcholine is a depolarizing neuromuscular blocker that binds to the alpha subunits of the nicotinic acetylcholine receptors leading to depolarization and muscle contraction, as evidenced by fasciculations. Succinylcholine remains attached to the nicotinic receptors leading to a prolonged depolarization and subsequent muscle relaxation, known as a phase I blockade. Giving multiple doses of succinylcholine can cause a phase II blockade, which resembles a nondepolarizing block with a train-of-four in a fade pattern. It is thought that pure phase II blockade results from tachyphylaxis and can potentially be reversed with neostigmine [39, 43].

Succinylcholine's effect is terminated by redistribution to the plasma where it is metabolized by butyrylcholinesterase (BChE), also known as plasma cholinesterase or pseudocholinesterase. A patient with an **atypical BChE** can have a prolonged block by succinylcholine, causing apnea for longer than expected with a typical induction dose. The activity of BChE can be qualitatively assessed by the dibucaine number, which is related to the percent of BChE inhibited by the local anesthetic dibucaine. Since dibucaine normally inhibits 80% of the activity of normal BChE and 20% of the activity of homozygous atypical BChE, a normal dibucaine number is 80 and fully atypical is 20. There is age-related variation in BChE activity. BChE is 50% as active in infants from birth to age 6 months as nonpregnant adults, 70% as active by age 6, and normal adult level at puberty [39, 42].

As a result of the depolarization caused by the phase I block, succinylcholine causes potassium excretion into the extracellular space leading to hyperkalemia. Disease states that upregulate the junctional and extrajunctional cholinergic receptors can exacerbate hyperkalemia to lethal levels – these include burns, trauma, upper motor neuron diseases such as multiple sclerosis, and muscular dystrophy. Under-dosing succinylcholine can cause laryngospasm because patients are not completely paralyzed. Bradycardia caused by succinylcholine is difficult to treat, highlighting the importance of pre-treatment with atropine IV 2 mg/kg or IM 4 mg/kg. The pediatric dose of atropine is higher because children have an increased volume of distribution.

The most significant side effect of succinylcholine is malignant hyperthermia. Other adverse effects are postoperative myalgia, rhabdomyolysis (especially in patients with muscular dystrophy), bradycardia, increased intraocular pressure, increased intragastric pressure, increased lower esophageal sphincter tone, and increased intracranial pressure. Giving a defasciculating dose of a nondepolarizing neuromuscular blocker does not mitigate hyperkalemia or the rise in intragastric pressure, but it does decrease fasciculations and attenuates a rise in ICP [39, 42].

Nondepolarizing Neuromuscular Blockers (NDNMBs)

These drugs are structurally either benzylisoquinolines (atracurium, cisatracurium, mivacurium) or aminosteroids (rocuronium, vecuronium, pancuronium) and are competitive antagonists against the nicotinic acetylcholine receptor (nAChR) alpha-subunit. Muscle relaxation by a NDNMB differs from a depolarizing blockade by succinylcholine phase I block in that the former is associated with tetanic fade, a train of four ratios of T4/T1 less than 1, and no fasciculations. Nondepolarizing blockade is also terminated by the use of an acetylcholinesterase inhibitor which raises the level of ACh to outcompete the NDNMB at the nAChR alpha subunit. Upregulation of the nAChR, as seen in burns for instance, can raise the ED50 of NDNMBs. In contrast, concomitant use of volatile anesthetics, local anesthetics, diuretics, aminoglycosides, magnesium, and lithium can increase the effect of NDNMBs. This enhanced blockade is also seen physiologically with acidosis, hypokalemia, and hypothermia and in disease states such as myasthenia gravis. Anaphylaxis during anesthesia is often caused by neuromuscular blockers. Intubating dose is 2 x ED95 dose and RSI dose is 4 x ED95 dose [42].

Of note, pancuronium is a poor choice for patients with renal failure and is associated with a vagolytic effect leading to a rise in blood pressure and heart rate. Pancuronium can also inhibit butyrylcholinesterase. Atracurium is metabolized both by Hofmann elimination (spontaneous nonenzymatic breakdown) and also by nonspecific plasma esterases to an active metabolite, laudanosine which is associated with seizures at high concentrations. Atracurium can also cause histamine release leading to hypotension. Cisatracurium also undergoes Hofmann elimination but does not have an active metabolite, rendering it safe for patients with hepatic and renal dysfunction. Hofmann elimination is enhanced by high pH and high temperature. Mivacurium is also associated with histamine release and concomitant hypotension but is no longer available in the US [39, 42, 45].

Reversal of Neuromuscular Blockade

Sugammadex

Sugammadex is a gamma-cyclodextrin that can selectively reverse the blockade of aminosteroids like rocuronium, vecuronium, and pancuronium by encapsulating the NDNMB, rendering it unable to bind the nicotinic AChR at the neuromuscular junction. Sugammadex can not reverse the blockade caused by benzylisoquinolinium NDNMBs or succinylcholine. Because Sugammadex does not affect acetylcholinesterase like neostigmine, it does not have the risk of muscarinic side effects. Adverse effects of Sugammadex include nausea, vomiting, pain, hypotension, headache, anaphylaxis, and binding of hormonal contraceptive drugs. Consequently, nonhormonal contraception should be used for at least 1 week for those patients reliant on systemic hormonal contraceptives following sugammadex administration. The Sugammadex-NDNMB complex is renally excreted and administration of Sugammadex is not recommended in severe renal impairment (creatinine clearance <30 mL/min) [20, 39, 42, 44]. Sugammadex is dosed based on train-of-four, as detailed in Table **7**.

Table 7. Dosing of Sugammadex [20, 39, 42, 44].

Twitches	Dose (mg/kg)
At least 2/4 twitches on TOF	2
No twitches on TOF but presence of post-tetanic twitch	4
No post-tetanic twitches or rapid reversal after RSI	16

RSI – rapid sequence induction, TOF – train-of-four stimulation

Acetylcholinesterase Inhibitors (AChEi)

Neostigmine inhibits acetylcholinesterase and prevents the breakdown of ACh to choline and acetate. It thereby raises the level of ACh available to outcompete the neuromuscular blocker at the nAChR alpha subunit. Neostigmine is 50% renally excreted and has an elimination half life of 76 minutes. The recommended dose is 0.05-0.07 mg/kg (max dose of 5mg) after the return of ¾ twitches on TOF.

Edrophonium is also an AChEi. Edrophonium is 67% renally excreted and has an elimination half life of 66 minutes. The recommended dose is 1 mg/kg after the return of three out of four twitches on TOF.

To avoid the undesirable increase in the muscarinic effects (bradycardia, increased secretions, bronchospasm) by the rise in ACh caused by administration of an AChEi, an antimuscarinic like glycopyrrolate or atropine should be paired with administration of the AChEi. **Glycopyrrolate** has an onset of 1 minute, and a half-life of 45-60 minutes. Its reversal dose is 0.01-0.15 mg/kg IV.

Unlike glycopyrrolate, which is a quaternary amine, **atropine** is a tertiary amine and can cross the blood-brain-barrier. This leads to CNS effects like central anticholinergic toxicity in elderly patients, confusions, disorientation, visual disturbances, tachycardia, and other antimuscarinic effects. Atropine undergoes rapid redistribution, hepatic metabolism, and is about 50% excreted renally unchanged.

Residual neuromuscular blockade with inadequate reversal can lead to prolonged apnea, desaturation, respiratory collapse, and reintubation. Of note, volatile anesthetics can prolong the neostigmine-reversal of NMB (desflurane > sevoflurane > isoflurane > halothane > nitrous oxide) [39, 42].

Opioids

Opioids work at the level of the mu, delta, and kappa opioid receptors which are **G-protein coupled receptors** that activate a secondary messenger cascade when activated, resulting in a rise in cyclic adenosine monophosphate (cAMP). The observed effects of these different receptor types are organized in Table **8**. Short-acting opioids are less habit-forming than other opioids and better at preventing addiction than long-acting opioids [33]. Opioids that are more lipid soluble have a faster onset and shorter duration of action. Most opioids undergo hepatic metabolism and renal elimination. The commonly used opioids and their unique properties are charted in Table **9**.

Table 8. Systemic Effects of Opioid Receptor Activation [32].

Opioid Receptor	Effect
Mu-1	sedation, bradycardia, pruritus, nausea, vomiting, supraspinal analgesia
Mu-2	respiratory depression, constipation, pruritus, physical dependence, euphoria
Kappa	spinal analgesia, respiratory depression, miosis, and sedation
Delta	spinal analgesia and respiratory depression

Table 9. Opioid Agonists [38, 46 - 48].

Opioid	Receptor Site	Metabolism	Dose	Unique Properties
Fentanyl	Mu agonist	Hepatic, inactive metabolites	IV Bolus 1-2 mcg/kg Intranasal 1-2 mcg/kg OTFC 5-15 mcg/kg	50 times as potent as morphine. Neonates can have suppressed baroreceptor reflex, long CSHT.
Sufentanil	Mu agonist	Hepatic, desmethyl sufentanil active metabolite with 10% activity	IV Loading dose: 1-2 mcg/kg Infusion dose: 0.1-0.2 mcg/kg/hr	Shorter CSHT than fentanyl, analgesic tail useful after painful surgeries in PACU
Alfentanil	Mu agonist	Hepatic inactive metabolites	IV Bolus 25 mcg/kg IV Loading dose 50-100 mcg/kg Infusion 0.5-2 mcg/kg/min	Almost entirely protein bound to AAG, more rapid onset than fentanyl, (pK$_a$ 6.5)
Remifentanil	Mu agonist	Non specific tissue and plasma esterases	IV Loading dose 1 mcg/kg Infusion 0.25-3 mcg/kg/min	Short CSHT regardless of infusion time, opioid induced hyperalgesia
Methadone	L-methadone Mu agonist D-methadone NMDA antagonist	Hepatic, inactive metabolites	Neonatal abstinence syndrome: IV 0.05-0.2 mg/kg Q12-24 h IV Analgesic dose 0.1mg/kg/dose for 2-3 doses given Q4-6 h.	QTc prolongation Long half life (19 hr) Safe for renal insufficiency
Tramadol	Mu agonist, SNRI	Hepatic, desmethyl-tramadol active metabolite	PO 1-2 mg/kg IV 2-2.5 mg/kg Up to 4-6 times/day	Can potentiate serotonin syndrome if given with MAO inhibitors. No significant respiratory depression
Hydrocodone	Mu agonist	Hepatic, CYP2D6 to hydromorphone, CYP3A4 to norhydrocodone	PO 0.05-0.1 mg/kg	Often paired with acetaminophen
Oxycodone	Mu agonist	Hepatic O-methylation to oxymorphone *active metabolite	PO, IV, IM administration is 0.1 mg/kg with a max dose of 5 mg/kg.	Clearance reaches adult levels by age 2-6 months.
Codeine	Mu agonist	Hepatic, O-demethylation to morphine	PO or IM: 1 mg/kg Max dose 3 mg/kg/day	Ultrarapid metabolizers can be predisposed to morphine overdose

CSHT: context-sensitive half time, Oral transmucosal fentanyl citrate (OTFC), SNRI: serotonin and norepinephrine reuptake inhibitor, AAG: alpha-1 acid glycoprotein

Pain transmission originates in the periphery where noxious stimuli transmit pain signals *via* A-beta, A-delta, and C fiber neurons. These neurons synapse with the second-order neurons in the dorsal horn of the spinal cord (layers 4 and 5 of the substantia gelatinosa). These second-order neurons travel through the dorsal columns and spinothalamic tract and synapse with third-order neurons at the level of the thalamus, which sends signals to the cerebral cortex where the pain is processed [32, 39]. The systemic effects common to most opioids are organized in Table **10** by organ system.

Table 10. Systemic Effects of Opioids [39, 42, 50].

Organ System	Systemic Opioid Effects
Central Nervous System	• Increase postoperative nausea and vomiting • Cause sedation at higher doses • Reduce $CMRO_2$, ICP, CBF* • Meperidine can lower the seizure threshold • Remifentanil can increase opioid induced-hyperalgesia • Decrease MAC of volatile anesthetics
Pulmonary	• Dose-dependent depression in ventilatory response to CO_2 • Blunt ventilatory response to hypoxemia • Decrease respiratory rate and minute ventilation • Meperidine and morphine-6-glucuronide cause histamine release which can trigger bronchospasm
Musculoskeletal	• Decrease chest wall compliance and increase skeletal muscle rigidity • Meperidine can decrease postoperative shivering
Cardiac	• Can cause dose-dependent bradycardia and decrease cardiac output • Baroreceptor reflex inhibition, arteriolar and venous dilation • Meperidine, structurally similar to atropine, can cause tachycardia • Meperidine and methadone can prolong QTc
Gastrointestinal	• Increase smooth muscle tone in bowel, decrease gastric motility • Contract Sphincter of Oddi
Genitourinary	• Inhibit urethral sphincter relaxation, leading to urinary retention
Endocrine	• Inhibit gonadotropin-releasing hormone and corticotropin-releasing hormone to decrease release of cortisol to blunt the stress response to surgery

$CMRO_2$ is cerebral metabolic requirement of O_2 consumption, CBF is cerebral blood flow, ICP is intracranial pressure

Opioid Agonist-Antagonist Nalbuphine

Nalbuphine is an opioid derivative that is equipotent with morphine. It is a mupartial antagonist and kappa agonist, thus giving it a ceiling effect with analgesia which is typically seen at 150-300 mcg/kg. Nalbuphine can treat pruritus induced by opioid administration without reversing analgesia as would naloxone. A 2006 study found that nalbuphine could be used to decrease the incidence of postoperative delirium in children who had general anesthesia without prolonging PACU stay [49].

Opioid Antagonists

Naloxone

Naloxone is an opioid antagonist at the mu, kappa, delta opioid receptors. Naloxone can be used to reverse opioid overdose in boluses of 0.01 mg/kg given every 2-3 minutes. In neonates, IM and IV naloxone administration achieved similar serum concentrations. Low-dose naloxone infusions have been used to treat opioid induced nausea, vomiting and pruritus at a dose of 0.25 mcg/kg/hr [39].

Naltrexone

Naltrexone is also an opioid antagonist at the mu, kappa, delta opioid receptors. Naltrexone has better PO bioavailability than naloxone and has a long duration of action. Methylnaltrexone is a new opioid antagonist that has been approved for opioid-induced constipation in adults and children [39, 51].

Local Anesthetics

Local anesthetics are weak bases (-ester or -amide) that cross the neuron cell membrane and inactivate the alpha-subunit of the intracellular voltage-gated Na^+ channel, stopping nerve conduction. Because local anesthetics must be nonionized to cross the lipid bilayer of the cell membrane, the potency of the local anesthetics depends on the degree of lipid solubility.

A serum pH be close to the pKa of the local anesthetic allows for a greater nonionized fraction of local anesthetic to cross the lipid membrane and result in a faster block, but an acidic environment will increase the gradient between the pH and pKa leading to a greater fraction of ionized local anesthetic, resulting in a slower block onset. Therefore, the speed of onset depends on the pKa of local anesthetic and its concentration. The pKa values and dosing of commonly used local anesthetics are charted in Table **11**. This relationship is characterized with the Henderson-Hasselbalch Equation:

Table 11. Local Anesthetic Properties [38, 52].

Local Anesthetic	Class	pK$_a$	Max Dose (mg/kg)	Max Dose with Epinephrine (mg/kg)	Onset
Lidocaine	Amide	7.9	4.5	7	Fast
Mepivacaine	Amide	7.6	4.5	7	Moderate
Bupivacaine	Amide	8.1	3	3	Slow
Ropivacaine	Amide	8.1	4	4	Slow
Chloroprocaine	Ester	8.7	12	15	Fast
Tetracaine	Ester	8.5	3	3	Slow

Of note, amides have two "i" in their name and esters only have one "i"

$$pH = pK_a + \log [A\text{-}]/[HA]$$

[A-] is the concentration of the weak base and [HA] is the concentration of its conjugate acid.

Local anesthetics are cleared by redistribution and protein binding to alpha-1 acid glycoprotein (AAG) in the plasma. The duration of action of local anesthetics depends on the degree of protein binding. Infants have immature hepatic clearance and decreased levels of AAG, predisposing them to a higher risk of local anesthetic toxicity than adults.

Ester local anesthetics are metabolized by plasma pseudocholinesterase and RBC esterase. Amide local anesthetics are hepatically metabolized by amide hydrolysis, N-dealkylation, and hydroxylation. Absorption of local anesthetics is dependent on the vascularity at the site of injection [42]. This mnemonic is helpful for stratifying local anesthetic absorption: IV > tracheal > intercostal > caudal > epidural > brachial plexus > axillary > lower extremity (femoral) > subcutaneous.

Mnemonic is "ICE BALLS"

Benzodiazepines

Benzodiazepines are sedative-hypnotic agents that increase the affinity of GABA for the GABA-A receptor. Benzodiazepines have mostly displaced barbiturates because of their lower risk of fatal CNS depression. Most common adverse effects include lightheadedness, motor incoordination, confusion, impairment of mental functions, respiratory depression at high doses, prolonged anesthesia recovery [39]. Notably, suddenly stopping the administration of benzodiazepines after chronic use can precipitate withdrawal. This typically manifests with sweating, tremors, irritability, dysphoria, and anxiety. Benzodiazepines undergo hepatic metabolism with renal elimination [53]. The commonly used benzodiazepines and their unique properties are described in Table **12**.

Table 12. Benzodiazepines [38, 54 - 56].

Benzodiazepine	Duration	Sedation Dose	Metabolism	Side Effects
Diazepam	Long	0.05-0.3mg/kg IV 0.05-0.3mg/kg IM	Hepatic, desmethyldiazepam and oxazepam metabolites	Pain on injection, reduced BP, CO. Decreased slope of CO_2 ventilatory response curve
Lorazepam	Long	0.05mg/kg PO *Limited dosing data in children	Phase 2 hepatic glucuronidation to inactive metabolites *safe for renal dysfunction	More potent than diazepam or midazolam, pain on injection
Midazolam	Short	age 6 month to 5 years: 0.05-0.1 mg/kg IV (max 6mg) age 5 to 12 years: 0.025-0.05mg/kg IV (max 10mg) 0.1-0.15mg/kg IM 0.1-0.15mg/kg IN 0.1mg/kg PR 0.5-0.75mg/kg SL	Rapid hepatic metabolism	Metabolites can accumulate in renal failure

Flumazenil

Flumazenil is an antagonist of the GABA-A channel at the benzodiazepine binding site. Because flumazenil has such a short duration of action (30-60 minutes), flumazenil can clear faster than the benzodiazepine it is trying to antagonize. This situation can lead to a reemergence of the action of a benzodiazepine and its associated toxicity leading to seizures, arrhythmias, and death. Flumazenil initial dosing is 0.01 mg/kg (max dose 0.2 mg) which can be repeated at 1 minute intervals up to 4 additional doses. The max dose is 1 mg or 0.05 mg/kg, whichever is lower [34].

NSAIDS

Nonsteroidal anti-inflammatory agents (NSAIDs) such as ketorolac and ibuprofen are analgesics that can be used to decrease the use of opioids in the perioperative period. Their mechanism of action is inhibition of cyclooxygenase 1 and 2 (COX-1, COX-2) which are involved in the metabolism of arachidonic acid to prostaglandins, prostacyclins, thromboxane, and leukotrienes. NSAID toxicity can lead to GI bleeding, decreased renal blood flow, liver injury, and other bleeding complications. More specifically, adverse effects of COX-1 inhibition include GI side effects like bleeding, perforation, and ulceration which occur in susceptible patients or those with chronic use. COX-1 inhibition also predisposes to bleeding complications secondary to inhibition of the thromboxane A2 synthesis, which is involved in platelet aggregation. COX-2 inhibitors, such as celecoxib, are rarely used in the pediatric population but are linked to an increased risk of stroke or MI [39, 57].

Acetaminophen

Acetaminophen is used as an anesthetic adjuvant for its analgesic and antipyretic effects, with less GI and antiplatelet side effects than NSAIDs. Analgesia is secondary COX-3 inhibition, reduction of nitric oxide in the spinal cord, NMDA antagonism and reduction of substance P. Acetaminophen can be given IV (10-15 mg/kg), PR (20 mg/kg), or PO as in Table **13** below.

Table 13. Maximum daily dose of PO acetaminophen is age dependent [39, 58].

Age	PO Acetaminophen Max Dose
Neonate 28-32 weeks gestational age	40 mg/kg/day
Infants 33-37 weeks gestational age	60 mg/kg/day
Infants, children, adolescents	75 mg/kg/day, not to exceed 4000 mg/day

Acetaminophen and NSAIDs can be used for closure of a patent ductus arteriosus in premature infants [59]. Acetaminophen undergoes hepatic metabolism to a toxic intermediate NAQPI (N-acetyl-p-benzoquinone imine) which subsequently is conjugated by glutathione. In acetaminophen toxicity, glutathione is depleted leading to a buildup of NAQPI which leads to hepatotoxicity [39].

Antiemetics

Postoperative nausea and vomiting (PONV) can prolong PACU stay and is very common in the pediatric population. The risk of PONV for children over age 3 years old can be characterized by the Erbhart risk stratification. Children who had surgery greater than 30 minutes, strabismus surgery, personal or family history of PONV had a 70% risk of PONV [60]. In addition to decreasing the use of noxious agents, antiemetics from a series of drug classes can be utilized to decrease the risk of PONV (Table **14**). Antiemetics have greater efficacy when at least two different drug classes are given.

Table 14. Commonly used antiemetics and PONV prophylaxis [22, 42, 60 - 64].

Antiemetic	Mechanism	Dose	Metabolism	Side Effects
Ondansetron	5-HT3 antagonist at CTZ	IV 0.05- 0.1mg/kg up to 4mg total PO 4mg or 8mg	Hepatic	QTc prolongation, headache
Metoclopramide	5-HT3 antagonist D2-antagonist Increase GI motility	IV 0.15 mg/kg	Hepatic	Antidopaminergic, EPS (*treat with anticholinergic), tardive dyskinesia, diarrhea
Promethazine	H-1 antagonist, antimuscarinic, D2 antagonist	PO 25 mg (age >2 year old) Rectal: 12.5 mg or 25 mg suppository at 4-6hr intervals	Hepatic	Black box warning in children <2 yr old for seizures, EPS, NMS, respiratory depression
Droperidol	Antidopaminergic at CTZ	IV 0.015- 0.025 mg/kg	Hepatic	Sedation, dysphoria,hypotension, QTc prolongation
Dexamethasone	Glucocorticoid and mineralocorticoid receptor agonist	IV 0.1 mg/kg	Hepatic	Studies showed that a single dose does **not** increase risk of adrenal suppression, hyperglycemia, or delayed wound healing
Aprepitant	Substance P antagonist on neurokinin-1 receptor	No official recommendations regarding the use of neurokinin-1 antagonists in the pediatric population	Hepatic	Multiple retrospective studies have shown that aprepitant is well-tolerated in children

EPS extrapyramidal symptoms, NMS neuroleptic malignant syndrome, CTZ chemoreceptor trigger zone

Anticholinergics

In addition to being used as a pretreatment for acetylcholinesterase inhibitor administration in the reversal of neuromuscular blockade, anticholinergics are frequently used in pediatric anesthesia as antisialogogues, bronchodilators, and as PONV prophylaxis. Anticholinergic agents can cause decreased secretions, bronchospasm, tachycardia, dizziness, blurry vision, constipation, and urinary retention.

Atropine

Atropine is an antimuscarinic tertiary amine that crosses the blood-brain barrier, unlike glycopyrrolate. Atropine has a fast onset of 1 minute and duration of 30-60 minutes. Atropine is commonly used to treat and prevent bradycardia which is common in the pediatric population. The recommended IV dose is 10-20 mcg/kg and IM dose is 20 mcg/kg [39, 42].

Glycopyrrolate

Glycopyrrolate is an antimuscarinic that is a quaternary amine and does not cross the blood-brain-barrier. It is mainly used to prevent the vagally-mediated bradycardia that would result from neostigmine. The recommended dose of IV glycopyrrolate is 10 mcg/kg when given with neostigmine.

Antihistamines

Diphenhydramine is an antihistamine H1-antagonist that can treat nausea and vomiting with the vestibular system, making it useful for middle ear and strabismus surgeries. It can lead to sedation and dyskinesia from its anticholinergic effects. It has a recommended IV dose of 0.5-1mg/kg, with a max dose of 50mg [39].

Dimenhydrinate

Dimenhydrinate is a combination of diphenhydramine and 8-chlorotheophylline that is an effective antiemetic but causes less sedation than diphenhydramine. The recommended PO dose is 0.5-1 mg/kg, with a maximum dose of 50 mg every 6 hours [39].

PHARMACOGENETIC VARIATIONS

Morphine

Morphine is a widely used analgesic in the pediatric population. *OCT1* is an organic cation transporter found in the liver that is involved in morphine clearance. Children who were homozygous for defective *OCT1* alleles were found to have decreased morphine clearance compared to children who were heterozygous or homozygous for active *OCT1* alleles [23].

Codeine

Codeine is an opioid prodrug used to treat mild-to-moderate pain and undergoes hepatic metabolism by CYP2D6 to morphine. There exists inter-individual differences in its metabolism based on the presence of homozygous or heterozygous active CYP2D6 alleles. Children who are homozygous for defective CYP2D6 alleles have significantly decreased codeine metabolism to morphine and experience low levels of analgesia. In contrast, children can also have more than two copies of the functional CYP2D6 alleles making them "ultra-rapid metabolizers" leading them to metabolize codeine to morphine more rapidly than children with two normal copies of CYP2D6 alleles. These ultra-rapid metabolizers can consequently experience morphine overdose leading to drowsiness, lethargy, and the potential for life-threatening respiratory depression [24].

Acetaminophen

Acetaminophen is an analgesic and antipyretic widely used in the pediatric population. Acetaminophen can cause hepatotoxicity, secondary to a buildup of the intermediate NAQPI (N-acetyl-p-benzoquinone imine) from metabolism by cytochrome P450 enzymes. NAQPI is normally metabolized by glutathione, which is formed by glutathione synthetase. Consequently, children with glutathione synthetase deficiency have low levels of glutathione and have decreased metabolism of NAQPI, leading to hepatotoxicity [25].

FLUID AND ELECTROLYTE REQUIREMENTS IN HEALTHY CHILDREN

Fluid Compartments

Infants have a greater percentage of total body water (TBW) than older children, as they have a larger ratio of extracellular fluid (ECF) to intracellular fluid (ICF). Normally in adults, ICF = 2/3 TBW and ECF = 1/3 TBW. However, in term neonates the ECF is up to 60% of TBW and declines with age. ECF is composed of interstitial fluid and intravascular fluid. The latter includes plasma (blood cells, platelets, blood proteins). Circulating blood volume also declines with age, see Table **15**. Interstitial fluid has a similar solute composition to plasma but has less proteins [64, 65].

Table 15. Fluid Compartment Variation with Age [64, 65].

Age	TBW (% of bodyweight)	Blood Volume (mL/kg)
Premature Neonate	80	90-100
Term infant < 6 months	75	80-90
Age	**TBW (% of bodyweight)**	**Blood Volume (mL/kg)**
Infants > 6 months and adolescents	60	60-75

Fluid and Electrolyte Requirements in Children and Infants

Infants have a higher fluid requirement than older children, as illustrated in Table **16**. Infants have an increased rate of metabolism compared to older children and adults. Infants also have a larger ratio of body-surface-area to weight resulting in a higher proportion of insensible fluid loss through evaporation. Increased energy expenditure also leads to an increase in fluid and electrolyte requirements (Table 17). Furthermore, premature infants have immature skin that leads to even more evaporative heat loss than term infants [66 - 68].

Table 16. Daily pediatric fluid requirement [66 - 68].

Age, Weight	Fluid Requirement (mL/kg/day)
0-3 postnatal days	40-60
Preterm, >10kg	150
Preterm <10kg	100-125
Term, 11-20kg	50
Term, >20kg	20

Table 17. Electrolyte requirements based on energy expenditure in children [66 - 68].

Electrolyte	Requirement per 100 kcal Energy Expenditure
Sodium	2.5 mmol
Potassium	2.5 mmol
Chloride	5 mmol
Dextrose	25 g

Homeostatic Mechanisms and Maturation

Maturation of Renal Function

Nephrons of mature kidneys are formed by 36 weeks gestation and continue hyperplasia until postnatal month 6. Afterwards, cells undergo hypertrophy instead of hyperplasia until they reach adult levels. RBF in children 6 months to 1 year of age is about 50% of adult values, normalizes to adult levels by age 3 years, and then begins to decline after age 30 years [14].

GFR levels reach adult levels at 2 years of age but rise more slowly for premature infants. Term neonates can still conserve sodium despite their low GFR. This phenomenon is due to glomerulotubular balance, which allows each successive segment of the proximal tubule to reabsorb a constant fraction of glomerular filtrate and sodium, across a range of GFR.

Urine concentrating ability also increases with age, and is lower for premature infants than term infants. This is due to a hypotonic renal medulla due to an immature development of the length of the loop of Henle, collecting ducts, decreased Na^+ reabsorption in the ascending limb of the Loop of Henle, low accumulation of medullary urea, and decreased sensitivity of the collecting duct to ADH. Urine diluting ability matures by postnatal week 3-5 [39, 69].

PARENTERAL FLUIDS AND ELECTROLYTES

Children are at risk for dehydration and electrolyte disturbance in the perioperative period, and are commonly given IV fluids to prevent this. NPO guidelines are similar to those for adults with the addition of breast milk NPO time (see Table **18**).

Table 18. Perioperative Fasting Guidelines [70].

Item	Fasting Before Surgery (hours)
Regular meal	8
Light meal, formula, non-human milk	6
Breast milk	4
Clear fluids	2

Choice of Fluids

Berry's formulas from 1986 are used to calculate the rate of IV fluid administration on an hourly basis and depend on age-based caloric expenditure, the preoperative fasting volume deficit, severity of trauma in surgery, and blood and fluid losses. The goal of fluid management is to maintain intravascular volume without causing hyponatremia, which children are predisposed to due to prehydration with hypotonic fluids, GI losses through nausea, vomiting, and stress of surgery stimulating excess ADH release postoperatively. Neonates also have limited urinary excretion, predisposing them to be volume overloaded with excessive IV fluid administration. Hyponatremia, especially acute, can lead to cerebral edema, which can be physically manifest by constitutional symptoms like nausea, vomiting, headache, and muscle weakness [14, 39].

Crystalloids

Crystalloids such as normal saline or lactated ringers are used before colloids in the treatment of volume deficits perioperatively. Normal saline when given in excess can lead to hyperchloremic metabolic acidosis because the strong ion difference induced by hyperchloremia leads to bicarbonate loss in the urine and concomitant acidosis. Compared to colloids, crystalloids are cheaper, do not affect coagulation (like hetastarch), and have less risk of infection or anaphylaxis.

Sodium, bicarbonate, and calcium should be appropriately supplemented but potassium should be used with caution because of the predisposition to hyperkalemia.

During the perioperative period, isotonic fluid administration is recommended unless there is a free water deficit with balanced electrolyte solutions such as Plasmalyte or lactated ringer being superior to 0.9% normal saline due to a less risk of causing an acidosis [38].

Glycemic Control

Perioperative hypoglycemia and hyperglycemia should be avoided in pediatric patients. Hypoglycemia triggers a stress response that affects cerebral blood flow and prolonged hypoglycemia can lead to neurocognitive impairment. To prevent intraoperative hypoglycemia, a dextrose-containing isotonic maintenance fluid solution such as 2.5% or 5% dextrose in lactated ringers can be used. Dextrose-solutions should not be used for fluid resuscitation or replacement of insensible surgical third-space losses to avoid causing hyperglycemia. Hyperglycemia can lead to lactic acidosis, cell death, osmotic diuresis, and dehydration, especially in the setting of ischemia [39, 71].

Colloids

Colloids are classified as either naturally occurring proteins such as albumin or synthetic compounds such as hydroxyethyl starch (hetastarch), gelatins, and dextrans. Five percent albumin is equivalent to blood plasma in a 1:1 ratio. Of note, colloids should be used with extreme caution in pediatric patients who have disease states with increased intravascular permeability such as sepsis and burns where colloids can traverse to the interstitial space and exacerbate edema [39, 72].

Electrolyte Disturbances

There is a predisposition to hyponatremia in the pediatric population with excessive IV fluid administration. Neonates have immature Na^+ reabsorption mechanisms, smaller tubular length in nephrons, decreased responsiveness to aldosterone, immature urine concentrating ability, and lower levels of ADH than adults. Furthermore, preterm neonates have a higher fractional excretion of Na^+ (FENa) than term-neonates, making them even more prone to hyponatremia and subsequent neurologic deficits. The other consequence of an immature aldosterone responsiveness in the distal tubule is a reduced ability to appropriately excrete potassium, predisposing both term and preterm neonates to hyperkalemia [39, 42, 73].

Fluid Replacement

Maintenance Fluid

The "4/2/1" rule developed by Holliday and Segar in 1957 can be used to calculate the hourly fluid requirements. Usually 100 mL of water can be used to metabolize 100 kcal. The following rules can be used to calculate the maintenance fluid requirement.

For children <10 kg, multiple body weight (kg) x 4.

For children 10-20 kg, the hourly need is 40 mL + (weight – 10 kg) x 2.

For children >20 kg, fluid is 60 mL + (weight – 20 kg) x 1

For example, the maintenance fluid for a child weighing 15 kg would be 40 mL + (15 kg – 10 kg) x2 = 50 mL/hr. In the past, children were often given 5% dextrose with 0.25% saline but because of the risk of hyponatremia and increased ADH secretion, which can lead to encephalopathy and neurological damage, intraoperative fluid management is usually replaced with an isotonic solution like lactated ringers [74].

Fluid Deficit

The fluid deficit is a product of fluid loss during preoperative fasting, gastrointestinal loss or other fluid deficits. These deficits can be replaced by one-third in the first hour, and the remainder can be spread out over the remainder of surgery [39, 74].

Intraoperative Replacement of Insensible Loss

Because neonates have a larger ratio of ECF to ICF than older children and adults, they can have a higher rate of third-space insensible losses. The severity of the surgery and tissue trauma is related to insensible losses and should be replaced by the dosing guidelines in Table **19**, added to the maintenance hourly fluid requirement in the intraoperative period [39, 42].

Table 19. Insensible fluid loss based on the type of trauma [39, 42].

Type of Trauma	Insensible Loss Requirement (mL/kg/hr)
Mild	2-6
Moderate	4-8
Severe	6-10

Dehydration

Decreased volume status in neonates can be assessed by delayed capillary refill, decreased skin turgor, lethargy, tachycardia, oliguria, weight loss and sunken fontanelles. Neonates can tolerate dehydration to a large degree before having overt symptoms due to their large TBW to body-weight ratio, but when they do become symptomatic, dehydration can progress very quickly. Preterm neonates are particularly susceptible to dehydration due to skin immaturity, phototherapy, undergoing convection in non humidified incubators, hyperthermia, and tachypnea.

The main determinants of the magnitude of ECF volume depletion are fluid deficit, electrolyte deficit and the rate at which dehydration occurs. Dehydration is classified based on sodium levels, with the most common being isonatremic > hyponatremic > hypernatremic dehydration. Free water loss can cause hypernatremic dehydration in infants in whom water intake is limited due to decreased access or GI losses such as vomiting and diarrhea. During hypernatremic dehydration, children can have preservation of ECF volume and a reduction in ICF volume and the severity of dehydration can be underestimated. Older children who can drink more fluids in response to dehydration can have excess free water intake that can cause hyponatremia.

Rehydration is aimed at intravascular volume expansion to restore hemodynamic stability and perfusion of tissues. Correction of 1% dehydration requires 10 mL/kg of fluids. Severely dehydrated infants should receive intravenous boluses of 20-40 mL/kg LR or normal saline until hemodynamically stable. Hypotonic fluids should be used in the case of hypernatremia following rehydration therapy. Hypotonic fluids should be avoided until dehydration is corrected and ADH secretion is not further stimulated. Usually 5% dextrose is co administered with IV fluids to avoid ketosis [39, 75].

Electrolyte Disorders

Hyponatremia

Hyponatremia (defined by serum Na^+ <135 mEq/L) is a multifactorial disorder that occurs usually secondary to changes in fluid balance, weight loss, diuretic use, and medical disease. The manifestations of hyponatremia are organized by disease state in Table **20**.

Table 20. Complications of Hyponatremia [39, 42].

Hyponatremia Complication	Manifestation
Hyponatremic Encephalopathy	Water shifted from ECF to ICF down the solute concentration gradient. Leads to cerebral edema. Children higher risk due to large brain: intracranial volume ratio
Symptom of inappropriate ADH production (SIADH)	High levels of ADH leads to water retention. Can be primary CNS disorder or secondary to metabolic or iatrogenic etiologies. Treat underlying cause, use hypertonic or isotonic fluids, diuretics. Use demeclocycline for SIADH refractory to these modalities.
Cerebral Salt Wasting (CSW)	Believed to occur due to release of natriuretic peptides, inhibition of RAAS system, decreased relative ECF volume compared to SIADH. Treat volume depletion with IV fluids in symptomatic patients.

RAAS – renin-angiotensin-aldosterone system, ADH antidiuretic hormone, ECF extracellular fluid, ICF intracellular fluid

Complications of Hyponatremia in Children

Serum sodium concentration <120 mEq/L is associated with increased mortality and rapid correction of hyponatremia can lead to neurologic damage in the form of central pontine myelinolysis. Severe hyponatremia should be corrected slowly at a rate of 1-2 mEq/L/hr until serum Na^+ concentration reaches 125-130 mEq/L. Children have multiple stimuli for ADH production compared to adults. Furthermore, even mild hyponatremia (Na^+ >130 mEq/L) can be associated with cerebral herniation so hypotonic fluids should be avoided in the postoperative period and isotonic fluids should be used instead.

Hypernatremia

Hypernatremia (Na^+ >145 mEq/L) is commonly seen in patients who are fluid depleted, especially those with decreased ADH release or impaired thirst response. With the increased ECF solute concentration, fluid shifts from the ICF to ECF compartment resulting in brain volume reduction, leading to hemorrhages secondary to tears of bridging veins from the separation of the brain from meninges. The free water deficit which should be replaced can be calculated as:

Free Water Deficit (L) = (0.6 x weight kg) x ($[Na^+]/140 - 1$)

Where $[Na^+]$ is serum sodium concentration

Correcting hypernatremia too quickly can lead to cerebral edema. The rate of correction should be 1 mEq/hour or 15 mEq/24 hours while carefully monitoring for the development of neurologic signs such as seizures and encephalopathy. If these occur, the correction rate should be slowed [76].

Diabetes Insipidus (DI)

Decreased ADH secretion by the posterior pituitary can lead to hypernatremia in DI. Patients with DI can present with polydipsia, polyuria, and decreased urine osmolality. Etiology of central DI can be due to brain trauma, intracerebral hemorrhage, stroke, CNS infections, brain malignancy, and neurosurgery. Patients who can secrete ADH normally but have decreased effect of ADH at the V2-receptor can have nephrogenic diabetes insipidus. Desmopressin is a V2-receptor agonist that can be administered to distinguish the two etiologies, such that in central DI patients clinically improve with desmopressin administration but there is no change in response in patients with nephrogenic DI [42, 77, 78].

Shock States

Decreased blood perfusion to organs and tissues resulting in cell injury characterizes shock, of which there are four principal types, see Table **21** [12, 37].

Table 21. Shock States [12, 37].

Shock	Mechanism	Example	SVR	MAP	PCWP	CVP	CO
Hypovolemic	Reduced circulating blood volume	Hemorrhage	↑	↓	↓	↓	↓
Cardiogenic	Pump failure	Myocardial infarction	↑	↓	↑	↑	↓
Obstructive	Blockage of forward flow	Pericardial tamponade	↑	↓	↑	↑	↓
Distributive	Systemic vasodilation	Septic shock	↓	↓	↓	↓	↑ or ↓

SVR systemic vascular resistance, MAP mean arterial pressure, PCWP pulmonary capillary wedge pressure, CVP central venous pressure, CO cardiac output

Blood Transfusion

Children are more sensitive to the metabolic changes associated with blood transfusion than adults so have to go through a thorough evaluation regarding the necessity of transfusion. Packed red blood cells (PRBCs) contain additives such as citrate, phosphate, dextrose, and adenine and can be stored for up to 35 days. Immunocompromised children should receive irradiated blood. PRBCs can also be packed with a solution of adenine, saline, dextrose, and mannitol which allows storage up to 42 days [79, 80].

Complications of PRBCs

The most common complications of PRBC transfusion are hyperkalemia, hypothermia, and hypocalcemia. The risk of hyperkalemia with blood transfusion is increased with large volumes of PRBCs, rapid transfusion rate, use of a central line, transfusion in a neonate rather than older child, and increased acidosis and tissue injury. PRBCs are stored cold and if given without a fluid warmer, can cause hypothermia. Hypothermia is detrimental to PRBC transfusion because it left-shifts the oxyhemoglobin dissociation curve and can lead to coagulopathy. Citrate used in PRBC storage can chelate calcium and cause hypocalcemia. This is seen more commonly with fresh frozen plasma (FFP) and whole blood transfusion than with PRBCs [39, 81, 82].

Electrolyte Disorders

Potassium

Unlike sodium, potassium is mostly concentrated in the ICF. Normal serum potassium concentration is in the range of 3.5-5.5 mEq/L. Total body potassium content is proportional to muscle mass, body weight, and height and increases with age in children.

Hypokalemia is serum $[K^+]$ less than 3.5 mEq/L. In conditions without a total body potassium deficit, intracellular shift of potassium can occur during alkalosis where there can be a 0.6 mmol/L drop in $[K^+]$ for every 0.1 unit rise in serum pH. Insulin and beta-agonists such as epinephrine can activate Na^+/K^+ ATPase which causes increased K^+ uptake intracellularly. Hypokalemia is usually secondary to a nutritional deficiency, renal or extrarenal etiologies. Loop or thiazide diuretics can increase urine potassium excretion [83].

Hyperchloremia can impair the chloride-linked sodium reabsorption in the distal tubule by increasing sodium reabsorption and potassium excretion. Other causes of hypokalemia include hypomagnesemia, high renin states, Conn syndrome, and direct damage to the renal epithelium which can be mediated by infections, toxins and drugs such as amphotericin. Licorice can cause hypokalemia because it contains glycyrrhizic acid which impairs 11-beta-hydroxysteroid dehydrogenase which metabolizes glucocorticoids. The buildup of glucocorticoids can activate mineralocorticoid receptors leading to an aldosterone-like mediated hypokalemia [39, 42].

Hyperkalemia occurs when $[K^+] > 5.5$ mEq/L and can be caused by increased potassium ingestion, transcellular shifts, impaired renal excretion, or drug side effects. Hydrogen ions are buffered with potassium ions, so in cases of metabolic acidosis, H+ can shift intracellularly leading to an extracellular K^+ shift (a 0.1 unit drop in pH is associated with a $[K^+]$ increase of 0.6 mEq/L). Other causes of hyperkalemia include adrenal insufficiency, potassium-sparing diuretics like spironolactone and amiloride, ACE inhibitors, angiotensin II receptor blockers, succinylcholine, beta-blockers, digoxin, and penicillin G. Severe hyperkalemia can be treated by producing transcellular shifts such as activation of the Na^+/K^+ ATPase as mediated by beta-agonists, and insulin (which should be given with glucose) [39]. Hyperventilation and giving sodium bicarbonate can induce an alkalosis which can cause an intracellular K^+ shift *via* the H/K^+ exchange buffer. To prevent life threatening cardiac abnormalities, IV calcium gluconate 100-200 mg/kg can be given. Further K^+ excretion can be achieved by loop and thiazide diuretics, kayexalate, and dialysis [84].

Calcium

Normal serum calcium (Ca) levels are maintained at 9-10.5 mg/dL and ionized calcium (Ca^{2+}) is about 4-5 mg/dL. Acidosis can lead to a reduction in albumin-bound calcium and promote hypercalcemia and in contrast, alkalosis can promote calcium-albumin binding and lead to hypocalcemia (as seen with large blood transfusions and hyperventilation). Calcium absorption occurs in the small intestine and by 1,25-dihydroxy vitamin D3 which activates basolateral calcium transporters. Infants can have high serum calcium levels as lactose can stimulate calcium absorption. In the kidneys, parathyroid hormone (PTH) increases Ca^{2+} excretion at the proximal tubule but increases Ca^{2+} reabsorption at the distal tubule and collecting duct, resulting in a net increase in serum Ca^{2+} concentration.

Hypocalcemia is defined as a total serum Ca concentration < 7, 8, and 8.8 mg/dL in preterm, term newborn, and children respectively. Young children are susceptible to hypocalcemia because of decreased PTH secretion in preterm infants as well as decreased calcium intake. Additionally hypomagnesemia, as seen in infants of diabetic mothers, can lead to hypocalcemia. Hypocalcemia is treated with calcium repletion at 15 mg calcium/kg body weight over 4-6 hours. In emergencies, IV calcium gluconate can be given at 2-4 mg/kg and 2-3 mg/kg in newborns and children respectively. **Hypercalcemia** is defined as a serum Ca concentration > 10.5 mg/dL and usually occurs iatrogenically from excess calcium intake, and also from vitamin D intoxication, thiazide diuretic use, hyperparathyroidism, hypophosphatemia, multiple fractures, acute renal failure, and milk alkali syndrome. Hypercalcemia should be treated by first stopping the administration of agents that increase calcium and vitamin D and starting IV fluids. Though diuretics such as loop diuretics can promote calciuria, thiazides should be avoided as they can cause hypercalcemia. Other treatment modalities include glucocorticoids, bisphosphonates, parathyroidectomy, and in severe cases, dialysis [39, 42, 85, 86].

Magnesium

Magnesium is located mostly intracellularly and normal serum magnesium (Mg^{2+}) levels are 1.7-2.5 mg/dL. Almost half of magnesium in the body is absorbed in the intestines. In the kidneys, the majority of magnesium reabsorption occurs in the thick ascending limb of the loop of Henle, mediated by the NKCC2 cotransporter and the Na^+/K^+ ATPase. **Hypomagnesemia** is defined as a serum Mg^{2+} concentration < 1.7 mg/dL and can occur due to dietary deficiency and losses by the GI tract or kidneys. **Hypermagnesemia** is defined as a serum Mg^{2+} concentration > 2.5 mg/dL and is usually iatrogenic due to excessive magnesium supplementation. Hypermagnesemia can manifest as hypotension, lethargy, respiratory depression, decreased deep tendon reflexes, and bradycardia and can be treated by IV calcium, diuretics, and in severe cases, dialysis [87, 88].

Phosphorus

Most of the body's phosphorus content is in bone, teeth, soft tissues and only a small amount (0.1%) of phosphorus is in the extracellular fluid. Normal serum phosphorus concentration ranges from 3-8.5 mg/dL and is the highest in neonates and infants because of an increase in growth hormone. Parathyroid hormone (PTH) causes phosphorus excretion Phosphorus absorption occurs in the ileum and jejunum and is enhanced by vitamin D3. Of the phosphorus that is renally filtered, most reabsorption occurs in the proximal tubule and about 10-20% is excreted. **Hypophosphatemia** increases calcitriol production which stimulates intestinal calcium and phosphate absorption and decreases calcitonin release. Excess PTH can stimulate the sodium-phosphate antiporter in the proximal tubule to cause phosphaturia which can lead to hypophosphatemia [25]. Hypophosphatemia decreases 2,3 diphosphoglycerate and left-shifts the oxyhemoglobin dissociation curve, decreases phosphorus available to form ATP, and can lead to muscle weakness and rhabdomyolysis. Hypophosphatemia can be treated with sodium or potassium phosphate and in severe cases (<1.5 mg/dL phosphorus), IV phosphorus can be used. **Hyperphosphatemia** can occur from transcellular shifts, increased phosphorus intake, hypoparathyroidism or decreased renal excretion. High phosphate ingestion can stimulate release of parathyroid hormone which promotes renal excretion of phosphate. Hyperphosphatemia can present with seizures, arrhythmias, laryngospasm, and renal failure and can lead to formation of calcium-phosphate (hydroxyapatite) crystals throughout the body [39, 89].

Anesthetic Agents and the Kidneys

Fluid losses through fasting deficit, insensible losses, blood loss, urine output in conjunction with the stress of surgery stimulate the renin-angiotensin-aldosterone system as well as increase ADH secretion to promote fluid retention. This collectively can reduce GFR, increasing the half-life of biologically active compounds that rely on renal excretion. Neonates and infants younger than age 6 months can have decreased renal clearance of propofol metabolites because of the short length of their nephron tubules and underdeveloped secretory systems. Though it is not used in practice anymore, methoxyflurane is a volatile anesthetic that highlights the impact of fluoride toxicity on the kidneys. After degradation in soda lime, sevoflurane was found to form Compound A which was nephrotoxic in rats, though the clinical significance of this in humans is still being studied [26].

Postoperative Pulmonary Edema

Postoperative pulmonary edema has many etiologies including excessive perioperative fluid administration with coexisting cardiac disease, acute respiratory distress syndrome, neurogenic pulmonary edema, sepsis, hyponatremia, anaphylaxis, burns, and negative pressure pulmonary edema (NPPE). NPPE often occurs in intubated patients who bite down on an endotracheal tube and inspire against a closed glottis. Any instance of inspiration against an upper airway obstruction has the potential to precipitate NPPE. This can cause an acute negative intrathoracic pressure (up to 50 to -100 cm H_2O) which causes a large increase in venous return and increase in left ventricular end-diastolic volume. The combination of increased pulmonary vascular resistance from hypoxia due to the airway obstruction and increased preload contributes to pulmonary edema. Treatment of postoperative pulmonary edema should be directed at the underlying cause and includes different modalities such as diuretics (outlined in Table **22**), beta agonists, steroids, and noninvasive positive pressure ventilation to decrease work of breathing [27].

Table 22. Diuretics [42, 90 - 92].

Diuretic	Nephron Site of Action	Mechanism	Pediatric Dose	Unique Indications	Side Effects
Mannitol	Proximal convoluted tubule, descending limb, collecting duct	Decreases gradient for NaCl reabsorption in distal tubule	0.5-1 g/kg/day	Reduce ICP, IOP	Reduces ICF volume, increase ECF volume, can precipitate heart failure

(Table 22) cont.....

Diuretic	Nephron Site of Action	Mechanism	Pediatric Dose	Unique Indications	Side Effects
Acetazolamide	Proximal convoluted tubule	Carbonic anhydrase inhibitor, reduce HCO3 reabsorption	5-7 mg/kg/day	Altitude sickness, refractory hydrocephalus, Meniere's disease, alkalinize urine	Metabolic acidosis, hypokalemia, hyperphosphaturia and hypercalciuria predispose to calcium phosphate nephrolithiasis
Loop diuretics Furosemide Torsemide Bumetanide Ethacrynic acid	Thick ascending limb of Loop of Henle	Mostly inhibit NKCC2 cotransporter in TAL and partly inhibit NaCl transporter in PCT and distal tubule	<u>Furosemide</u> PO 2-6mg/kg/day IV 1-6mg/kg/day	Unlike other loop diuretics, ethacrynic acid is safe in sulfa allergy	Hypokalemia, ototoxicity, neonatal jaundice *(furosemide is highly protein bound, displaces bilirubin from albumin in neonates), avoid in sulfa allergy
Thiazide HCTZ Chlorthalidone	Distal tubule	Block NaCl cotransporter	<u>HCTZ</u> IV 1-2mg/kg/day	Hyperkalemia, HTN, hypercalciuria	Hypercalcemia, hyperglycemia, hyperuricemia, hypokalemia
Spironolactone	Distal tubule	Competitive antagonist at mineralocorticoid receptor	1-3.3 mg/kg PO (max 100mg/day)	Hypokalemia, heart failure, hyperaldosteronism	Hyperkalemia, hypomagnesemia, hyponatremia
Amiloride Triamterene	Collecting duct	ENaC inhibitor	*	Hypokalemia, heart failure, hyperaldosteronism	Hyperkalemia Thrombocytopenia with amiloride

ICF intracellular fluid, ECF extracellular fluid, HCTZ hydrochlorothiazide, *no official pediatric dose recommendations

CONCLUSION

Pediatric anesthetic medication management and fluid resuscitation differ in many key ways from adult management. Although many of the drugs and core principles remain the same, the pediatric patient's unique metabolic pathways, differences in body size and composition, immature organ systems, altered enzymatic pathways, and particular childhood pathologies complicate the picture. Pediatric patients present differently in shock states and illness, and respond to treatment differently than the typical adult. The proper application of this knowledge of the alterations in physiology and drug response will give pediatric patients the best perioperative experience possible, and can be lifesaving.

CONSENT FOR PUBLICATION

Not applicable.

CONFLICT OF INTEREST

The author declares no conflict of interest, financial or otherwise.

ACKNOWLEDGEMENTS

Declared none.

REFERENCES

[1]   Hinderliter P, Saghir SA. 2014.https://www.sciencedirect.com/science/article/pii/B97801238645 4300419X

[2]   Ford JB, Wayment MT, Albertson TE, Owen KP, Radke JB, Sutter ME. Elimination kinetics of ethanol in a 5-week-old infant and a literature review of infant ethanol pharmacokinetics. Case Rep Med 2013; 2013: 250716.
[http://dx.doi.org/10.1155/2013/250716] [PMID: 24368917]

[3]   Greenblatt DJ. Elimination half-life of drugs: value and limitations. Annu Rev Med 1985; 36(1): 421-7.
[http://dx.doi.org/10.1146/annurev.me.36.020185.002225] [PMID: 3994325]

[4]   Krishna S, White NJ. Pharmacokinetics of quinine, chloroquine and amodiaquine. Clinical implications. Clin Pharmacokinet 1996; 30(4): 263-99.
[http://dx.doi.org/10.2165/00003088-199630040-00002] [PMID: 8983859]

[5]   Thomson A. Examples of dosage regimen design. Pharm J 2004; 273(7311): 188-90.

[6]   Bailey JM. Context-sensitive half-times: what are they and how valuable are they in anaesthesiology? Clin Pharmacokinet 2002; 41(11): 793-9.
[http://dx.doi.org/10.2165/00003088-200241110-00001] [PMID: 12190329]

[7]   Kapila A, Glass PS, Jacobs JR, *et al.* Measured context-sensitive half-times of remifentanil and alfentanil. Anesthesiology 1995; 83(5): 968-75.
[http://dx.doi.org/10.1097/00000542-199511000-00009] [PMID: 7486182]

[8]   Davis PJ, Cladis FP. The use of ultra-short-acting opioids in paediatric anaesthesia: the role of remifentanil. Clin Pharmacokinet 2005; 44(8): 787-96.
[http://dx.doi.org/10.2165/00003088-200544080-00002] [PMID: 16029065]

[9]   Fernandez E, Perez R, Hernandez A, Tejada P, Arteta M, Ramos JT. Factors and mechanisms for pharmacokinetic differences between pediatric population and adults. Pharmaceutics 2011; 3(1): 53-72.
[http://dx.doi.org/10.3390/pharmaceutics3010053]

[10]   Rasmussen GE, Grande CM. Blood, fluids, and electrolytes in the pediatric trauma patient. Int Anesthesiol Clin 1994; 32(1): 79-101.
[PMID: 8144255]

[11]   Holzman RS, Mancuso TJ, Polaner DM. A practical approach to pediatric anesthesia. Philadelphia, PA: Lippincott Williams and Wilkins 2015.

[12]   Kliegman RM, Stanton BF. Nelson textbook of pediatrics. Elsevier 2020.

[13]   Allen AM, Zhuo J, Mendelsohn FA. Localization of angiotensin AT1 and AT2 receptors. J Am Soc

Nephrol 1999; 10 (Suppl. 11): S23-9.
[PMID: 9892137]

[14] Hayton WL. Maturation and growth of renal function: dosing renally cleared drugs in children. AAPS PharmSci 2000; 2(1): E3.
[http://dx.doi.org/10.1208/ps020103] [PMID: 11741219]

[15] Waldman SA. Does potency predict clinical efficacy? Illustration through an antihistamine model. Ann Allergy Asthma Immunol 2002; 89(1): 7-11. quiz 11–2, 77
[http://dx.doi.org/10.1016/S1081-1206(10)61904-7]

[16] Allegaert K, Peeters MY, Verbesselt R, *et al.* Inter-individual variability in propofol pharmacokinetics in preterm and term neonates. Br J Anaesth 2007; 99(6): 864-70.
[http://dx.doi.org/10.1093/bja/aem294] [PMID: 17965417]

[17] Bradley AED, Tober KES, Brown RE. Use of propofol in patients with food allergies. Anaesthesia 2008; 63(4): 439.
[http://dx.doi.org/10.1111/j.1365-2044.2008.05505.x] [PMID: 18336502]

[18] Kam PCA, Cardone D. Propofol infusion syndrome. Anaesthesia 2007; 62(7): 690-701.
[http://dx.doi.org/10.1111/j.1365-2044.2007.05055.x] [PMID: 17567345]

[19] Vanlander AV, Okun JG, de Jaeger A, *et al.* Possible pathogenic mechanism of propofol infusion syndrome involves coenzyme q. Anesthesiology 2015; 122(2): 343-52.
[http://dx.doi.org/10.1097/ALN.0000000000000484] [PMID: 25296107]

[20] Schaller SJ, Fink H. Sugammadex as a reversal agent for neuromuscular block: an evidence-based review. Core Evid 2013; 8: 57-67.
[PMID: 24098155]

[21] Khurmi N, Patel P, Kraus M, Trentman T. Pharmacologic considerations for pediatric sedation and anesthesia outside the operating room: A review for anesthesia and non-anesthesia providers. Paediatr Drugs 2017; 19(5): 435-46.
[http://dx.doi.org/10.1007/s40272-017-0241-5] [PMID: 28597354]

[22] Shillingburg A, Biondo L. Aprepitant and fosaprepitant use in children and adolescents at an academic medical center. J Pediatr Pharmacol Ther 2014; 19(2): 127-31.
[http://dx.doi.org/10.5863/1551-6776-19.2.127] [PMID: 25024673]

[23] Fukuda T, Chidambaran V, Mizuno T, *et al.* OCT1 genetic variants influence the pharmacokinetics of morphine in children. Pharmacogenomics 2013; 14(10): 1141-51.
[http://dx.doi.org/10.2217/pgs.13.94] [PMID: 23859569]

[24] Krasniak AE, Knipp GT, Svensson CK, Liu W. Pharmacogenomics of acetaminophen in pediatric populations: a moving target. Front Genet 2014; 5: 314.
[http://dx.doi.org/10.3389/fgene.2014.00314] [PMID: 25352860]

[25] Tsukamoto Y. The effects of parathyroid hormone (PTH) on ca transportNephrology. Berlin, Heidelberg: Springer Berlin Heidelberg 1991; pp. 1509-16. [http://dx.doi.org/10.1007/978-3-6-2-35158-1_157]

[26] Mazze RI, Jamison R. Renal effects of sevoflurane. Anesthesiology 1995; 83(3): 443-5.
[http://dx.doi.org/10.1097/00000542-199509000-00001]

[27] Bajwa SS, Kulshrestha A. Diagnosis, prevention and management of postoperative pulmonary edema. Ann Med Health Sci Res 2012; 2(2): 180-5.
[http://dx.doi.org/10.4103/2141-9248.105668] [PMID: 23439791]

[28] Roberts F, Freshwater-Turner D. Pharmacokinetics and anaesthesia. Contin Educ Anaesth Crit Care Pain 2007; 7(1): 25-9.
[http://dx.doi.org/10.1093/bjaceaccp/mkl058]

[29] Batchelor HK, Marriott JF. Paediatric pharmacokinetics: key considerations. Br J Clin Pharmacol

2015; 79(3): 395-404.
[http://dx.doi.org/10.1111/bcp.12267] [PMID: 25855821]

[30]   Sebel PS, Bovill JG, van der Haven A. Cardiovascular effects of alfentanil anaesthesia. Br J Anaesth 1982; 54(11): 1185-90.
[http://dx.doi.org/10.1093/bja/54.11.1185] [PMID: 6128013]

[31]   Redhu S, Jalwal GK, Saxena M, Shrivastava OP. A comparative study of induction, maintenance and recovery characteristics of sevoflurane and halothane anaesthesia in pediatric patients (6 months to 6 years). J Anaesthesiol Clin Pharmacol 2010; 26(4): 484-7.
[PMID: 21547175]

[32]   Barash PG, Cahalan MK, Cullen BF, Stock MC, *et al.* Clinical anesthesia, 8e: Print + ebook with multimedia. Philadelphia, PA: Lippincott Williams and Wilkins 2017.

[33]   Manchikanti L, Kaye AM, Knezevic NN, *et al.* Responsible, safe, and effective prescription of opioids for chronic non-cancer pain: American society of interventional pain physicians (ASIPP) guidelines. Pain Physician 2017; 20(2S): S3-S92.
[http://dx.doi.org/10.36076/ppj.2017.s92] [PMID: 28226332]

[34]   Sharbaf Shoar N, Bistas KG, Saadabadi A. FlumazenilStatPearls. Treasure Island, FL: StatPearls Publishing 2020.

[35]   Bergendahl H, Lönnqvist P-A, Eksborg S. Clonidine in paediatric anaesthesia: review of the literature and comparison with benzodiazepines for premedication. Acta Anaesthesiol Scand 2006; 50(2): 135-43.
[http://dx.doi.org/10.1111/j.1399-6576.2006.00940.x] [PMID: 16430532]

[36]   Mitra S, Kazal S, Anand LK. Intranasal clonidine *vs.* midazolam as premedication in children: a randomized controlled trial. Indian Pediatr 2014; 51(2): 113-8.
[http://dx.doi.org/10.1007/s13312-014-0352-9] [PMID: 24277961]

[37]   Sethuraman U, Bhaya N. Pediatric shock. Therapy 2008; 5(4): 405-23.
[http://dx.doi.org/10.2217/14750708.5.4.405]

[38]   Lobo DN, Awad S. Should chloride-rich crystalloids remain the mainstay of fluid resuscitation to prevent 'pre-renal' acute kidney injury?: con. Kidney Int 2014; 86(6): 1096-105.
[http://dx.doi.org/10.1038/ki.2014.105] [PMID: 24717302]

[39]   Davis PJ, Cladis FP. Smith's Anesthesia for Infants and Children Ninth. Philadelphia, PA: Elsevier 2018.

[40]   Chidambaran V, Costandi A, D'Mello A. Propofol: a review of its role in pediatric anesthesia and sedation. CNS Drugs 2015; 29(7): 543-63.
[http://dx.doi.org/10.1007/s40263-015-0259-6] [PMID: 26290263]

[41]   Skibiski J, Abdijadid S. Barbiturates.StatPearls. Treasure Island, FL: StatPearls Publishing 2020.http://www.ncbi.nlm.nih.gov/books/NBK539731/

[42]   Coté CJ, Lerman J, Anderson BJ, Eds. A practice of anesthesia for infants and children. 6th ed., Philadelphia, PA: Elsevier 2019.

[43]   Donati F, Bevan DR. Antagonism of phase II succinylcholine block by neostigmine. Anesth Analg 1985; 64(8): 773-6.
[http://dx.doi.org/10.1213/00000539-198508000-00004]

[44]   Yang LPH, Keam SJ. Sugammadex: a review of its use in anaesthetic practice. Drugs 2009; 69(7): 919-42.
[http://dx.doi.org/10.2165/00003495-200969070-00008] [PMID: 19441874]

[45]   Embree PB. Long-acting nondepolarizing neuromuscular blocking agents. AANA J 1993; 61(4): 382-7.
[PMID: 8397465]

[46]   Manjushree R, Lahiri A, Ghosh BR, Laha A, Handa K. Intranasal fentanyl provides adequate postoperative analgesia in pediatric patients. Can J Anaesth 2002; 49(2): 190-3.
[http://dx.doi.org/10.1007/BF03020494] [PMID: 11823399]

[47]   Ziesenitz VC, Vaughns JD, Koch G, Mikus G, van den Anker JN. Pharmacokinetics of fentanyl and its derivatives in children: a comprehensive review. Clin Pharmacokinet 2018; 57(2): 125-49.
[http://dx.doi.org/10.1007/s40262-017-0569-6] [PMID: 28688027]

[48]   Andrews CM, Krantz MJ, Wedam EF, Marcuson MJ, Capacchione JF, Haigney MC. Methadone-induced mortality in the treatment of chronic pain: role of QT prolongation. Cardiol J 2009; 16(3): 210-7.
[PMID: 19437394]

[49]   Dalens BJ, Pinard AM, Létourneau D-R, Albert NT, Truchon RJY. Prevention of emergence agitation after sevoflurane anesthesia for pediatric cerebral magnetic resonance imaging by small doses of ketamine or nalbuphine administered just before discontinuing anesthesia. Anesth Analg 2006; 102(4): 1056-61.
[http://dx.doi.org/10.1213/01.ane.0000200282.38041.1f] [PMID: 16551898]

[50]   Baldini A, Von Korff M, Lin EHB. A review of potential adverse effects of long-term opioid therapy: a practitioner's guide. Prim Care Companion CNS Disord 2012; 14(3)
[http://dx.doi.org/10.4088/PCC.11m01326]

[51]   Rodrigues A, Wong C, Mattiussi A, Alexander S, Lau E, Dupuis LL. Methylnaltrexone for opioid-induced constipation in pediatric oncology patients. Pediatr Blood Cancer 2013; 60(10): 1667-70.
[http://dx.doi.org/10.1002/pbc.24615] [PMID: 23766091]

[52]   Peedikayil FC, Vijayan A. An update on local anesthesia for pediatric dental patients. Anesth Essays Res 2013; 7(1): 4-9.
[http://dx.doi.org/10.4103/0259-1162.113977] [PMID: 25885712]

[53]   Goodchild CS. GABA receptors and benzodiazepines. Br J Anaesth 1993; 71(1): 127-33.
[http://dx.doi.org/10.1093/bja/71.1.127] [PMID: 8393687]

[54]   McGhee B, *et al.* Pediatric drug therapy handbook and formulary Department of Pharmacy. 6th ed., Children's Hospital of Pittsburgh of UPMC 2011.

[55]   Spear RM, Yaster M, Berkowitz ID, *et al.* Preinduction of anesthesia in children with rectally administered midazolam. Anesthesiology 1991; 74(4): 670-4.
[http://dx.doi.org/10.1097/00000542-199104000-00009] [PMID: 2008948]

[56]   Henry DW, Burwinkle JW, Klutman NE. Determination of sedative and amnestic doses of lorazepam in children. Clin Pharm 1991; 10(8): 625-9.
[PMID: 1934919]

[57]   Gillis JC, Brogden RN. Ketorolac. A reappraisal of its pharmacodynamic and pharmacokinetic properties and therapeutic use in pain management. Drugs 1997; 53(1): 139-88.
[http://dx.doi.org/10.2165/00003495-199753010-00012] [PMID: 9010653]

[58]   Sullivan JE, Farrar HC. Fever and antipyretic use in children. Pediatrics 2011; 127(3): 580-7.
[http://dx.doi.org/10.1542/peds.2010-3852] [PMID: 21357332]

[59]   Oncel MY, Yurttutan S, Erdeve O, *et al.* Oral paracetamol versus oral ibuprofen in the management of patent ductus arteriosus in preterm infants: a randomized controlled trial. J Pediatr 164(3): 510- 4.e1. 2014; 164(3): 510-4.e1.

[60]   *A Guide for the Non-Pediatric Anesthesia Provider Ahmad and Dippo* patent ductus arteriosus in preterm infants: a randomized controlled trial. J Pediatr 2014; 164(3): 510-4.e1.
[http://dx.doi.org/10.1016/j.jpeds.2013.11.008] [PMID: 24359938]

[60]   Eberhart LHJ, Geldner G, Kranke P, *et al.* The development and validation of a risk score to predict the probability of postoperative vomiting in pediatric patients. Anesth Analg 2004; 99(6): 1630-7.

[http://dx.doi.org/10.1213/01.ANE.0000135639.57715.6C] [PMID: 15562045]

[61] Charbit B, Albaladejo P, Funck-Brentano C, Legrand M, Samain E, Marty J. Prolongation of QTc interval after postoperative nausea and vomiting treatment by droperidol or ondansetron. Anesthesiology 2005; 102(6): 1094-100.
[http://dx.doi.org/10.1097/00000542-200506000-00006] [PMID: 15915019]

[62] Madan R, Bhatia A, Chakithandy S, *et al.* Prophylactic dexamethasone for postoperative nausea and vomiting in pediatric strabismus surgery: a dose ranging and safety evaluation study. Anesth Analg 2005; 100(6): 1622-6.
[http://dx.doi.org/10.1213/01.ANE.0000150977.14607.E1] [PMID: 15920184]

[63] Diemunsch P, Gan TJ, Philip BK, *et al.* Single-dose aprepitant *vs* ondansetron for the prevention of postoperative nausea and vomiting: a randomized, double-blind phase III trial in patients undergoing open abdominal surgery. Br J Anaesth 2007; 99(2): 202-11.
[http://dx.doi.org/10.1093/bja/aem133] [PMID: 17540667]

[64] Hill LL. Body composition, normal electrolyte concentrations, and the maintenance of normal volume, tonicity, and acid-base metabolism. Pediatr Clin North Am 1990; 37(2): 241-56.
[http://dx.doi.org/10.1016/S0031-3955(16)36865-1] [PMID: 2184394]

[65] Kagan BM, Stanincova V, Felix NS, Hodgman J, Kalman D. Body composition of premature infants: relation to nutrition. Am J Clin Nutr 1972; 25(11): 1153-64.
[http://dx.doi.org/10.1093/ajcn/25.11.1153] [PMID: 5086038]

[66] Wu PY, Hodgman JE. Insensible water loss in preterm infants: changes with postnatal development and non-ionizing radiant energy. Pediatrics 1974; 54(6): 704-12.
[http://dx.doi.org/10.1542/peds.54.6.704] [PMID: 4431668]

[67] Winters RW. Principles of pediatric fluid therapy. 2nd ed., Boston: Little, Brown 1982.

[68] Avner ED, Ed. Pediatric nephrology 6, completely rev, updated and enl. Berlin: Springer 2009.
[http://dx.doi.org/10.1007/978-3-540-76341-3]

[69] Fawer CL, Torrado A, Guignard JP. Maturation of renal function in full-term and premature neonates. Helv Paediatr Acta 1979; 34(1): 11-21.
[PMID: 429191]

[70] Practice guidelines for preoperative fasting and the use of pharmacologic agents to reduce the risk of pulmonary aspiration: application to healthy patients undergoing elective procedures. Anesthesiology 2017; 126(3): 376-93.
[http://dx.doi.org/10.1097/ALN.0000000000001452] [PMID: 28045707]

[71] McCaig WD, Patel PS, Sosunov SA, *et al.* Hyperglycemia potentiates a shift from apoptosis to RIP1-dependent necroptosis. Cell Death Discov 2018; 4(1): 55.
[http://dx.doi.org/10.1038/s41420-018-0058-1] [PMID: 29760953]

[72] 5 human albumin. Transfus Med Hemother 2009; 36(6): 399-407.
[http://dx.doi.org/10.1159/000268061] [PMID: 21245971]

[73] Schwartz GJ, Brion LP, Spitzer A. The use of plasma creatinine concentration for estimating glomerular filtration rate in infants, children, and adolescents. Pediatr Clin North Am 1987; 34(3): 571-90.
[http://dx.doi.org/10.1016/S0031-3955(16)36251-4] [PMID: 3588043]

[74] Holliday MA, Segar WE. The maintenance need for water in parenteral fluid therapy. Pediatrics 1957; 19(5): 823-32.
[http://dx.doi.org/10.1542/peds.19.5.823] [PMID: 13431307]

[75] Winters RW. Principles of pediatric fluid therapy. 2nd ed., Boston: Little, Brown 1982.

[76] Adrogué HJ, Madias NE. Hypernatremia. N Engl J Med 2000; 342(20): 1493-9.
[http://dx.doi.org/10.1056/NEJM200005183422006] [PMID: 10816188]

[77]   Oiso Y, Robertson GL, Nørgaard JP, Juul KV. Clinical review: Treatment of neurohypophyseal diabetes insipidus. J Clin Endocrinol Metab 2013; 98(10): 3958-67.
[http://dx.doi.org/10.1210/jc.2013-2326] [PMID: 23884783]

[78]   Wise-Faberowski L, Soriano SG, Ferrari L, *et al.* Perioperative management of diabetes insipidus in children. J Neurosurg Anesthesiol 2004; 16(3): 220-5.
[http://dx.doi.org/10.1097/00008506-200407000-00006] [PMID: 15211159]

[79]   D'Alessandro A, Liumbruno G, Grazzini G, Zolla L. Red blood cell storage: the story so far. Blood Transfus 2010; 8(2): 82-8. [Internet].
[PMID: 20383300]

[80]   Goel R, Johnson DJ, Scott AV, *et al.* Red blood cells stored 35 days or more are associated with adverse outcomes in high-risk patients. Transfusion 2016; 56(7): 1690-8.
[http://dx.doi.org/10.1111/trf.13559] [PMID: 27062463]

[81]   Smith HM, Farrow SJ, Ackerman JD, Stubbs JR, Sprung J. Cardiac arrests associated with hyperkalemia during red blood cell transfusion: a case series. Anesth Analg 2008; 106(4): 1062-9. [table of contents.].
[http://dx.doi.org/10.1213/ane.0b013e318164f03d] [PMID: 18349174]

[82]   Raza S, Ali Baig M, Chang C, *et al.* A prospective study on red blood cell transfusion related hyperkalemia in critically ill patients. J Clin Med Res 2015; 7(6): 417-21.
[http://dx.doi.org/10.14740/jocmr2123w] [PMID: 25883703]

[83]   Rastegar A, Soleimani M. Hypokalaemia and hyperkalaemia. Postgrad Med J 2001; 77(914): 759-64.
[http://dx.doi.org/10.1136/pgmj.77.914.759] [PMID: 11723313]

[84]   Mushiyakh Y, Dangaria H, Qavi S, Ali N, Pannone J, Tompkins D. Treatment and pathogenesis of acute hyperkalemia. J Community Hosp Intern Med Perspect 2012; 1(4)
[http://dx.doi.org/10.3402/jchimp.v1i4.7372] [PMID: 23882341]

[85]   Matkovic V, Heaney RP. Calcium balance during human growth: evidence for threshold behavior. Am J Clin Nutr 1992; 55(5): 992-6.
[http://dx.doi.org/10.1093/ajcn/55.5.992] [PMID: 1570810]

[86]   Moore EW. Ionized calcium in normal serum, ultrafiltrates, and whole blood determined by ion-exchange electrodes. J Clin Invest 1970; 49(2): 318-34.
[http://dx.doi.org/10.1172/JCI106241] [PMID: 4983663]

[87]   Konrad M, Weber S. Recent advances in molecular genetics of hereditary magnesium-losing disorders. J Am Soc Nephrol 2003; 14(1): 249-60.
[http://dx.doi.org/10.1097/01.ASN.0000049161.60740.CE] [PMID: 12506158]

[88]   Cole DEC, Quamme GA. Inherited disorders of renal magnesium handling. J Am Soc Nephrol 2000; 11(10): 1937-47.
[http://dx.doi.org/10.1681/ASN.V11101937] [PMID: 11004227]

[89]   Knochel JP. The pathophysiology and clinical characteristics of severe hypophosphatemia. Arch Intern Med 1977; 137(2): 203-20.
[http://dx.doi.org/10.1001/archinte.1977.03630140051013] [PMID: 836118]

[90]   Imbs JL, Schmidt M, Giesen-Crouse E. Pharmacology of loop diuretics: state of the art. Adv Nephrol Necker Hosp 1987; 16: 137-58.
[PMID: 3101419]

[91]   Warren SE, Blantz RC. Mannitol. Arch Intern Med 1981; 141(4): 493-7.
[http://dx.doi.org/10.1001/archinte.1981.00340040089023] [PMID: 6782963]

[92]   Maren TH. Carbonic anhydrase: General perspective and advances in glaucoma research. Drug Dev Res 1987; 10(4): 255-76.
[http://dx.doi.org/10.1002/ddr.430100407]

CHAPTER 3

Pediatric Operating Room Setup

Bharathi Gourkanti[1,*], **Marlo DiDonna**[1] and **Rosemary De La Cruz**[1]

[1] Department of Anesthesiology, Cooper Medical School of Rowan University, Cooper University Health Care, Camden, NJ, USA

Abstract: The pediatric population presents many unique challenges to the anesthesia care team. A well-organized pediatric anesthesia room setup is essential to facilitate a smooth induction, maintenance, and emergence. Infants and children have a greater metabolic rate and increased oxygen consumption. Although the child's functional residual capacity (FRC) is similar to an adult's, the child's ability to compensate during periods of hypoxia is limited due to these compounding factors. As a result, rapid oxygen desaturation is more prevalent in the pediatric population, and limits the amount of time the anesthesia provider has to rectify these conditions. A thorough operating room setup includes precise drug calculations, ventilator settings and airway equipment, IV and colloid infusions, and thermoregulation considerations. Knowledge of these considerations allows the non-routine pediatric anesthesia provider an opportunity to provide safe, efficient, and optimal care to the pediatric population during the intraoperative period.

Keywords: Airway equipment, Anesthesia setup, Anesthesia cart, Anesthesia machine, Bleeding tonsil, Blood transfusion, Cleft lip/palate, Difficult airway, Epiglottitis, Fiberoptic intubation, Fiberoptic intubation blocks, Handoff communication, Neonatal anesthesia, Obesity, Pediatric drug dosing, Pediatric laryngoscopes, Pediatric trauma, Postoperative transport, Pyloromyotomy, Sleep apnea, Thermoregulation and warming devices, Tracheostomy, Transport ventilator, Videolaryngoscopy.

INTRODUCTION

A seasoned pediatric anesthesia provider follows a methodical checklist when preparing for the administration of anesthesia to a pediatric patient. It is important to stress that children have unique characteristics that distinguish them from adults.

---

* **Corresponding author Bharathi Gourkanti:** Department of Anesthesiology, Cooper Medical School of Rowan University, Cooper University Health Care, Camden, NJ, USA; E-mail: gourkantibharathi@ cooperhealth.edu

Bharathi Gourkanti, Irwin Gratz, Grace Dippo, Nathalie Peiris and Dinesh K. Choudhry (Eds.)
All rights reserved-© 2022 Bentham Science Publishers

Even an adult-sized teenager can present challenges that need to be anticipated when considering a plan of care.

Children have an uncanny ability to compensate; however, when their reserves are depleted, decompensation is abrupt and often dire. Anesthesia providers are aware of this and use their checklist in combination with their clinical skills to recognize ominous situations and react swiftly to prevent decompensation. We will modify an acronym commonly used in all areas of anesthesia OR setup and adapt it to create a basic pediatric checklist (Fig. **1**) that will enable all anesthesia providers to be prepared and ready for induction, maintenance, and successful emergence of pediatric patients.

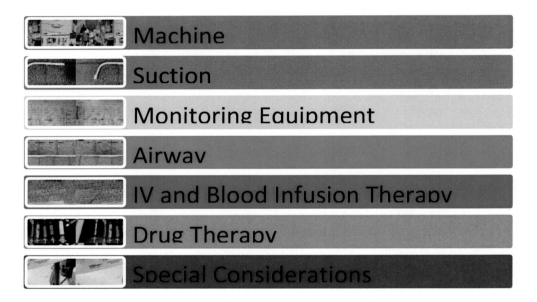

Fig. (1). MSMAIDS mnemonic commonly used for anesthesia operating room setup [1].

The pediatric anesthesia setup checklist is a step-by-step document [1]. A precise checklist enables the anesthesia provider to quickly ascertain the equipment and adjuncts required to initiate a safe anesthetic. This is especially relevant in current pediatric anesthesia practice, as outside locations such as MRI, CT scan, interventional radiology, endoscopy, and radiation therapy, are now common treatment sites [2].

Machine

The anesthesia machine allows oxygen, air, nitrous oxide and inhalational agents to be delivered to the patient while providing an outlet for exhaled carbon dioxide. Modern anesthesia circuits are unidirectional, semi-closed circle systems. They maintain heat and humidity while decreasing the amount of exhaled gasses with an adjustable scavenger system device and carbon dioxide absorbent [3]. A reservoir bag allows for spontaneous or assisted ventilation and an adjustable pressure limiting (APL or "pop-off") valve controls the amount of positive pressure delivered to the patient's lungs. Another key component of the modern anesthesia machine (Fig. **2**) is the ventilator. Modern machines are technologically advanced and have internal electronics to monitor patient status, allowing for precise delivery of tidal volumes and minute ventilation through a variety of modes [3].

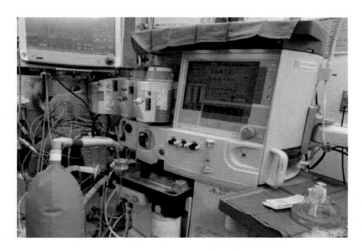

Fig. (2). Modern anesthesia machine (Photo taken by Marlo DiDonna).

In 1993, the FDA published an anesthesia machine checklist to ensure the correct functioning of the equipment prior to the induction of anesthesia. It was updated in 2008 to reflect the increasing sophistication and diversity of anesthesia delivery systems [4].

After the machine checklist is completed, the ventilator should be programmed according to the patient's weight and age prior to induction. By entering these values, modern machines may give preset volumes and pressures to ensure that safe minute ventilation is delivered to the patient. If adjustments for weight and age parameters are not available, the ventilator can be set to Pressure Control Ventilation (PCV) between 12-15cm H_2O with the respiratory rate adjusted to the age of the patient to ensure a safe minute ventilation.

Pediatric circle systems come in smaller diameters and lengths with lower volume reservoir bags. These circuits can be used in conjunction with passive HMEs (heat and humidity exchangers) which will maintain better heat and humidity preservation but will increase dead space within the system. During the machine check, one should elongate the corrugated circuit entirely to accurately prepare the machine to deliver accurate minute ventilation. If the circuit is adjusted after the initial machine check, the internal computer of modern anesthesia machines may not be able to compensate for the narrow safety margin in pediatric tidal volumes in the smallest patients [5]. Choosing an appropriately sized reservoir bag (Fig. **3**) is important to ensure that an appropriate amount of positive pressure can be maintained. Pediatric circuits typically come with a 1-liter reservoir bag (larger infants, toddlers, and young children); however, 0.5L (< 3kg patient) and 2L (school-aged children) are also available.

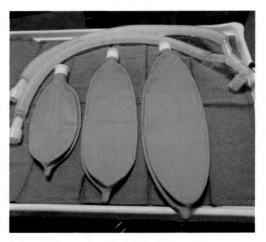

Fig. (3). Different sized reservoir bags (Photo taken by Marlo DiDonna).

The pipeline and backup cylinder pressures of oxygen, nitrous oxide, and air should always be checked. It is optimal to have a pipeline pressure of >1000 PSI. In the event of machine failure, unexpected malignant hyperthermia, or pipeline failure, a separate oxygen source should also be available in the room. Often these oxygen cylinders are mounted on the back of the anesthesia machine or the pediatric anesthesia cart. An appropriately sized bag-mask valve (AMBU) should also be available to deliver positive pressure ventilation in an emergency.

Most young children (less than 8 years old) do not tolerate the placement of an intravenous catheter prior to induction, therefore inhalation induction is preferred. Sevoflurane is the most widely used pediatric inhalational induction agent and should be checked and refilled prior to induction.

The CO_2 absorbent should be monitored for exhaustion. Exhausted CO_2 absorbent can cause elevated end-tidal CO_2, rebreathing, and delayed emergence. Baralyme and other strongly alkaline CO_2 absorbents were discontinued because of the increased risk of carbon monoxide toxicity and Compound- A buildup leading to renal and hepatic issues [6]. These complications are no longer an issue with the advent of NaOH-free and KOH-free desiccants. Color indicators are a way to ascertain CO_2 absorbent exhaustion, but not always reliable. If you notice a violet color in the CO_2 absorbent coupled with a rise above baseline in the $ETCO_2$ tracing, replace the CO_2 absorbent.

Suction

An available and working suction apparatus is imperative when anesthetizing patients. The suction canister can be found attached to the anesthesia machine, mounted on the wall, or be free-standing.

The suction apparatus consists of a collection container, a vacuum source that sometimes is controlled by a vacuum regulator, and tubing that extends to some type of suction catheter. Suction catheters can either be rigid or flexible depending on what types of secretions need to be removed. The standard yankauer suction is a large, rigid catheter; this can be useful to remove large amounts of secretions, and is used for larger children and teenagers approaching adult size. A flexible salivary ejector is used in the younger pediatric population for gentle, yet effective suctioning. It is softer than a traditional rigid yankauer, so teeth and oral tissue will be better protected from damage. Soft suction catheters are useful in infants to clear oral secretions and suction the endotracheal tube (ETT). Soft suction catheters come in a variety of sizes. An 8F soft suction catheter is small enough to suction a 3.0 endotracheal tube ETT. These catheters often have a suction port that needs to be occluded for suction to ensue.

Monitoring Equipment

Monitoring equipment recommended by the American Society of Anesthesiologists (ASA) is the standard of care. Heart rate, pulse oximetry, blood pressure, temperature, and end tidal carbon dioxide are monitored and documented. The electronic health record (EHR) (Fig. **4**) uses computer software to integrate data from the anesthesia machine into the electronic record. The electronic filing of patient data may erroneously record aberrancies, for example, when the surgeon leans on a BP cuff, and it can inaccurately portray the current status of the patient. This is particularly common in the pediatric population, and anesthesia providers should document the reason for any aberrancies to reflect the patient's condition more accurately.

We will explore the different types of monitoring equipment (Fig. **5**) that are available for the pediatric population, focusing on the pillars of basic monitoring.

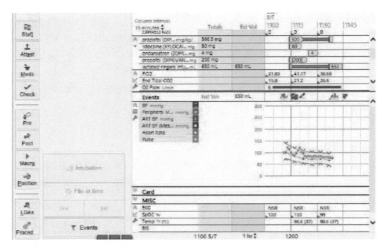

Fig. (4). Example of the modern electronic anesthesia chart (Permission: Cooper University Hospital; Camden, NJ).

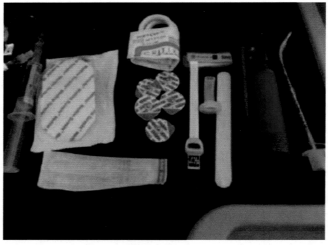

Fig. (5). Basic pediatric monitors and equipment (Original photo taken by Marlo DiDonna).

Electrocardiogram (ECG) Five lead ECG monitoring is the standard in anesthesia. In the general pediatric population, three lead ECG monitoring is acceptable. Small ECG electrodes are helpful when monitoring the smallest of patients. Drying and preparing the area with an alcohol swab may help with electrode adherence and allow for a better ECG tracing.

Non-invasive blood pressure As with all patients, a properly fitting blood pressure cuff covers two-thirds of the upper arm length. Calf and thigh NIBP monitoring is frequently used in the pediatric population and should also be sized to two-thirds of the limb. Every five minutes is the standard of care for blood pressure monitoring during the operative period. Most monitors can be set to adult, child, or infant mode; this allows for appropriate inflation/deflation times that limit the risk of nerve compression and venous stasis. In the neonate, automated NIBP cuffs are available in sizes 1-5 that loosely correlate to the weight of the patient in kilograms. These types of cuffs come with a separate tubing hose that can be interchanged into the monitoring manifold.

Pulse oximetry Because the pulse oximetry reading is not affected by electrocautery, it should be chosen as the beat source on your monitor. Bandage-type probes work well on infants and toddlers. They can be wrapped entirely around the foot or hand of a neonate to obtain a pulse oximetry reading. It is prudent to have either a second pulse oximeter or place a second probe that can quickly be switched to in the case of monitoring aberrancies.

End tidal carbon dioxide End tidal carbon dioxide ($ETCO_2$) is a standard monitor. Pediatric nasal cannulas and face masks have ports for $ETCO_2$ and respiratory rate monitoring. $ETCO_2$ monitoring aids in the early detection of hypoventilation prior to desaturation.

Temperature An underdeveloped physiological ability to compensate for heat loss in addition to an increased metabolic demand puts neonates and infants at a greater risk of hypothermia [7]. Hyperthermia can also be indicative of malignant hyperthermia when coupled with increasing $ETCO_2$. The esophageal stethoscope is a good indicator of core temperature and comes in pediatric sizes. A temperature-sensitive sticker placed on a patient's forehead or a probe placed under the axilla is a reliable non-invasive option for temperature monitoring in pediatrics.

Airway

Rapid desaturation is prevalent in pediatric anesthesia. While the functional residual capacity is similar on a per-kilogram basis across age groups, the FRC represents a larger percentage of the total lung capacity (TLC). During apnea, hypoxemia can develop rapidly. A variety of masks, endotracheal tubes (ETT), oral and nasal airways, and laryngeal mask airways (LMA), should be available in the anesthesia cart to facilitate a safe induction period. Video laryngoscopy, such as the GlideScope or the C-MAC, can complement the airway setup. We will present a variety of instruments and techniques for airway control, intubation, and ventilation.

Face Masks

The mask is a plastic device with an inflatable cushioned rim available in a variety of sizes. It is useful to follow the manufacturer's recommendations for size fit. Alternative sizes should be available if quick adjustments need to be made as pediatric anatomy varies [3]. A properly fitting mask fits over the bridge of the nose and extends comfortably down to the angle of the mandible with minimal pressure to the orbital area, nose, and mouth to provide a seal.

Oropharyngeal and Nasopharyngeal Airways

The pediatric anatomy is especially vulnerable to airway obstruction. A large tongue, a lack of fully formed teeth, and an infant's tendency for obligate nasal breathing make induction, sedation, and the emergence period challenging.

Oropharyngeal airways (Fig. **6**) are made of rigid, non-latex plastic materials that are shaped to open the airway and come in a variety of sizes. Improperly fitted oral airways can be a detriment and further compound airway obstruction. An oral airway that is too small for the patient can displace the posterior tongue further and worsen the obstruction. If the oral airway is too large, it may push the epiglottis into the glottic aperture and create airway obstruction or cause injury to the epiglottis and uvula [3]. The appropriate length of an oral airway can be approximated by the distance from the bottom of the earlobe or just above the mandibular angle to the mouth. Airways should always be inserted midline taking precautions to avoid teeth, compression of the tongue, and occlusion of soft tissue. Some airways have center openings that facilitate soft suctioning and ease ventilation.

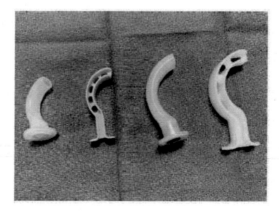

Fig. (6). Oropharyngeal airways.

Nasopharyngeal airways (Fig. **7**) are inserted into the nose and advanced to the posterior pharynx. They are useful in opening a compromised airway, but instrumenting the nasal cavity can cause epistaxis. Nasopharyngeal airways are composed of soft, pliant plastic materials. Lubrication with either Lidocaine jelly or water-soluble ointment and pretreatment with Oxymetazoline spray to the nares can decrease the incidence of epistaxis. Nasopharyngeal airways come in a variety of sizes, from 12F to 38F. An approximation of correct size can be made by placing the trumpet from the tip of the nose to the bottom of the earlobe or just above the mandibular angle [3].

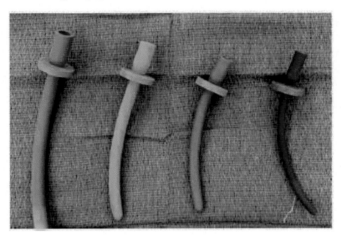

Fig. (7). Nasopharyngeal airways. (Original photo by Marlo DiDonna.)

Nasopharyngeal airways are better tolerated than oral airways in conscious, spontaneously breathing patients. In cases of airway obstruction, nasopharyngeal airways can be helpful in maintaining airway patency in the immediate post-operative period.

Supraglottic Airway Devices

Supraglottic airway devices (Fig. **8**) are useful in emergent difficult airway situations, but also have a role in routine, pediatric surgeries when general anesthesia is indicated.

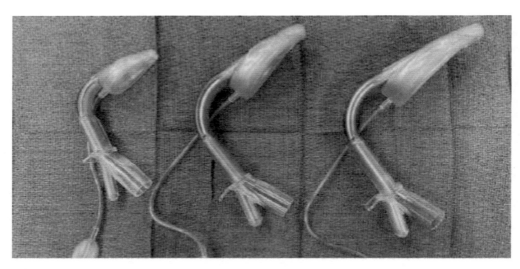

Fig. (8). Pediatric supraglottic airway devices (Photo taken by Marlo DiDonna).

The LMA Supreme is a disposable supraglottic device that is shaped into the optimal curve to allow for ease of insertion along the patient's hard palate. It is made of a harder plastic than seen in earlier generations of LMAs, has a reinforced tip to prevent it from folding onto itself in the hypopharynx, and has a secondary port that can be used to vent excess gastric air and to suction gastric contents [8]. The rigid plastic composition makes it even more useful in the pediatric population than previous generations, as it stabilizes the LMA in edentulous infants. The LMA Supreme is available in a variety of sizes, and sizing is weight-based as depicted in Table **1**.

Table 1. Laryngeal mask size based on patient weight and maximum oral endotracheal tube sizes.

LMA Size	Weight (kg)	Maximum Endotracheal Tube Size (ID in mm)
1	< 5	3.0 uncuffed
1.5	5- 10	4.0 uncuffed, 3.5 cuffed
2	10- 20	4.5 uncuffed, 4.0 cuffed
2.5	20- 30	4.5 cuffed
3	30- 50	5.5 cuffed
4	50- 70	5.5 cuffed
5	70- 100	6.5 cuffed
6	> 100	6.5 cuffed

Laryngoscopy Equipment and Endotracheal Tubes

In pediatrics, laryngoscopy and endotracheal intubation present unique challenges due to major anatomical differences in the pediatric airway which are most pronounced in neonates and in children less than one year of age [9]. See Chapter 1 for further details on anatomical differences.

Laryngoscopes

A variety of laryngoscopes (Fig. **9**) with different blade shapes and sizes should be available. Because of an infant's rigid, u-shaped epiglottis, the Miller laryngoscope blade is a better option for intubation in infants. It exposes the vocal cords more effectively, as it lifts the epiglottis rather than resting in the vallecula. Macintosh blades can be used in older children and can also be useful in palate surgery as the curved blade is less likely to become caught in an open palate, obscuring the view. The Wis-Hipple blade is also commonly used in infants and toddlers. It is considered a straight blade, but the tip for lifting the epiglottis is wider than a traditional straight blade.

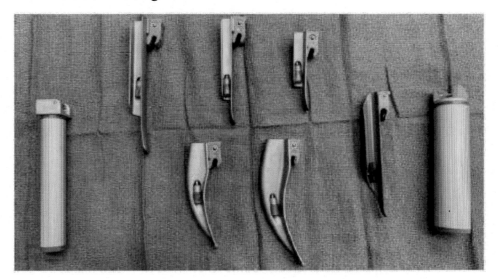

Fig. (9). Various pediatric blades and laryngoscope handles; Clockwise from upper left (Miller 2, 1, 0; Wis-Hipple 1.5; Mac 2, 1) shown with pediatric laryngoscope handle (left) and stubby laryngoscope handle (right); (Photo taken by Marlo DiDonna).

Endotracheal Tubes

Choosing the correct size of endotracheal tube is important, as the pediatric trachea is funnel-shaped rather than cylindrical as in adults. The funnel-shaped trachea in young children can lead to damage to the subglottic mucosa and subglottic stenosis if the endotracheal tube is too large. Historically, it was recommended that uncuffed endotracheal tubes be used in all children less than eight years of age. With the advent of high-volume, low-pressure cuffed endotracheal tubes, the argument over the safety and efficacy of uncuffed *versus* cuffed endotracheal tubes in pediatrics has ensued.

The Microcuff® endotracheal tube (Fig. **10**) was originally intended for use in the critical care environment where long term intubation is common and ventilator-associated pneumonia from micro-aspiration can occur. Soon, the potential for use in pediatric anesthesia became apparent, as the material used to create the cuff is ultrathin but still provides a safe, adequate seal. The Murphy eye has been eliminated, which has allowed the cuff to be situated more distally on the tracheal tube shaft. When inflated, the cuff expands below the cricoid level, providing a seal with a cuff pressure <15 cm H_2O, thus decreasing the incidence of post-extubation stridor and mucosal damage [10].

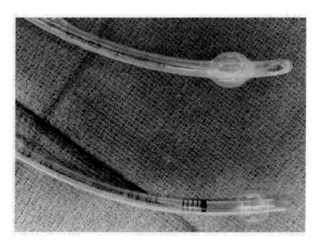

Fig. (10). (Top) Conventional pediatric 4.0 cuffed ETT with location of inflated cuff and presence of Murphy eye; (Bottom) Microcuff pediatric 4.0 cuffed ETT cuff with distally situated inflated cuff and absence of Murphy eye (Photo taken by Marlo DiDonna).

Vigilant monitoring of cuff pressures should occur if a cuffed ETT is chosen. An acceptable audible leak should be heard at peak pressures <25cm H_2O; however, with the Microcuff® endotracheal tube an adequate seal can be produced at 10-15cm H_2O, so it appears to be a safer alternative especially in infants. Nonetheless, all cuff pressures should be monitored throughout the surgery, especially if nitrous oxide is used, as N_2O can diffuse into the cuff and increase its pressure. If an excessive air leak is noted after successful intubation, the use of a cuffed endotracheal tube allows the practitioner more flexibility in making an adjustment. Small amounts of air can be added to the cuff to adequately provide a seal without the need for further laryngoscopy.

Age-based formulas presented in Table **2** for determining ETT sizes should only serve as a starting point in choosing an appropriate size. The inner diameter is the only standardized sizing required of manufacturers; the outer diameter varies among manufacturers and can influence the choice.

Table 2. Commonly used formulas for sizing pediatric endotracheal tubes [11].

Uncuffed ETT		Microcuff® ETT Sizing	
		Inner diameter of ETT	Age of child
Modified Cole formula	ID(mm) = (age/4) + 4	3.0	Term (>3kg) - <8 months
Morgan & Steward formula	ID(mm) = (age + 16)/4	3.5	8 months - < 2 years
		4.0	2 years - < 4 years
Cuffed ETT (non- Microcuff®)		4.5	4 years - < 6 years
Motoyama formula	ID(mm) = age/4 + 3.5	5.0	6 years - < 8 years
Khine formula	ID(mm) = (age/4) + 3	5.5	8 years - <10 years
		6.0	10 years - <12 years

The following table shows the most commonly used formulas to determine the size for both uncuffed and cuffed endotracheal tubes [11]. These formulas are intended for children at least two years of age. For premature neonates, a 2.5 or 3.0 ETT is usually appropriate, whereas a 3.5 or 4.0 ETT would be chosen for a healthy 1 year old. Considerations need to be made based on the presence of a cuff, ease of insertion, length of surgery, and presence of air leak <25cm H_2O. Observation of these variables will help to guide the practitioner's choice of an endotracheal tube.

When choosing an endotracheal tube, it is useful to have an endotracheal tube 0.5mm size smaller and 0.5mm larger to accommodate for differences in individual anatomy. If a cuffed endotracheal tube is used, choosing a tube that is 0.5mm size smaller can allow for the additional bulk of the cuff. Additionally, the Microcuff endotracheal tube has a larger outer diameter and the company has set forth their own recommendations on tube size based on age, however differences in anatomy are still to be considered based on laryngoscopy and ease of placement.

The endotracheal tube depth should always be evaluated through bilateral auscultation of the lungs and reexamined after head extension/flexion and positioning changes. A good rule of thumb is to multiply the size of the endotracheal tube by 3 to ascertain an approximate depth. Correct placement is confirmed with auscultation.

Difficult Airway

Emergencies arising from airway complications constitute 25% to 36% of all reported anesthesia closed claims. Of those reported respiratory events, 43% of complications occur in children, and 30% occur in adults [12]. Pediatric patients suffer a higher mortality rate of 50%, compared to 35% seen in adult patients [13]. The review of difficult airway algorithms (*e.g.* The American Society of Anesthesiology Difficult Airway Algorithm) can assist the anesthesia provider in the preparation of a reasonable airway management plan.

Laryngeal Mask Airways (LMA)

LMAs have gained widespread use and are available for all age groups from neonates < 5 kg to adolescents and adults weighing more than 90 kg [14]. The appropriate size is selected by guidelines based on the patient's weight as shown in Table **1** [15].

There are several different types of LMAs available (Fig. **11**), including the classic LMA, LMA Flexible (soft, malleable wired neck), LMA ProSeal (with a second channel to direct gastric contents away from the airway), LMA Supreme (is similar to the Proseal with a built-in bite block), I-gel and the intubating LMA.

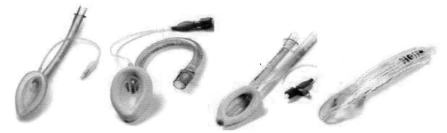

Fig. (11). Classic LMA, LMA Flexible, LMA Proseal, and I-gel (Illustrated by Rosemary De La Cruz).

There is a lack of high-quality data comparing advantages and disadvantages of the different types of LMAs in children. However, the LMA is a lifesaving device for ventilation in the emergency and nonemergency pathways of the ASA difficult airway algorithm [16].

Video-assisted Laryngoscopy Video-assisted laryngoscopy has revolutionized the ease of handling a potentially disastrous difficult airway situation. The GlideScope and the C-MAC are two widely used video-assisted laryngoscopy systems. They simulate traditional laryngoscopy without the need for excessive head extension where cervical instability is a concern and in severely anterior airways. In teaching institutions, these devices allow the instructor and trainee to share the same magnified view of the airway, granting better identification of the anatomy, and helping the instructor to guide the trainee. It is imperative to have one of these devices available in your setup if a difficult intubation is predicted or if a neonate or small infant is having surgery.

Multiple studies have shown that although "time to best view" was shorter, "time to intubation" was longer, most notably in infants, when compared to traditional laryngoscopy [17]. This can be especially problematic in a pediatric patient where desaturation can occur quickly. Factors that may contribute to this delay have been suggested but not definitively studied in the pediatric population. A suboptimal acute angle that inhibits the passage of the endotracheal tube due to an infant's natural cephalad position of their vocal cords and omega-shaped epiglottis has been discussed as a potential factor. It has been suggested that withdrawing the video laryngoscope to produce a Grade 2 view instead of a Grade 1 view and molding the endotracheal tube at an acute angle with a flexible stylet can aid in the successful passage of the endotracheal tube [18].

Video-assisted laryngoscopy has been instrumental in the management of pediatric airways in cases of anticipated difficult intubation because of increased first-attempt success rates and better laryngoscopy views [19]. However, in certain circumstances, fiberoptic bronchoscopy continues to be the most effective, and for this reason, anesthesia providers should still be proficient in this technique. The simultaneous use of video-assisted laryngoscopy and fiberoptic bronchoscopy has been used successfully in difficult airway situations [20].

There are a variety of video laryngoscopy devices available for intubation in the pediatric population, however the clinical advantages of the different devices have not been well evaluated in children, particularly those with a difficult airway [21]. The GlideScope and the C-MAC are the most widely used in the pediatric population, and we will focus on these systems in our discussion.

GlideScope

The GlideScope is an intubating instrument with a hyper-curved blade (60-degree angulation) that includes a camera with a built-in antifog system connected to a high-resolution monitor [22]. The blades are offered in various sizes to meet the patient's requirements as shown in Table **3**.

Table 3. Appropriate GlideScope blade size based on patient weight.

Blade Size	Weight
GVL 0	1.5 kg
GVL 1	1.5 - 3.8 kg
GVL 2	1.8 - 10 kg
GVL 2.5	10 - 28 kg
GVL 3	10 kg – adult
GVL 4	40 kg - large adult

For a successful intubation, a styletted endotracheal tube (ETT) should be curved to mimic the shape of the selected GlideScope blade. The manufacturer offers a rigid stylet [23], which can accommodate tubes as small as size 3.0. The GlideScope blade should be inserted into the mouth in a midline approach, the blade tip is positioned in the vallecula and at this point, the elevation of the blade exposes the glottis. Once a good view is seen in the monitor, the styletted ETT is inserted into the mouth with direct visualization to avoid injuries to mucosa. As soon as the ETT is visible on the GlideScope® monitor, the tip of the tube is directed to the glottic inlet and inserted through the vocal cords. The stylet should be removed to facilitate the advancement of the ETT down the trachea.

Occasionally difficulties with ETT insertion are encountered despite a good view of the glottic opening in the GlideScope monitor. Providers should practice with normal airways to develop good hand-eye coordination. The GlideScope blades can be bigger than other laryngoscopes which limits the space available for the insertion and manipulation of the ETT.

The GlideScope has several advantages: 1) the skill set required to operate the GlideScope is similar to traditional direct laryngoscopy, 2) tongue displacement is not necessary, therefore the visualization of the glottic inlet should not be affected in cases such as macroglossia, 3) the airway view is displayed in a portable monitor, allowing visualization to other operators, 4) the 60-degree angulation in the blade decreases the motion of the cervical spine by 50% when compared to direct laryngoscopy [24]. This particular design allows visualization of the cords without the need to align the 3 airway axes, which can be advantageous in several situations like tongue swelling, pharyngeal obstruction, or cervical spine immobilization.

C-MAC Videolaryngoscope

The C-MAC is a video-assisted laryngoscope with an integrated straight or curve blade attached to a conventional handle [25]. It has a combined camera and light bundle located close to the tip of the blade. The image can be displayed on a separate monitor or a monitor attached to the handle. There are several sizes suitable for different pediatric airways, ranging from neonates to teenagers [15]. The appropriate size will be selected based on weight as shown in Table **4**.

Table 4. Appropriate C-MAC® blade size based on patient weight.

Blade Size	Weight
C-MAC Miller 0	< 2.5 kg
C-MAC Miller 1	2.5- 5 kg
C-MAC Miller 1	5- 15 kg
C-MAC Macintosh 2	15- 30 kg
C-MAC Macintosh 3	30- 70 kg
C-MAC Macintosh 4	> 70 kg

The design of the C-MAC is unique among video-assisted laryngoscopes, as it allows for its use as an indirect laryngoscope while simultaneously functioning as a direct laryngoscope [25]. In other words, it allows the laryngoscope operator to visualize the glottic opening under direct vision or on a monitor. This feature may be useful in the case of video failure or secretions obstructing the camera lens.

When using the C-MAC for direct laryngoscopy, the intubation procedure is the same as conventional laryngoscopy. The device is introduced into the right side of the mouth, the tongue is swept to the left by the blade flange, and the blade tip is advanced into the vallecula. However, if the intention is to use the video features of the device, a midline insertion technique without sweep of the tongue is sufficient to achieve an unobstructed view of the larynx [25].

The tip of the blade can be positioned in the vallecula; however due to the magnified lens of the camera, the view may be obstructed by the epiglottis. In that situation, the tip of the blade is best used to lift the epiglottis in order to obtain visualization of the glottic inlet. Once a good view of the airway is obtained, the ETT is placed along the shaft of the video blade, allowing for immediate visualization of the ETT in the camera avoiding injury to airway soft tissues.

A rigid stylet is not necessarily required for intubation with a C-MAC, a malleable stylet can be used instead. A styletted ETT with a slight bend at the tip can be very helpful for bringing the tube tip up to the glottis, especially in the case of anticipated difficult airway.

To obtain a good view of the airway, the use of C-MAC has some disadvantages, including the frequent need for alignment of the pharyngeal, laryngeal, and tracheal axes. In patients with cervical spine disorders and immobilization, Glidescope and C-MAC video-assisted laryngoscopes provide comparable laryngeal views, but the C-MAC device has a higher first-attempt failure rate and requires significantly more intubation attempts and optimizing maneuvers [24]. The C-MAC also lacks an anti-fog mechanism, which can impair visualization.

Flexible Intubation Scopes/Fiberoptic Bronchoscopy Techniques

The flexible fiberoptic bronchoscope (FOB) is one of the most versatile tools available in a difficult airway situation. There are different models available, however the fundamental elements consist of an insertion cord with a directable tip controlled by 2 wires traveling from the control lever down to the distal end and a long-glass-fiber bundle also running inside of an insertion cord. Along with the imaging elements, there is also a light source to visualize the distal tip of the insertion cord. Some flexible scopes contain an accessory lumen or working channel that can be used for suction, administration of oxygen or medications (*e.g.* local anesthetics). This accessory lumen can also be used to insert a guide wire for airway exchange techniques. However, pediatric-sized flexible bronchoscopes are usually too small and do not have this channel [22].

Flexible FOBs are available in various sizes; the smallest 2.2 mm in diameter, can fit an endotracheal tube as small as 3.0 mm ID (inside diameter). In general, the FOB should be at least 1 mm smaller in outside diameter compared to the ID of the endotracheal tube [15].

The ideal position of the child for fiberoptic bronchoscopy is different from the position for rigid laryngoscopy. The head should be flat on the table and slightly extended at the atlanto occipital joint to prevent the epiglottis from obstructing a view of the glottic opening [26]. If an oral approach is selected for intubation, an intubating oral airway can serve as a conduit to direct the FOB in the midline. A nasal approach can facilitate midline placement and it also avoids the risk of the child biting the FOB or ETT [26]. With both approaches, an assistant should perform a jaw thrust to open the posterior pharyngeal and supraglottic spaces. Traction of the tongue can also be helpful for optimization of the view. This may be achieved by grasping the tongue with a gauze, forceps, or application of high suction to the tip of the tongue.

Before starting the procedure, the ETT should be loaded onto the scope with the bevel facing down for oral intubation and bevel facing up for nasal intubation [26]. The tip of the FOB should be introduced midline under direct vision until identifiable airway structures are visualized. The tip of the FOB is advanced down the trachea and the airway structures must be appropriately identified before any attempts are made to pass the ETT through the nose or oropharynx. If resistant to ETT passage is encountered, the ETT should be rotated 90 to 180 degrees to facilitate the passage through the vocal cords [26].

One of the alternatives for flexible fiberoptic intubation is an LMA. The LMA provides an excellent channel directly to the vocal cords by shielding the bronchoscope from secretions and blood, and at the same time allows for continuous oxygenation and ventilation [21]. An observational study in 14 centers demonstrated that fiberoptic intubation through a supraglottic airway and videolaryngoscopy have similar rates of first-attempt success in children with difficult airways. However, selecting fiberoptic intubation through a supraglottic airway as the first technique was associated with significantly fewer intubation attempts and changes in airway management strategies [21]. Furthermore, hypoxemia was less common during the fiberoptic through supraglottic airway technique when continuous ventilation was used throughout the intubation attempt.

In cases where the FOB is too large to pass through the appropriately sized ETT, an exchange guidewire can be employed to perform fiberoptic intubation. The wire is advanced through the working channel of the FOB into the trachea, the FOB is then removed leaving the guidewire in place [26]. At that point, the ETT is threaded over the guidewire, which is then removed.

Regardless of the approach chosen for fiberoptic intubation, multiple studies have concluded that the intubating time is slightly greater compared to videolaryngoscopy; thus, it is important to have extensive practice in simulations and normal airways before attempting this technique in an anticipated difficult airway.

Infants and children are unlikely to cooperate with awake fiberoptic intubation. If there is concern for difficult ventilation, the anesthesia provider should maintain spontaneous ventilation and provide oxygen. The administration of neuromuscular blocking agents can improve viewing conditions by decreasing movement and fogging of the bronchoscope [15]. While performing fiberoptic intubation, it is essential to monitor depth of anesthesia as well as oxygen saturation.

To provide oxygen continuously during the procedure, a nasal cannula can be used. Another helpful technique is using an endoscopy mask which has an adapter to pass the fiberoptic scope while being able to deliver oxygen to a spontaneously breathing child or to ventilate a child that has been paralyzed with neuromuscular blocking agents. Another option is to insert a nasal trumpet into the nasal cavity and then attach a connector from a tracheal tube, this will allow positive pressure ventilation throughout the procedure.

Though the flexible bronchoscope can be useful in a variety of abnormal airways conditions, it has a limited field of vision that can be obstructed with blood or secretions. Furthermore, some institutions still use standard FOBs, which are quite fragile and require careful handling and manipulation to prevent damage.

Awake fiberoptic intubation is usually challenging to perform in pediatric patients as they are less likely to be cooperative during the procedure. The anesthesia provider should formulate a plan that includes the administration of antisialogogues, topical vasoconstrictors for nasal intubation, sedation and topical local anesthetics. Glycopyrrolate should be administered at least 15 minutes before beginning the procedure. A topical vasoconstrictor such as phenylephrine 0.5% or oxymetazoline 0.05% should be applied to the nasal mucosa to reduce the chance of bleeding with passage of the bronchoscope and the ETT.

The decision to use sedation during awake intubation is made on a case-by-case basis, and the goal is to provide anxiolysis, amnesia, and analgesia. Minimal sedation should be used in patients with concerns for aspiration or respiratory decompensation, and medications that can be reversed or have a short duration of action are preferred. Benzodiazepines, opioids, hypnotics, and alpha-2 agonists can be used alone or in combination. Standard monitors should always be applied prior to initiating sedation.

Additionally, topical anesthesia and nerve blocks have been developed to blunt the protective airway reflexes and provide analgesia. The therapy is directed to anesthetize the nasal cavity/nasopharynx, the pharynx, the base of the tongue, the oropharynx, the hypopharynx, and the trachea.

Nasal Cavity Block

The nasal cavity is innervated by the greater and lesser palatine nerves and the anterior ethmoidal nerve which are distal branches of the trigeminal nerve (cranial nerve V) [22]. To block these nerves through a noninvasive nasal approach, cotton-tipped applicators soaked with local anesthesia are passed through the nasal cavity until the posterior wall of the nasopharynx is reached and left there for 5 to 10 minutes. In the invasive oral approach, a needle is introduced into the greater palatine foramen, which can be palpated in the posterior-lateral aspect of the hard palate. 1 to 2 ml of 1% lidocaine is injected carefully avoiding intravascular injection.

Glossopharyngeal Nerve Block

The glossopharyngeal nerve supplies sensory innervation to the posterior third of the tongue, the tonsils, walls of the pharynx, vallecula and the anterior surface of the epiglottis [22]. This nerve also provides the afferent limb of the gag reflex. The simplest technique to anesthetize this area is by aerosolized local anesthetic solution in the back of the throat, or a voluntary local anesthetic "swish and swallow". Another noninvasive technique is the application of cotton-tipped applicators soaked with local anesthetic in the inferior aspect of the palatoglossal folds for 5 to 10 minutes. If these techniques are inadequate, local anesthetic can be injected in this same location.

Superior Laryngeal Nerve Block

The superior laryngeal nerve is a branch of the vagus nerve (cranial nerve X). The internal branch of the superior laryngeal nerve provides sensory innervation to the base of the tongue, posterior aspect of the epiglottis, aryepiglottic folds, and arytenoids [22]. The external branch of the superior laryngeal nerve supplies motor innervation to the cricothyroid muscle and has no sensory component.

For a noninvasive technique, forceps loaded with anesthetic soaked cotton swabs are slid over the lateral tongue into the pyriform sinuses bilaterally. The swabs are then held in place for 5 to 10 minutes. For an invasive block, the clinician identifies the greater cornu of the hyoid bone beneath the angle of the mandible. A needle is then inserted over the greater cornu and walked off the bone in an inferomedial direction until it can be passed through the thyrohyoid ligament. 1 to 2 ml of local anesthetic is then injected in the space between the thyrohyoid membrane and the pharyngeal mucosa.

Recurrent Laryngeal Nerve Block

The recurrent laryngeal nerve is another branch of the vagus (cranial nerve X), as it provides sensory innervation to the vocal cords and the trachea [22]. Transtracheal injection of local anesthetic is a simple technique that can produce adequate analgesia. To perform this block, a syringe is inserted through the cricothyroid membrane perpendicular to the plane of the cervical spine. Constant retraction on the syringe plunger will result in air aspiration when the trachea is entered, and then two to four milliliters of local anesthetic is injected. Another effective technique for tracheal and vocal cord topicalization is to inject local anesthetic through the working channel of the fiberoptic scope.

IV and Blood Transfusion

The goal of intraoperative intravenous therapy is to maintain hourly maintenance fluids and to replace deficits that arise due to oral fasting, blood loss, and insensible losses during surgery. The appropriate catheter gauge depends on age, expected blood loss, and type of surgery. In routine surgeries where massive fluid shifts or blood loss is not expected, one reliably functioning IV is adequate.

Flow rate depends on catheter gauge and length, and for this reason, shorter IV catheters are preferred. 24-gauge catheters are typically adequate in infants, 22-gauge catheters are best suited for toddlers and young children, and 20-gauge catheters are optimal beginning in adolescence for routine surgeries. During emergence, pediatric patients may be dysphoric or confused. It is important to secure the IV either on an arm board or have it wrapped with Coban ™ (Fig. **12**). A pulse oximeter placed on a distal finger is recommended to assess for perfusion and the IV insertion site should be easily accessible to evaluate.

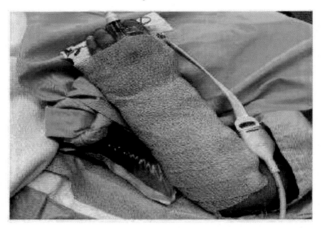

Fig. (12). IV wrapped with Coban™ and secured on an arm board (Photo taken by Marlo DiDonna).

To avoid unintentional rapid volume administration, the IV tubing should be placed on a pump, or the provider may use a microdrip infusion set or a Buretrol. Luer-lock access points should be as close as possible to the entry point of the IV, so excess fluids are not necessary to flush medications. All ports must have air removed from them prior to connecting to the patient. This is of utmost importance in neonates, infants, and children with congenital heart disease. Triple stopcocks are useful in gaining access points proximal to the patient and will not slow flow rate like small-bore extension sets can.

Avoidance of Dehydration

In 2011, the American Society of Anesthesiologists reexamined their stance on NPO guidelines for fasting patients [27]. By following these updated guidelines, the need for large volume fluid replacement is reduced, post-operative hydration status is improved, and hypoglycemia is avoided. See Chapter 4 for details of preoperative fasting guidelines.

A Lactated Ringer's or Normal Saline bolus of 10-20 mL/kg up to 40-50 mL/kg will increase BP, restore intravascular volume and is well tolerated in most pediatric patients [28]. Although 0.9% Normal Saline is isotonic, it has a large amount of chloride, and in excessive amounts can lead to a hyperchloremic metabolic acidosis. Lactated Ringers may be more appropriate if large amounts of volume are being administered.

Research has shown that only excessively long fasting times of 8-19 hours will put children at risk for hypoglycemia, therefore, glucose-free isotonic solutions are preferred with frequent intraoperative glucose monitoring, even in healthy neonates [28]. Neonates born to mothers with gestational diabetes, those receiving long-term hyperalimentation, and those with endocrine pathologies are particularly at risk for hypoglycemia. A low concentration of dextrose (1-3%) can be administered in the maintenance fluids. Boluses of fluid should not contain dextrose, and frequent glucose checks should be done [29].

Pediatric Blood Transfusion

The Society for Pediatric Anesthesia recommends that anesthesia providers anticipate intraoperative blood loss prior to hemodynamic compromise, so that they may transfuse early in order to avoid rapid delivery [30]. Rapid delivery of blood is associated with hyperkalemia which can lead to cardiac arrest. Delivery through a peripheral IV over a central IV is preferred; the speed of delivery should never exceed 1.5-2 mL/kg/minute. The blood bank should make their best attempt to use RBC units that are within 7 days of collection, washing the units if possible, and minimizing the time between irradiation and transfusion. If these measures are taken, the amount of potassium that is leaked into the banked blood during storage is reduced. Blood banks can often prepare several aliquots from one unit of blood. When this method is used, the child is only exposed to a single donor, and each aliquot can be infused as needed. Blood should be warmed to avoid hypothermia and the patient's temperature and vital signs should be closely monitored.

Maximum Allowable Blood Loss (MABL)

Prior to surgery, maximum allowable blood loss (MABL) should be calculated. Most healthy children will tolerate a hematocrit (Hct) of 25-30% [31, 32]. In Table **5**, 27% is used as the lowest acceptable hematocrit in this example to calculate MABL.

In the example provided in Table **5**, 28.3 mL of PRBC are needed and it would be appropriate to request that the blood be split into aliquots for potential future transfusions. Blood should be prepared through a fluid warmer and the IV line should be primed with normal saline. In order to maintain aseptic conditions, the system should not be breached once the infusion has begun. This can be accomplished by using a three-way stopcock to draw the appropriate volume into a syringe after the blood has been filtered through an appropriate 170-260 micron filter to remove aggregates.

Table 5. Calculating Maximum Allowable Blood Loss (MABL) and blood replacement [32].

A 4-week-old full term child is having open abdominal surgery. He weighs 4 kg (8.8 lbs.). His starting hemoglobin is 13g/dL with a hematocrit of 40%. Using 27% as the lowest acceptable hematocrit (LAH), what is the Maximum Allowable Blood Loss (MABL) in this surgery?

Estimated Blood Volume (EBV) = 85ml/kg (85 X 4kg)

= 340ml is the child's EBV

MABL = EBV X (child's Hct - LAH) ÷ child's Hct

$$= \frac{340ml \times (40 - 27)}{40}$$

$$= \frac{340 \times 13}{40}$$

= 111mL is the Maximum Allowable Blood Loss (MABL)

If 111mL is the Maximum Allowable Blood Loss (MABL) when we are using 27% as the Lowest Acceptable Hematocrit (LAH), how many mL of Packed Red Blood Cells (PRBC) would be required to restore an estimated Hct of 32%?

$$\text{Volume (cc) of PRBC} = \frac{\text{(Desired Hct - Current Hct)} \times \text{Estimated Blood Volume}}{\text{Estimated Average Hematocrit of PRBC}}$$

$$= \frac{(32-27) \times 340\text{mL}}{60}$$

$$= \frac{5 \times 340}{60}$$

$$= 28.3\text{mL of PRBC would be required}$$

Drug Therapy

Medication errors are possible in the care of pediatric patients. Decimal place errors can occur, especially when the medication is available in multiple concentrations [33]. Each drug should be labeled with dose concentration, initialed, timed, and dated. Open communication with other providers who also are involved in administering drugs is vital. When caring for very small patients that require miniscule dosing, it is useful to draw up drugs in 1ml syringes for easier administration, as each 0.1ml is marked and dosing is as accurate as possible. Certain frequently used drugs should be diluted with extreme caution, as this is a time when medication errors and a communication breakdown between providers can happen. Many drugs are now available in commercially prepared pre-filled syringes. As always, check the drug concentrations and expiration dates of these pre-filled syringes. Table **6** shows a simple way to dilute epinephrine for more accurate dosing and Table **7** provides a list of basic anesthetic drugs used in pediatric practice.

Table 6. Epinephrine dilution often used in pediatrics.

Epinephrine is often diluted to prepare an appropriate concentration in pediatrics.

Epinephrine (supplied in 1mg/mL vial)

Step 1: *Dilute 1mg/mL in 9mL of NSS to make a 0.1mg/mL concentration.*
Step 2: *Place 1mL of the 0.1mg/mL concentration in a 1mL Luer Lock syringe*
Each graduated mark (0.1mL) = 10mcg (0.01mg) Epinephrine

The appropriate dose of Epinephrine is 0.01mg/kg. A 6kg infant would require 0.06mg in an emergency.

0.06mg = 60 mcg = 0.6mL of final Epinephrine concentration prepared in 1mL Luer Lock syringe

Table 7. Basic Anesthetic Drug Setup used at Cooper University Hospital; Camden, NJ.

Basic Anesthetic Drug Setup	Recommended Available Dose
Atropine *(supplied in 1mg/mL and 0.4mg/mL vials)* 0.12mg)	0.02mg/kg (minimum
(Use a 24G needle in case there is a need for emergent IM injection prior to obtaining an IV)	
Succinylcholine *(supplied in 20mg/mL vial)*	2-4mg/kg
(Higher dosing range required for IM injection in laryngospasm prior to obtaining an IV; 24G needle attached)	
Propofol *(supplied in 10mg/mL vials and bottles)*	3mg/kg
Fentanyl *(supplied in 50mcg/mL vial)*	1-3mcg/kg
or	
Morphine *(supplied in 2, 4, 8, 10mg/mL vials)* CHECK CONCENTRATION PRIOR TO DILUTING!	0.1-0.2mg/kg
Rocuronium *(supplied in 10mg/mL vial)* RSI)	0.5mg/kg (1.2mg/kg for
Glycopyrrolate *(supplied in 0.2mg/mL vial)*	0.01mg/kg
IV prep pack, IV extension set, 2 pre-packaged NSS flushes	
Other Meds to Consider	Recommended Available Dose
Toradol *(supplied in 30mg/mL vial)*	0.5-0.6mg/kg
Zofran *(supplied in 4mg/mL vial)*	0.1-0.15mg/kg
Decadron *(supplied in multiple concentrations)*	0.25-0.5mg/kg

Special Considerations

Environmental Conditions & Maintaining Normothermia in the Pediatric Patient

Heat is lost through four mechanisms: radiation, evaporation, convection, and conduction. Due to a large surface area to body mass ratio, infants and small children lose heat primarily through radiation and convection. Non-shivering thermogenesis is a method of heat production seen in neonates. This process involves the release of norepinephrine which stimulates the breakdown of brown fat. Unfortunately, this process causes an increase in oxygen consumption, glucose utilization, and acid production in the neonate [34]. A warm operating room between 23-25 degrees Celsius (73-77 degrees Fahrenheit) reduces the risk of hypothermia (<36 degrees Celsius), thus preventing these detrimental factors. Using head coverings, plastic wrap around exposed areas, and warm blankets is also beneficial.

Cutaneous warming systems are the most common types of active warming systems. Forced-air systems, such as the BAIR Hugger, use warmed air to actively heat the patient, in addition to providing passive insulation. Electric warming blankets, such as the HotDog® Patient Warming System, also provide passive insulation in addition to utilizing conductive warming [35]. It is important to use warming devices according to the manufacturer's directions and to have a routine maintenance plan in order to prevent burns or electrical malfunctions.

Heating intravenous fluids will not effectively increase a patient's temperature but can help to prevent hypothermia when large volumes of IV fluid and blood are administered.

Handoff and Safe Transport of the Postoperative Child

At the end of surgery, the child is transported to the Post Anesthesia Care Unit (PACU) or to an intensive care unit. Children can be dysphoric and restless upon emergence, so a crib provides the safest environment for an infant or toddler. Stretchers and beds may be used for children >3 years of age. In either case, the child should be centered on the bed and positioned away from hard bed rails. Additional personnel may be needed to restrain or redirect the child during transport. The child can be placed on their side in the "rescue position" to facilitate better airway patency and a safer position in case of vomiting or coughing during transport. Two rolled blankets can be placed on both sides of the child which serve as "bumpers" to prevent excess motion while in transit.

It is prudent to give a phone report before arriving at the intensive care unit and completing a final handoff prior to leaving the unit. This ensures that necessary equipment, such as suction, oxygen and monitors, are available for the child's care at arrival. The final handoff should involve the entire team, including surgeons, anesthesia providers, the pediatric intensivist, and registered nurse. The handoff should include a systems overview, a description of the surgery performed, any notable intraoperative events, and any follow up recommendations. This provides an opportunity to ask questions and discuss any concerns. Many institutions have created standardized handoff checklists that have reportedly decreased patient care errors. A standardized handoff allows for a more organized, succinct dialogue and it allows the handoff recipient an opportunity to ask questions [36]. At the minimum, a portable pulse oximeter should be used to monitor the child during transport. If a child is transported to a critical care unit, EKG, blood pressure, and capnometry should also be monitored. Standardized emergency drug cards (Table **8**) with weight-adjusted doses are a useful aid in the event of an emergency. Parents and caregivers should be educated on the typical postoperative behaviors of children, including emergence delirium, and encouraged to offer support to their children. Lastly, a quiet, soothing environment with dimmed lighting can improve patient satisfaction and decrease anxiety.

Table 8. Pediatric emergency drug list used at Cooper University Hospital, Camden, NJ.

Pediatric Emergency Drug Sheet

PLACE PATIENT LABEL HERE   Patient's weight (kg): **10 kg**

Medication	Concentration	Dosage	Patient Dose	Volume
Atropine	0.4mg/ml	0.02mg/kg	0.2mg	0.5ml
Succinylcholine	20mg/ml	2mg/kg	20mg	1ml
Propofol	10mg/ml	3mg/kg	30mg	3ml
Etomidate	2mg/ml	0.3mg/kg	3mg	1.5ml
Ketamine	10mg/ml	2mg/kg	20mg	2ml
Midazolam	1mg/ml	0.1mg/kg	1mg	1ml
Fentanyl	50mcg/ml	2mcg/kg	20mcg	0.4ml
Rocuronium	10mg/ml	0.6mg/kg	6mg	0.6ml
Vecuronium	1mg/ml	0.1mg/kg	1mg	1ml
Lidocaine (2%)	20mg/ml	1.5mg/kg	15mg	0.75ml
Glycopyrrolate	0.2mg/ml	0.01mg/kg	0.1mg	0.5ml
Naloxone	0.4mg/ml	0.1mg/kg	1mg	2.5ml
Flumazenil	0.1mg/ml	0.02mg/kg	0.2mg	2ml

Transporting to the Neonatal Intensive Care Unit

The goal of transport is to prevent complications during transit and to maintain patient safety. The anesthesia providers, surgeons, and surgical staff will give a verbal handoff report upon arrival to the NICU. The transport isolette ideally should be an integrated unit with built-in mechanisms to ventilate and monitor the child. Manually bag-ventilating a child in an incubator during transport is difficult and impractical. A stand-alone transport ventilator that is separate from the isolette is not recommended either, because of the greater risk of dislodgement and extubation. Once the team reaches the unit and the child is safely situated, the anesthesia provider will check vital signs and ensure that the airway is intact. At this time, the receiving team should address updates and follow-up concerns before the anesthesia team departs.

Special Setup/Unique Considerations

The Neonatal Intensive Care Unit (NICU) Baby

Effective evaluation, preparation, and anesthetic management of the neonate depends on the appropriate knowledge of neonatal physiology. Major factors in planning the anesthetic include 1) monitoring requirements, 2) intravenous access, 3) airway equipment, 4) induction and maintenance of anesthesia, 5) fluid management and anticipated blood loss, and 6) postoperative recovery and need for postoperative ventilation requirements. The suggested equipment is shown in Table **9**.

Observation of the neonate's color, capillary refill, fontanelle fullness and chest expansion are useful monitors, however they are difficult to assess once the patient is covered in surgical drapes; consequently, there is dependence on electronic monitors during the majority of the procedure. Standard monitors include pulse oximeter, blood pressure monitor, electrocardiograph, temperature probe, end-tidal carbon dioxide, and agent analyzer.

Table 9. Suggested equipment for the operating room setup for the NICU baby.

Monitors	Environment	Intravenous access
Pulse oximeter	Room temperature 80° – 85° F	20 G, 22G and 24 G IV catheters
Blood pressure monitor	Underbody warming blanket with forced warm air delivery device	Ultrasound
Electrocardiograph		
Temperature		
End-tidal carbon dioxide		
Agent analyzer		

Airway	Fluids	Medications
Facemask	Infusion pumps	Anesthetic drugs
Oral airways 30 mm and 40 mm	Fluids and blood warmer	Neuromuscular blocking agents
Cuffed and uncuffed endotracheal tube 3.0 and 3.5	Isotonic crystalloid	Epinephrine
Miller blades 0 and 1	Albumin	Atropine
	Blood products if indicated	

Pulse oximetry monitor placement is sometimes difficult in neonates because of their small fingers. In those circumstances, it may be necessary to place the probe across the web space between the thumb and the first finger or around the lateral aspect of the hand or foot. It is recommended to limit the use of oxygen in neonates and keep oxygen saturation between 93% and 95% in order to decrease oxidative stress [37].

Proper **non-invasive blood pressure** cuff size is 1/2 to 2/3 of the length of the upper arm. The cuff should not be cycled more frequently than every 3 minutes to prevent venous stasis.

Invasive arterial blood pressure monitoring offers the advantage of accurate blood pressure readings; however, placement should be decided on a case by case basis. Ultrasound guidance is a valuable tool in the placement of arterial access in neonates. Some patients may present to the operating room with an umbilical arterial line in place. Although these can be used for monitoring, umbilical lines have infectious and embolic risks and may be in the way of the surgical field [37].

The **electrocardiogram** is primarily useful to assess heart rate and rhythm. In neonates ST-T wave abnormalities may be an indicator of electrolyte abnormalities rather than abnormalities related to myocardial ischemia. Wiping the skin with alcohol can be helpful to adhere the leads properly.

Capnography and $PaCO_2$ correlate well in studies done in intensive care unit (ICU) ventilators; however, this is not necessarily true in anesthesia machines where the anesthesia circuits tend to carry significantly more dead space [37]. Despite this difference, the shape of the waveform can give significant information about changes in ventilation, obstruction and rebreathing.

A **nerve stimulator** may be used if a neuromuscular blocking agent was administered, however the train-of-four response may be decreased in patients less than 2 months old [38].

Intravenous Access

Most neonates who come to the operating room will have vascular access in place, if not, the first task before induction is to establish adequate intravenous (IV) access. Obtaining IV access in a neonate can be difficult and may require multiple IV punctures. It is appropriate to have ultrasound available to assist with venous puncture. It is mandatory to establish IV access before induction in the newborn who is preterm, medically unstable, has a full stomach, has a potential for difficult airway, or has ongoing fluid losses. Rarely, it may be appropriate to use inhalational induction if vascular access is difficult in the older newborn close to one month of age.

Central venous catheters are utilized in hemodynamically unstable patients who are likely to require continuous vasopressors or when central venous monitoring is necessary. However, the benefits of placement must outweigh the risk associated with use. Ultrasound guided puncture minimizes the risks associated with placement of central venous access.

Airway Equipment

Airway management in a neonate requires understanding the differences between the newborn and adult airway. Considerations include: 1) avoidance of gastric distention by delivering gentle mask ventilation. Insufflation of the stomach may create challenging intubating conditions, can impair the movement of the diaphragm and ventilation may become difficult. If this occurs the stomach must be suctioned to allow adequate ventilation. 2) A shoulder roll (Fig. **13**) may be used for extension of the neck to improve visualization of the airway structures during laryngoscopy.

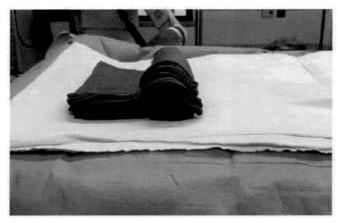

Fig. (13). Shoulder roll (Photo taken by Rosemary De La Cruz).

It is critical to identify intubating techniques with a high first pass successful attempt rate to minimize adverse events leading to hypoxemia and potential cardiac arrest. Different equipment and approaches for airway management have been discussed previously in this chapter. Preemptive strategies that are used with the equipment available in each institution will decrease complications associated with airway management.

Fluid and Blood Product Management

The appropriate type of maintenance depends on several factors. Patients arriving from the NICU should continue the same IV solution, usually this is a calcium- and/or glucose-containing solution or a hyperosmolar glucose or dextrose (10%) parenteral nutrition solution. In both cases, these solutions should not be discontinued [37]. Isotonic crystalloids should be used for boluses and most maintenance needs. Frequent glucose monitoring is required, and if hypoglycemia is a risk, dextrose may be added to the maintenance solution.

Most of the basic principles of blood component therapy are the same in newborns and older children and adults. In neonates, it is especially important to calculate estimated blood volume (EBV) and then maximum allowable blood loss (MABL) as discussed earlier in the chapter.

Method of induction and maintenance for neonates will be dependent on the medical condition, the surgical procedure, blood losses, gestational age, fasting status and plan of care after the procedure. It is important to dilute medications according to age appropriate doses. There is a detailed discussion of pharmacology in neonates in Chapter 2.

Tracheostomy

Patients with persistent respiratory failure or intermittent airway obstruction with failed extubation will force the need to secure the airway *via* tracheostomy [39]. In other cases, tracheostomy is performed on an emergency basis.

The surgeon performs a diagnostic laryngoscopy and possible bronchoscopy before proceeding with the tracheostomy. In that event, the endotracheal tube is removed; the airway examined with a rigid bronchoscope, and then the trachea is reintubated for the procedure. Airway management might be complicated in these patients due to distorted airway structures or obstructive lesions. If there is a concern for potential airway problems, it is appropriate to maintain spontaneous ventilation, and equipment for emergent tracheostomy must be immediately available.

Prior to surgical incision the child is positioned supine, with the head extended over a shoulder roll. If the patient is not intubated anesthesia is induced and maintained with inhalational agents to preserve spontaneous respiration. In patients who are intubated, anesthesia is maintained with volatile agents and muscle paralysis.

FIO_2 of 100% should be administered in case the airway is lost at any point; but during the use of electrocautery, the FIO_2 must be lowered to 30% or less to minimize the risk of fire as the trachea is surgically entered. The endotracheal tube should remain in the tracheal lumen, because if difficulty is encountered while passing the tracheostomy tube, the ETT can be readily advanced. After the correct position is confirmed by capnography and chest auscultation, the original endotracheal tube is removed, and the tracheal incision is closed.

Once the patient is positioned for postoperative care, it is good practice to perform flexible fiberoptic bronchoscopy through the new tracheostomy tube to confirm the position of the tip of the tracheostomy tube above the carina [39].

Cleft Lip and Cleft Palate

Cleft lip, with or without cleft palate, is one of the common congenital malformations. While most patients present with isolated cleft lip and/or palate, the list of associated anomalies is large. Primary cleft lip repair usually takes place at around 2 to 3 months of age, whereas primary cleft palate repair occurs at 6 to 10 months. Other procedures for lip or nose revision usually occur in early childhood, and palatal revision and alveolar bone grafts take place at approximately 10 years of age. Rhinoplasty and maxillary osteotomy to complete the repair may take place at 17 to 20 years of age [40]. For all of these procedures, the anesthetic goals and management are similar.

When preparing an anesthetic plan for the repair of cleft lip and/or cleft palate, potential difficult airway should be taken into account and you should prepare accordingly (refer to the difficult airway setup section). Induction of anesthesia *via* face mask is usually uncomplicated in patients with cleft lip and cleft palate, and thankfully, difficult ventilation with face mask is rare. However, a difficult view during laryngoscopy is a more common scenario. The frequency of difficult airways in children with cleft lip and palate ranges from 2.9% to 23% [40]. Micrognathia is an independent predictor of difficult intubation; the incidence of difficult direct laryngoscopy is around 50% in children with micrognathia but only about 4% in those without [40].

Laryngoscopy can be performed using a straight blade with direct laryngoscopy, alternatively, video laryngoscopy or fiberoptic intubation may be preferable. A piece of gauze packed into the cleft may help to avoid dropping the blade into the cleft. Different endotracheal tubes can be used for intubation of the airway in cleft lip and palate surgery, although the oral Ring-Adair-Elwyn (RAE) tube is ideally used to facilitate surgical access [40].

The addition of regional anesthesia with an infraorbital and external nasal nerve blocks after cleft lip repair is also a good alternative to provide pain relief in these patients [40]. Insertion of a nasopharyngeal airway (often placed by the surgeon) may be required to relieve upper airway obstruction after surgical procedure and enable suction without damaging the palate repair. These nasal trumpets are usually needed until the following day, by which time operative swelling has partially resolved. Additionally, intraoperative dexamethasone (0.5 mg/kg) may be administered to mitigate postoperative airway edema [41].

Postoperative attention must be paid for signs of airway obstruction. Close observation continues into the recovery period for approximately 48 hours and supplemental oxygen should be administered as needed.

Bleeding Tonsil

The most serious complication after tonsillectomy is postoperative hemorrhage, which occurs at a frequency of 0.1% to 8.1%. Approximately 75% of postoperative hemorrhage occurs in the first 6 hours, the remaining 25% occurs within 24 hours [42]. In the operating room the anesthesiologist may encounter several challenges due to a potentially difficult airway, hypovolemia, anemia, and a child with a full stomach.

To prepare for these cases, it is important to review the anesthetic record to collect information about difficulty with airway management or any other concerns. History of dizziness and the presence of orthostatic hypotension upon examination of the patient will provide important information about volume status and the need for aggressive fluid resuscitation and blood crossmatch before induction. Coagulation studies should be sent if required [39]. Intravenous access and vigorous fluid resuscitation (repeated boluses of 20 mL/kg of crystalloid and/or colloids) must be established before the induction of anesthesia [39].

A variety of intubating laryngoscopes, including video-laryngoscopes should be available. Blood in the airway may impair visualization during laryngoscopy, thus two suction circuits connected to a yankauer suction tip and/or a soft flexible suction catheter must be prepared before induction of anesthesia. A child presenting with a bleeding tonsil is considered full stomach due to a large volume of blood swallowed, therefore RSI is suggested. After application of routine monitors in the operating room, the child should be preoxygenated in the left lateral position and the head down to drain blood out of the mouth [39].

Epiglottitis

Epiglottitis usually presents in patients between 2-7 years of age, although it has been reported in younger children and adults [42]. In patients presenting with severe airway compromise, the safest approach is to take the patient from the emergency room directly to the operating room to secure the airway with tracheal intubation [42]. The anesthesia provider and the surgeon should always accompany the patient in case total airway obstruction occurs and premedication should be avoided; parental or caregiver presence may be necessary to keep the child calm. Excessive manipulation of the patient with blood drawing or intravenous catheter insertion should be avoided prior to the arrival to the operating room.

The operating room should be prepared with the equipment necessary for laryngoscopy, rigid bronchoscopy, and tracheostomy. The endotracheal tube chosen should be at least 0.5 mm smaller than the one normally chosen and should be styletted.

In the operating room, the child is kept in the sitting position while monitors are placed. The patient should undergo inhalation induction while still sitting up. After loss of consciousness, the child can be reclined in the supine position while maintaining spontaneous respiration. When the patient reaches a state of general anesthesia, intravenous access is established. A bolus of 20–40 mL/kg of an isotonic solution can be administered, because these children are often dehydrated [39]. Laryngoscopy followed by orotracheal intubation is then accomplished without the use of muscle relaxants.

Extubation is usually attempted 48 to 72 hours later in the operating room when a significant leak around the endotracheal tube is present and visual inspection of the larynx confirms the reduction of swelling of the epiglottis and surrounding tissue [42].

Obese Child

In children and adolescents, the Center of Disease Control (CDC) defines obesity as a body mass index at or above the 95th percentile for age [43]. When taking care of an obese child, these factors should be considered: 1) associated comorbidities such as obstructive sleep apnea, hypertension, insulin resistance and gastroesophageal reflux, 2) suitable size equipment, including operating tables, beds, and gowns, 3) recognize the need for additional time and personnel to position the patient.

Before induction of anesthesia, the patient should be in a ramped position with the tragus of the ear leveled with the sternum. This will improve oxygenation and ventilation, increasing the safe apnea time. The addition of PEEP and jaw thrust can be helpful in decreasing upper airway collapse during spontaneous ventilation, facilitating preoxygenation. Moreover, the ramped position has been demonstrated to improve laryngoscopy views in obese patients; therefore, it is the recommended default position during induction in all obese patients [43]. Any difficulty or failure of intubation should be promptly managed in accordance with the difficult airway guidelines [16]. Equipment for difficult intubation should be readily available prior to the induction of anesthesia.

Vascular access may also be challenging, hence long needles and ultrasound might be a useful adjunct. If the patient is identified as having a potentially difficult airway, it will be prudent to obtain intravenous access prior to induction of anesthesia.

Appropriately dosing medication is difficult as the pharmacokinetics of most anesthetics are affected by obesity. Unfortunately, there are limited studies in obese children to guide drug dosing. Consequently, it is wise to consider the use of easily reversible drugs, with fast onset and short duration.

The drug doses for several commonly used drugs in anesthesia might be estimated based on the patient's total body weight (TBW), ideal body weight (IBW), or lean body weight (LBW) as shown in Table **10**.

Table 10. Drug Dosing for Obese Children; (LBW = lean body weight; IBW = ideal body weight; TBW = total body weight).

Drug	Induction Dose	Maintenance Dose
Thiopental	LBW	-
Propofol	LBW	TBW
Synthetic opioids (fentanyl, alfentanil, sufentanil) *Morphine*	TBW IBW	LBW IBW
Remifentanil	LBW	LBW
Nondepolarizing neuromuscular blockers Succinylcholine	IBW TBW	IBW
Sugammadex	TBW	-

There is limited data to support the benefits of using total intravenous anesthesia (TIVA) *versus* inhalational agents for the maintenance of anesthesia. Fat-insoluble volatile agents such as desflurane or sevoflurane have a faster onset and shorter duration of action than isoflurane. There is evidence of faster return of airway reflexes with desflurane compared with sevoflurane in obese patients [44].

Before removal of the endotracheal tube, patients should be awake, and extubation should be performed with a 45° head-up tilt. In patients with obstructive sleep apnea, a nasopharyngeal airway before emergence helps mitigate airway obstruction.

Sleep Apnea

Children with known or suspected obstructive sleep apnea (OSA) present for all types of surgical and diagnostic procedures. The most studied procedure for this patient population is adenotonsillectomy, however perioperative complications are increased in OSA patients after all types of surgery, representing a challenge for anesthesia providers.

In children with severe OSA, consider the placement of intravenous access before induction of anesthesia. Premedication should be administered with caution in children with severe OSA as transient oxygen desaturation may occur.

The American Society of Anesthesiology practice guidelines for the management of patients with OSA recommends the use of local anesthesia or peripheral nerve blocks for superficial procedures, and spinal/epidural anesthesia for peripheral procedures [45]. If sedation is employed, ventilation should be continuously monitored by capnography. Continuous positive airway pressure (CPAP) should be considered if the patient uses a machine at home.

General anesthesia with a secure airway is preferable to deep sedation without a secure airway. If airway obstruction occurs during sedation or emergence from general anesthesia, jaw thrust maneuver, insertion of an oral or nasopharyngeal airway, and/or the application of continuous positive airway pressure (CPAP) may be required. Small increments in CPAP between 5 and 10 cm H_2O can significantly increase the dimension of the pharyngeal airway [39].

Full reversal of neuromuscular blockade guided by a nerve stimulator should be verified before extubation [39]. Unless there is a medical or surgical contraindication, children with OSA should be extubated while awake. When possible, extubation and recovery should be carried out in the lateral or semi-upright positions. Placing a nasopharyngeal or oropharyngeal airway before extubation should be considered to decrease supraglottic obstruction.

Trauma

Anesthesia providers should be familiar with the principles of pediatric trauma management. Patients often need immediate surgical intervention. Anesthesia providers, surgeons, and other personnel must work as a coordinated team to manage these patients. Table **11** includes a list of equipment recommended in the management of the pediatric trauma patient. Anesthesia considerations for the pediatric trauma patient are described in detail in Chapter 8.

Massive transfusion protocol is appropriate for patients who have profound hemorrhage or ongoing bleeding with an anticipated need to replace total blood volume over 24 hours. Use of such a transfusion protocol may be associated with better outcomes, although evidence is limited.

The placement of an arterial and/or central venous line should be selected on a case-by-case basis. Arterial catheters are useful adjuncts when there is a need to alter the blood pressure rapidly or when serial arterial blood gas testing is needed to assess changes in hematocrit, oxygenation and acid-base status.

Table 11. Suggested equipment for pediatric trauma setup (see Chapter 8).

Fluids	Medications	Other Equipment and Adjuncts
Isotonic crystalloid	Anesthetic drugs	Resuscitation cart
Albumin	Vasoactive drugs	Infusion pumps and rapid infusion devices
Blood products if indicated		Pressure bags
		Blood warming device
		External warming device

Monitors	Vascular Access	Airway
Pulse oximeter	Intravenous catheters	Self-inflating ventilating devices
Blood pressure monitor	Intraosseous catheters	Face mask, ETT, stylets, laryngoscopes, oral airways, nasal airways and LMA
Electrocardiograph	Central line kit	
Temperature	Arterial line kit	Difficult airway equipment: videolaryngoscope, fiberoptic bronchoscope and cricothyrotomy kits
End-tidal carbon dioxide	Tubing prepared for crystalloids IV fluids and blood products	
Transducers and monitors for arterial and central venous pressures	Ultrasound	Suction

CONCLUSION

It is advantageous for anesthesia providers to have an understanding of a basic pediatric OR setup. When caring for a pediatric patient, safety and efficiency are paramount. A methodical setup will also serve to improve your flexibility and resourcefulness outside of the operating room. Pediatric patients have unique needs, and these needs must be considered in an anesthesia provider's plan of care. This chapter's goal was to provide a basic understanding of these factors to the non-seasoned pediatric anesthesia provider. It is our hope that with this gained knowledge, all anesthesia providers will have the opportunity to carry out a safe and therapeutic anesthetic during the care of pediatric patients.

A thorough pediatric anesthesia room setup is multifactorial; precise drug calculations, ventilator settings and airway equipment, IV and colloid infusions, and thermoregulation considerations are at the core of a comprehensive setup. Table **12** summarizes the topics discussed and can be used as a general guide in your practice. Review of the chapter's details can further sharpen your overall clinical knowledge and ability to use this checklist.

Table 12. Pediatric operating room checklist; (Original table design by Marlo DiDonna, CRNA).

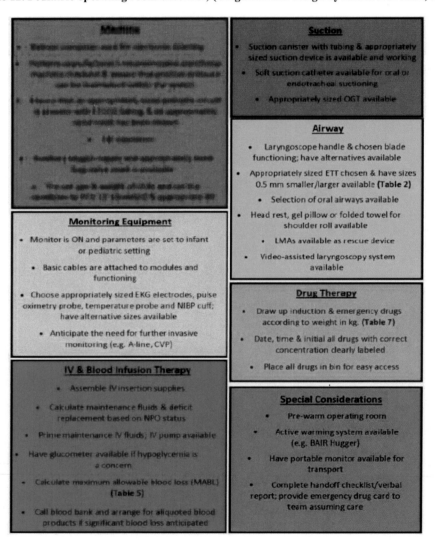

CONSENT FOR PUBLICATION

Not applicable.

CONFLICT OF INTEREST

The author declares no conflict of interest, financial or otherwise.

ACKNOWLEDGEMENTS

Declared none.

REFERENCES

[1]   Setting up the operating room for anesthesia (Internet). Rishi Kumar, MD; 2014 Jul (cited 2020 Apr 15) 2014.https://rk.md/2014/setting-operating-room-anesthesia/

[2]   Cravero JP, Landrigan-Ossar M. Anesthesia outside the operating roomA practice of anesthesia for infants and children. 6th ed. Philadelphia, PA: Elsevier 2019; pp. 1077-94.
        [http://dx.doi.org/10.1016/B978-0-323-42974-0.00046-X]

[3]   Ross PA, Lerman J, Coté CJ. Pediatric equipmentA practice of anesthesia for infants and children. 6th ed. Philadelphia, PA: Elsevier 2019; pp. 1175-203.
        [http://dx.doi.org/10.1016/B978-0-323-42974-0.00052-5]

[4]   Feldman JM, Olympio MA, Martin D, Striker A. New guidelines available for pre-anesthesia checkout 2008.https://www.apsf.org/newsletter/spring-2008/

[5]   Glenski TA, Diehl C, Clopton RG, Friesen RH. Breathing circuit compliance and accuracy of displayed tidal volume during pressure-controlled ventilation of infants: A quality improvement project Paediatr Anaesth (Internet). Sep (cited 2020 Apr 5); 2017; 27(9): 935-41.https://onlinelibrary.wiley.com/doi/abs/10.1111/pan.13164   DOI 10.1111/pan.1316410.1111/pan. 13164

[6]   Olympio MA. CO_2 absorbent desiccation safety conference convened by APSF APSF newsletter (Internet). 2005; 20(2): 25, 27-9.https://www.apsf.org/newsletter/summer-2005/

[7]   Soll RF. Heat loss prevention in neonates. J Perinatol 2008; 28 (Suppl. 1): S57-9.https://www.nature.com/articles/jp200851
        [http://dx.doi.org/10.1038/jp.2008.51] [PMID: 18446179]

[8]   Teleflex Medical Europe Ltd. LMA Supreme (Internet). (place unknown) (cited 2020 Apr 20). https://www.lmaco.com/products/lma%C2%AE-supreme%E2%84%A2-airway

[9]   Harless J, Ramaiah R, Bhananker SM. Pediatric airway management. International journal of critical illness and injury science 2014; 4(1): 65-70. http://www.ijciis.org/article.asp?issn=2229-5151; year=2014;volume=4;issue=1;spage=65;epage=70;a [http://dx.doi.org/10.4103/2229-5151.128015] [PMID: 24741500]

[10]   2006.https://investor.kimberly-clark.com/news-releases/ne-   s-release-details/kimberly-clark-laun-hes-microcuff-endotracheal-tube

[11]   Aker J. An emerging clinical paradigm: the cuffed endotracheal tube AANA Journal (Internet) 2008 Aug (cited 2020 Apr 21) 76(4): 293-300.https://www.aana.com/docs/default- source/aana-journa-
        -web-documents-1/jcourse3_0808_-
        293-300e0bf37731dff6ddbb37cff0000940c19.pdf?sfvrsn=38405ab1_6

[12]   Morray JP, Geiduschek JM, Caplan RA, Posner KL, Gild WM, Cheney FW. A comparison of pediatric and adult anesthesia closed malpractice claims. Anesthesiology 1993; 78(3): 461-7.

[http://dx.doi.org/10.1097/00000542-199303000-00009] [PMID: 8384428]

[13]   Dalesio NM. Planning Prevents Poor Performance: An Approach to Pediatric Airway Management Anesthesia Patient Safety Foundation 2018.https://www.apsf.org/article/planning- prevents-poo- -performance-an-approach-to-pediatric-airway-management/

[14]   Mathis MR, Haydar B, Taylor EL, *et al.* Failure of the Laryngeal Mask Airway Unique™ and Classic™ in the pediatric surgical patient: a study of clinical predictors and outcomes. Anesthesiology 2013; 119(6): 1284-95.
[http://dx.doi.org/10.1097/ALN.0000000000000015] [PMID: 24126262]

[15]   Klinger K, Infosino A. Airway ManagementMiller RD Basics of Anesthesia. 7th ed. Philadelphia: Elsevier 2018; pp. 239-70.

[16]   Apfelbaum JL, Hagberg CA, Caplan RA, *et al.* American Society of Anesthesiologists Task Force on Management of the Difficult Airway. Practice guidelines for management of the difficult airway: an updated report by the American Society of Anesthesiologists Task Force on Management of the Difficult Airway. Anesthesiology 2013; 118(2): 251-70.
[http://dx.doi.org/10.1097/ALN.0b013e31827773b2] [PMID: 23364566]

[17]   Sun Y, Lu Y, Huang Y, Jiang H. Pediatric video laryngoscope versus direct laryngoscope: a meta-analysis of randomized controlled trials 2014.https://onlinelibrary.wiley.com/doi/epdf/10.1111/pan.12458
[http://dx.doi.org/10.1111/pan.12458]

[18]   Fiadjoe JE, Kovatsis P. Videolaryngoscopes in pediatric anesthesia: what's new Minerva Anestesiol (Internet) 2014; 80(1): 76-82.https://www.minervamedica.it/en/freedownload.php?cod=R02Y2014N01A0076

[19]   Aziz MF, Dillman D, Fu R, Brambrink AM. . Comparative effectiveness of the C-MAC video laryngoscope versus direct laryngoscopy in the setting of the predicted difficult airway. Anesthesiology 2012; 116(3): 629-36.
[http://dx.doi.org/10.1097/ALN.0b013e318246ea34]

[20]   Moore A, Schricker T. Awake videolaryngoscopy versus fiberoptic bronchoscopy 2019.https://journals.lww.com/co-anesthesiology/Abstract/2019/12000/Awake
[http://dx.doi.org/10.1097/ACO.0000000000000771]

[21]   Burjek NE, Nishisaki A, Fiadjoe JE, *et al.* Videolaryngoscopy *versus* Fiber-optic Intubation through a Supraglottic Airway in Children with a Difficult Airway: An Analysis from the Multicenter Pediatric Difficult Intubation Registry. Anesthesiology 2017; 127(3): 432-40.
[http://dx.doi.org/10.1097/ALN.0000000000001758] [PMID: 28650415]

[22]   Rosenblatt WH, Abrons RO, Sukhupragarn W. Airway Management. In: Barash PG, Cahalan MK, Cullen BF, Stock MC, Stoelting RK Clinical Anesthesia. 8th ed. Philadelphia: Wolter Kluwer 2017; pp. 783-95.

[23]   Turkstra TP, Harle CC, Armstrong KP, *et al.* The GlideScope-specific rigid stylet and standard malleable stylet are equally effective for GlideScope use. Can J Anaesth 2007; 54(11): 891-6.
[http://dx.doi.org/10.1007/BF03026792] [PMID: 17975233]

[24]   Brück S, Trautner H, Wolff A, *et al.* Comparison of the C-MAC(®) and GlideScope(®) videolaryngoscopes in patients with cervical spine disorders and immobilisation. Anaesthesia. 2015.
[PMID: 25265994]

[25]   Xue FS, Li HX, Liu YY, Yang GZ. Current evidence for the use of C-MAC videolaryngoscope in adult airway management: a review of the literature. Ther Clin Risk Manag 2017; 13: 831-41.
[http://dx.doi.org/10.2147/TCRM.S136221] [PMID: 28740393]

[26]   Fiadjoe JE, Litman RS, Serber JF, Stricker PA, Cote CJ. The Pediatric Airway Cote C, Lerman J, Anderson B A Practice of Anesthesia for Infants and Children. 6th ed. Philadelphia: Elsevier 2018; pp. 307-38.

[27]   American Society of Anesthesiologists Practice Guidelines for Preoperative Fasting and the Use of Pharmacologic Agents to Reduce the Risk of Pulmonary Aspiration: Application to Healthy Patients Undergoing Elective Procedures: An Updated Report by the American Society of Anesthesiologists Committee on Standards and Practice Parameters (Internet) (place unknown): Lippincott Williams & Wilkins 2011 Mar (cited 2020 May 15).https://anesthesiology.pubs.asahq.org /article.aspx?articleid=1933410

[28]   Arya VK. Basics of fluid and blood transfusion therapy in paediatric surgical patients Indian J Anaesth (Internet)2012 Sep (cited 2020 May 5).
[http://dx.doi.org/10.4103/0019-5049.103960] [PMID: 3531000]

[29]   Sumpelmann R, Becke K, Zander R, Witt L. 2019.https://journals.lww.com/co-anesthesiology/Abstract/2019/06000/Perioperative_fluid_management_in_children can_we.20.aspx DOI 10.1097/ACO.0000000000000727 [http://dx.doi.org/10.1097/ACO.0000000000000727]

[30]   Society for Pediatric Anesthesia Wake up safe: the pediatric anesthesia quality improvement initiative (Internet) 2015 Jan (cited 2020 May 1).http://wakeupsafe.org/wp-content/uploads/2018/ 10/Hyperkalemia_statement.pdf

[31]   Kallos T, Smith TC. Replacement for intraoperative blood loss. Anesthesiology 1974; 41(3): 293-5.
[http://dx.doi.org/10.1097/00000542-197409000-00017] [PMID: 4854116]

[32]   Coté CJ, Grabowski EF, Stowell CP. Strategies for blood product management, reducing transfusions, and massive blood transfusion.A practice of anesthesia for infants and children. 6th ed. Philadelphia, PA: Elsevier. 2019; pp. 257-80.
[http://dx.doi.org/10.1016/B978-0-323-42974-0.00012-4]

[33]   Poole RL, Carleton BC. Medication errors: neonates, infants and children are the most vulnerable! J Pediatr Pharmacol Ther 2008; 13(2): 65-7.http://europepmc.org/article/PMC/3462059 DOI 10.5863/1551-6776-13.2.65
[http://dx.doi.org/10.5863/1551-6776-13.2.65] [PMID: 23055866]

[34]   CEUfast Nursing CE (Internet) Lake City, FL: CEUfast, Inc; Neonatal Thermoregulation 2017 (cited 2020 May 1).https://ceufast.com/course/neonatal-thermoregulation

[35]   McSwain JR, Yared M, Doty JW, Wilson SH. 2015.https://www.wjgnet.com/2218-6182/full/v4/i3/58.htm [http://dx.doi.org/10.5313/wja.v4.i3.58]

[36]   Boat AC, Spaeth JP. 2013.https://onlinelibrary.wiley.com/doi/abs/10.1111/pan.12199 DOI 10.1111/pan.1219 [http://dx.doi.org/10.1111/pan.12199]

[37]   Spaeth JP, Lam JE. The Extremely Premature Infant (micropremie) and Common Neonatal EmergenciesCote C, Lerman J, Anderson B A Practice of Anesthesia for Infants and Children. 6th ed. Philadelphia: Elsevier 2018; pp. 841-5.

[38]   Vadi M, Nour C, Leiter P, Carter H. 2017.https://www.intechopen.com/books/pediatric-and-neona--l-surgery/anesthetic-management-of-the-newborn-surgical-patient

[39]   Hannallah RS, Brown KA, Verghese ST. Otorhinolaryngologic ProceduresCote C, Lerman J, Anderson B A Practice of Anesthesia for Infants and Children. 6th ed. Philadelphia: Elsevier 2018; pp. 757-87.

[40]   Stricker PA, Fiadjoe JE, Lerman J. Plastic and Reconstructive SurgeryCote C, Lerman J, Anderson B A Practice of Anesthesia for Infants and Children. 6th ed. Philadelphia: Elsevier 2018; pp. 804-6.

[41]   Somerville N, Fenlon S. Anaesthesia for cleft lip and palate surgery. Contin Educ Anaesth Crit Care Pain 2005.
[http://dx.doi.org/10.1093/bjaceaccp/mki021]

[42]   Ferrari LR, Park RS. Anesthesia for OtorhinolaryngologyCahalan MK, Cullen BF, Stock MC, Stoelting RK Clinical Anesthesia. 8th ed. Philadelphia: Wolter Kluwer 2017; pp. 1357-72.

[43]   Peri-operative management of the obese surgical patient Anaesthesia

2015.https://www.ncbi.nlm.nih.gov/pmc/articles/PMC5029585/

[44] McKay RE, Malhotra A, Cakmakkaya OS, Hall KT, McKay WR, Apfel CC. Effect of increased body mass index and anaesthetic duration on recovery of protective airway reflexes after sevoflurane *vs* desflurane. Br J Anaesth 2010; 104(2): 175-82.
[http://dx.doi.org/10.1093/bja/aep374] [PMID: 20037150]

[45] Gross JB, Apfelbaum JL, Caplan RA, *et al.* Practice guidelines for the perioperative management of patients with obstructive sleep apnea: an updated report by the American Society of Anesthesiologists Task Force on Perioperative Management of patients with obstructive sleep apnea. Anesthesiology 2014; 120(2): 268-86.
[http://dx.doi.org/10.1097/ALN.0000000000000053] [PMID: 24346178]

CHAPTER 4

Preoperative Evaluation and Planning

Fatimah Habib[1] and **Kathleen Kwiatt**[1]

[1] *Department of Anesthesiology, Cooper Medical School of Rowan University, Cooper University Health Care, Camden, NJ, USA*

Abstract: This chapter will explore the basic principles of pre-anesthesia preparation and pre-operative planning for pediatric patients presenting to the operating room. This chapter discusses the general pediatric preoperative evaluation, including pertinent patient history, family history and exposures, along with psychological preparation of the child. Premedication often allows for a smoother induction; different options for premedication as well as types of induction will be explored. This chapter will conclude with planning for patients with special considerations and when transfer to a pediatric hospital for specialty care is indicated. The aim will be to provide safe and effective recommendations and guidelines for general anesthesiologists who provide care for children.

Keywords: Autism, Bronchopulmonary dysplasia (BPD), Developmental delay, Dexmedetomidine, Ketamine, Mask induction, Midazolam, Minors, NPO guidelines, Pediatric induction, Pediatric premedication, Pregnancy, Preoperative IV, Preoperative evaluation, Preoperative planning, Recent URI.

PREOPERATIVE EVALUATION

History and Physical Exam

In a pediatric patient, past medical history should include patient's comorbidities if any and their treatments, recent illnesses, travel history, vaccination status, allergic reactions, sick contacts, history of previous anesthetics and any associated complications, family history of anesthetic complications, history of perioperative emergence delirium and smoke exposure [1, 2]. Children are often at risk for upper respiratory infections, which can put them at risk for a reactive airway in the perioperative period.

* **Corresponding author Bharathi Gourkanti:** Department of Anesthesiology, Cooper Medical School of Rowan University, Cooper University Health Care, Camden, NJ, USA; E-mail: gourkantibharathi@cooperhealth.edu

Bharathi Gourkanti, Irwin Gratz, Grace Dippo, Nathalie Peiris and Dinesh K. Choudhry (Eds.)
All rights reserved-© 2022 Bentham Science Publishers

Smoke exposure (passive or active) can similarly cause them to have reactive airways, thus increasing their risk of pulmonary and airway complications such as bronchospasm or laryngospasm. A detailed evaluation of the severity of a patient's asthma should be obtained, such as triggers and recent exacerbations. Family history should be obtained to rule out genetic anesthesia- related disorders such as pseudocholinesterase deficiency, malignant hyperthermia, hematologic disorders, myopathies and history of postoperative nausea [1, 3]. The medical history of infants and neonates should include birth history, and any maternal complications during pregnancy or delivery, such as maternal substance abuse or maternal diabetes [3]. The most common allergies seen in young children are to antibiotics. Surgical procedures often require antibiotic prophylaxis, so inquiring into the reaction and identifying a true allergy helps guide appropriate surgical antibiotic prophylaxis [1]. Another common allergy in the pediatric population is a latex allergy, most commonly found in children with spina bifida, urinary tract malformations, or a history of multiple previous surgeries. In these children, latex exposure should be avoided [2, 3]. Reviewing a patient's current medications can help avoid any unwanted interactions with anesthetics or may have other anesthetic implications (*e.g.*, anti- epileptic medications decrease the duration of action of muscle relaxants) [2].

The physical exam should focus on the heart and lung exam and a basic airway exam. A basic heart exam includes an evaluation of the child's heart rate and blood pressure. Normal limits vary with age. Auscultation of the heart sounds is important to rule out cardiac murmurs [1]. Many childhood murmurs are benign and are often already part of the child's medical history. Benign murmurs tend to be systolic vibratory flow murmurs and are usually not louder than II/VI. If a murmur louder than II/VI is detected which was previously unknown, a decision needs to be made whether the situation allows for a cardiac evaluation prior to surgery [1]. If a pediatric cardiologist is not available at the institution, the child may need to be transferred to a facility where such resources are available. Other characteristics of a murmur requiring consultation include poor exercise capacity, oral cyanosis, abnormal or uneven pulses, syndromic features, congenital heart disease in the family, or diastolic murmur [1].

The lung exam includes baseline pulse oximetry and auscultation of lung sounds. In children with a history of asthma or any child with a recent upper respiratory illness, the finding of expiratory wheezing warrants treatment prior to surgery [1]. If the surgery is elective, uncontrolled asthma or acute symptomatic upper respiratory infection (pharyngitis, rhinitis, cough or fever) warrants rescheduling of the procedure.

An airway exam includes noting the facial characteristics of the child. Any abnormal facial characteristics that could be deemed "syndromic" should be further evaluated. Often pediatric syndromes are associated with difficult airways. Size and position of the child's chin, size of the tongue, shape and prominence of the maxilla, mobility of the mandible, along with loose or poor dentition can all be potential causes of difficult ventilation or difficult intubation [1]. Moderate scoliosis or kyphosis will hinder ideal positioning for a favorable airway.

Other systems should be reviewed and examined in more detail if the situation or the child's history deems them necessary. For example, a child with a broken arm should have a neurologic exam to determine function and sensation of the injured extremity for potential nerve damage [1]. A child with a history of cerebral palsy should have a neurological exam to determine the child's baseline spasticity, areas of contractures and extent of motor and cognitive delays. A child with a history of sickle cell disease should be examined for anemia and hypovolemia by examining capillary refill, and identifying any clubbing, cyanosis or pallor [3].

No laboratory work is indicated for routine procedures in healthy children, particularly in an outpatient setting [3]. Some surgeons, such as otolaryngologists may order basic labs such as a hemoglobin or hematocrit level or a coagulation profile prior to tonsillectomy/adenoidectomy to rule out any undiagnosed underlying bleeding disorders. All preoperative lab work should be ordered on a case by case basis based on the patient's comorbidities, complexity of the proposed procedure, anticipated blood loss, previous abnormal labs, and any new symptoms.

NPO (Nil per os) Guidelines

The risk of hypovolemia and its potentially catastrophic consequences in children allow for a slightly more relaxed NPO guideline in children *versus* adults. In fact, most children and infants especially are encouraged to have clear ups until 2 hours prior to surgery in order to avoid hypovolemia and hypoglycemia. Such a practice also increases parent satisfaction as they are able to assuage the patient's hunger somewhat by offering clear juice or water, and decrease the patient's irritability level [1]. The current NPO guidelines are shown below in Table **1** [1 - 3].

Table 1. Preoperative fasting guidelines.

Required NPO time prior to Anesthesia	Type of meal
2 hours	Clear fluids
4 hours	Breast milk
6 hours	Formula, citrus juices, *non-human milk
8 hours	Solids, *non-human milk

*Some references differ in NPO time recommendations for non-human milk.

Psychological Preparation

The anticipation prior to surgery can be a stressful time for both the child and the parents. It often falls on the anesthesiologist to alleviate the child and their parents' fears prior to the procedure [3]. The higher the level of anxiety preoperatively, the more likely the patient will emerge anxious or delirious [1]. Different methods of distraction have been used to assist in creating a less stressful perioperative environment, including playing a video on a tablet computer or iPhone or giving the child toys in the preoperative area, such as a stuffed animal that they can bring into the operating room with them. Most non-pharmacologic interventions have not been shown to be consistently effective, and further research is needed. Treatment with an anxiolytic medication is the only known proven way to effectively decrease preoperative anxiety in the child [1]. The parents also need anxiolysis. Witnessing the anesthesiologist develop a relationship with their child can provide them with confidence that their child is in experienced hands [1]. After introducing themselves to the parents, the anesthesiologist should introduce themselves to the child in a relatable way, such as with a high five or a fist bump. Also, making eye contact with the child during the interview instead of focusing on parents alone can help develop a relationship with the patient. Easy communication with the child can often provide parents with more comfort than can be given in lengthy explanations. Parental anxiety also revolves around the anesthetic more often than the surgery. When discussing risks of the anesthetic, one helpful approach is to put things into perspective for the parents. The likelihood of an adverse event occurring due to anesthesia in a healthy patient for a routine surgery is rare, approximately 1 in 200,000 [3].

Obtaining Consent

The simplest rule to follow is that consent is needed for all minors from a parent, guardian, or power of attorney. A minor typically means under the age of 18, not including emancipated minors. Each state is different in its definition of minors, as well as the rights of minors, so it is vital to be acquainted with the rules specific to your state. Some states, such as Nebraska and Alabama have the minor age defined as under 19. Mississippi and Pennsylvania consider minors to be under the age of 21. These states, however, have exceptions for medical consent, allowing "minors" to consent for their own medical care under certain circumstances. Therefore every practitioner needs to be familiar with their states' rules [4]. A good reference is the Centers for Adolescent Health and the Law, www.cahl.org.

Emancipated minors are usually minors who themselves are parents, pregnant, have been living without their parents and managing their financial affairs on their own, married, or in military service. An emancipated minor can provide their own consent for medical care. Many states require a formal court declaration for a minor to be officially considered emancipated. The concept of implied emancipation does exist, varies by state, and usually consists of military minors, minors who are parents, married, or pregnant minors. Every state has different definitions and criteria and therefore, every provider should be familiar with their state's laws [4].

In the situation where emergent care is required, consent does not need to be obtained. As with adults, if the care required is necessary to avoid serious morbidity or mortality, consent is implied. The consenting party, parents, or guardian should be notified as soon as possible.

A challenge arises when certain forms of potentially lifesaving treatment are denied by parents due to religious beliefs. A common example is when parents from the Jehovah's Witness community deny the consent for blood transfusion for their children. It is wise to involve the institutional ethics committee or risk management department with the care of these patients, and with other children in similar scenarios, from the initiation of care. The United States constitution allows for freedom of religion, and parents have the right to refuse medical care even for their children. However, when it comes to life-threatening circumstances, courts do not recognize or include the refusal of lifesaving care for a child as part of such rights. Traditionally, courts have favored providing blood to the patients against parents' wishes, and therefore hospitals will often seek a court order to provide treatment to a minor should parents refuse. Because the legality is complex, and varies by state, having risk management help with the discussion as early as possible is vital [5].

In practice, when confronted with such a situation, it is best to think of it in elective *versus* urgent/emergent terms. Notify risk management for all situations involving difficulty with obtaining consent. If the surgery is elective, and can safely be accomplished without the need for blood, all efforts to provide the service safely and in accordance with the parents' wishes should be made. A discussion of emergent medical necessities should still be had with parents or guardians and thoroughly documented. If blood may be needed in an elective surgery, the family should be directed to an institution with experience in all appropriate blood conservation strategies to comply with patient/family wishes while still offering a safe solution. Again, a discussion of all potential complications should be had and documented. In instances where the situation is urgent or emergent, courts often favor treatment first with a court order to follow.

This institution recommends involving the risk management department and ethics committee, and prioritizing the safety and protection of the child. Treatment should be provided as necessary, documented thoroughly, and then court orders obtained as soon as possible.

Pregnancy Testing

Early and unintended pregnancy rates have decreased in the US in recent years [2]; however, it is still a concern for patients presenting to the operating room due to unwanted potential anesthetic risks to a fetus. Teen pregnancy rates are considerably higher in the US than in other parts of the world. According to the CDC, in 2017, the birth rate for women between 15-19 years of age was 18.8 per 1000 women. It can be assumed that the unintended pregnancy rate was even higher.

Most institutions have a policy for pregnancy testing in all postmenarcheal females preoperatively. This takes the onus off of the anesthesiologist to determine the possibility of pregnancy in a patient under the age of 18 [2]. A positive pregnancy test can imply a sexually active patient or potential criminal activity by caretakers. Any concern for child safety then has to be reported. Also, according to the Health Insurance Portability and Accountability Act (HIPAA), if a pediatric patient is pregnant, the results must only be disclosed to her parents or caretakers with her permission. This makes the situation awkward and complicated, and there are potential legal ramifications. Therefore, the best option is to have a hospital-wide or institutional policy that calls for testing all postmenarchal patients [2].

Preoperative Intravenous Catheter (IV) Placement

The decision to place an IV preoperatively depends on comorbidities of the patient, patient age, and mental status. Most healthy patients under the age of 9-10 years coming for routine surgeries do not need preoperative IVs, and can safely be induced with an inhalational induction prior to IV placement. For younger patients, it is harder to obtain IV access while they are awake because of fear and lack of cooperation with placement. Usually, patients over the age of 9 or 10 years can be persuaded to get a preoperative IV, and with topical local anesthesia and some support from parents, they often tolerate it well.

If a patient has a potentially difficult airway or has had a known or suspected difficult intubation in the past, it is safest to obtain an IV preoperatively. If there is a concern for severe obstruction, such as in obstructive sleep apnea (OSA) patients who are overweight, coming for surgeries such as tonsillectomies, many practitioners will opt to get a preoperative IV. The potential for complications during mask induction is usually the deciding factor for proceeding with preoperative IV placement and an IV induction instead of mask induction. Other situations that may require a preoperative IV include patients with comorbidities that require preoperative hydration, such as sickle cell disease, or neonates. Often those patients are admitted the night before surgery, are made NPO at midnight, and an IV is placed the night before. They receive fluids overnight intravenously while remaining NPO which prevents the patient from presenting to the operating room in a dehydrated state. A patient with a full stomach, or in other situations with high aspiration risk, including acute abdomen, incarcerated hernia, or pyloric stenosis, should always be induced *via* rapid sequence induction (RSI), necessitating the need for obtaining preoperative IV access.

Triaging the Patient

When working in a setting that is not primarily created for pediatric care, an awareness of available resources and limitations can assist in the decision to transfer a patient to a facility with adequate and necessary pediatric resources. The decision is based on the limitations of the provider, the hospital, and the resources available. Anesthesia providers will likely only see patients in the preoperative setting. An emergent situation with no time for transfer is rare. Usually a pediatric patient with comorbidities will not arrive at a hospital with no pediatric resources, as they will be referred to the closest pediatric facility. It is possible that a patient may have an unknown underlying condition that only becomes evident on examination or preoperative review of systems and symptoms. If within history and physical exam, findings are evident of some perplexing disease process or complicated diagnosis, or expert consultation seems necessary, finding a better institution to care for the patient is reasonable. In a truly emergent situation with no time to spare, any lifesaving treatment should be provided as best as possible.

If a patient comes to the emergency room (ER) with clear evidence that transfer to a specialty pediatric hospital is best, as long as the patient is stable, that should be the goal of all teams involved before proceeding to surgery. If the patient is not stable, stabilizing the patient prior to transfer may still be the most appropriate course of events. An example is a patient who may have a foreign airway body presenting to an ER with no pediatric otolaryngologist. The patient may require stabilization or at least confirmation of stability before being transferred to a pediatric hospital with appropriate pediatric subspecialists available. Stabilization refers to supplemental oxygen, and no instrumentation of the airway if the patient is spontaneously ventilating with minimal distress. Similar indications apply for other surgical subspecialties, such as pediatric neurosurgery or thoracic surgery. If a general surgeon agrees to operate on a pediatric patient requiring a routine general surgery, but the patient happens to have an unrepaired congenital heart defect, a rare metabolic disease, or a syndrome that is associated with a known difficult airway, the decision to transfer to another hospital would be the decision of the anesthesiologist and his or her limitations. If the congenital heart disease is beyond the provider's scope of practice, and the patient would require advanced cardiac monitoring postoperatively, it is the anesthesia provider's responsibility to inform the surgeon that the patient would benefit from a pediatric team for intraoperative and postoperative care and monitoring. A healthy pediatric patient (not including neonates), who doesn't require access to other specialists either before or after surgery, and doesn't require expert opinion beyond the scope of practice of the anesthesiologist, can be safely managed in a non pediatric hospital setting. If post-operative management will require intensive care monitoring, a facility with a pediatric intensive care unit is better suited to take care of the patient.

Saettele *et al.* created a risk stratification tool to identify patients with congenital heart disease coming for noncardiac surgery as low risk, moderate risk, or high risk [6]. Based on the patient's history and condition, they were placed in a specific risk category. The low risk category patients were deemed safe to be taken care of in a freestanding ambulatory surgery center by pediatric anesthesiologists, with no particular extra training in cardiac anesthesia. The high risk patients were assigned to a pediatric cardiac anesthesia team. Both the moderate and high risk patients underwent surgery at a tertiary care children's hospital in which all subspecialist evaluations as well as postoperative pediatric specific care needs could be met [6]. Using this or similar criteria as a reference can help identify which patient with a congenital cardiac lesion could be safely done at a nonpediatric hospital. Examples of low risk, moderate risk and high risk lesions per Saettele *et al.* are shown in Table **2** below.

Table 2. Examples of cardiac lesions and associated anesthesia related cardiac risk as per Saettele *et al.* risk assessment tool [6].

Cardiac Condition ↓ / Risk →	Low Risk	Moderate Risk	High Risk
Structural Abnormalities	-repaired atrial septal defect -repaired ventricular septal defect -mild valvulopathy of single valve	-simple unrepaired atrial septal defect or ventricular septal defect -complex lesion, repaired -single ventricle patient s/p Glenn or Fontan, stable	-complex lesion, unrepaired -severe valvulopathy -systemic arterial to pulmonary arterial shunting
Conduction Abnormalities		-Wolff Parkinson White syndrome -Long QT syndrome -Pacemaker dependent	-
Pulmonary Hypertension		-Normal cardiac Index -NYHA functional Class 1	-Decreased cardiac index -Pulmonary pressures > systemic pressures -NYHA functional Class 3 or 4
Other		-Heart Transplant Recipient -Lung transplant Recipient	-Severe Heart Failure -Hypertrophic obstructive cardiomyopathy -William Syndrome

Expectations from Consultants

Pediatric consultants usually provide a more thorough plan of care and perioperative recommendations than adult consultants. Many pediatric conditions require close monitoring and long term management. Pediatric subspecialists often have a close relationship with their patients and are familiar with them, their families, and their disease process and progression. They can be an excellent resource to the anesthesia provider meeting a patient and their family for the first time and can provide meaningful insight and recommendations. For example, a pediatric hematologist caring for a patient with sickle cell anemia may already be aware of their patient presenting to the ER and requiring surgery. They often recommend preoperative hydration for a specific rate and time, pain management intraoperatively and postoperatively, as well as temperature management and other hemodynamic parameter recommendations. A pediatric cardiologist will often share imaging and diagnostic information and recommend preoperative antibiotic prophylaxis if necessary prior to surgery. They may warn against potential complications of increased pulmonary pressures and recommend postoperative monitoring strategies. If the patient has comorbidities that are well-managed, the expert consultants may only provide such information and recommend consultation postoperatively should any complications arise. In general, consultants tend to be a great resource in the pediatric population.

The primary care pediatrician can also provide a thorough summary of the patient's condition as well as help facilitate discussion between the anesthesiologist and subspecialists. Often, the pediatrician will be the initiator for requesting advice from a subspecialist preoperatively. A formerly healthy patient does not need subspecialty evaluation. A patient with a history of prematurity may see a pulmonologist for the history of bronchopulmonary dysplasia (BPD), or a patient with inborn errors of metabolism may see a metabolism and genetics expert. These subspecialists may recommend preoperative treatment such as preoperative bronchodilator therapy for a patient with known asthma or BPD, or preoperative intravenous glucose infusion and postoperative seizure monitoring in a patient with a metabolic disorder. A patient who is post-transplant would benefit from a consultation with the transplant team regarding continuation of immunomodulatory medication.

PREMEDICATION

The purpose of premedication in the pediatric population is to decrease preoperative anxiety, allowing for smooth separation from parents, facilitating induction, and decreasing postoperative behavioral disturbances [1, 2]. The age of onset for stranger anxiety and separation anxiety is 6-9 months of age. Prior to 6 months of age, most infants do not need an anxiolytic. Most premedications have the potential to produce respiratory depression, and therefore, close monitoring is required. Supplemental oxygen, monitoring, and ventilation support should be immediately available. In order to develop widely applicable recommendations, only commonly available anxiolytics and the most common routes of delivery will be discussed. The intramuscular route has fallen out of favor due to the pain associated with injection, which may create more anxiety in a patient returning for another procedure. Doses vary between patients, and so all doses mentioned are meant to act as guidelines only, and actual doses may be changed according to the anesthesiologist's judgment [2].

Midazolam

Midazolam is a fast onset, short-duration, water-soluble benzodiazepine that can be given *via* intravenous, nasal, rectal and oral routes. The most common method of administering midazolam is orally or intravenously. For ambulatory surgery pediatric patients, the oral route is preferred because it is easy and facilitates cooperation, alleviates anxiety, allows for separation from parents, and facilitates mask induction [2, 7]. It is also shown to decrease incidence of postoperative delirium [2]. It can be used in oral form to allow for preoperative IV placement if that is warranted. All routes of midazolam produce the same effects, decreasing anxiety, increasing patient cooperation, easing separation from the parents, creating temporary anterograde amnesia, and smoothing emergence without increasing postoperative recovery times [2]. A small group of patients may experience restlessness and agitation, often referred to as a paradoxical reaction, which can cause increased parental anxiety preoperatively [7]. If the patient has had a paradoxical reaction in the past, benzodiazepines should be avoided. The nasal route is utilized when the patient will not swallow liquids willingly, such in cases of disability, cognitive delay, or severe apprehension. The downside to the nasal route is discomfort of a nasal spray which requires the patient to be held firmly by the parents. Most patients find the nasal injection to be uncomfortable and irritating to the nasal passages. A special diffuser allows a small volume to be injected, but not all facilities are equipped with a nasal diffuser or the more concentrated version of the medication. Those patients who may not take oral or nasal midazolam may allow for rectal administration [2]. The rectal administration is challenging in that most patients may push it out if it is not injected properly. It is recommended for children 3 years of age and under, as older children may not tolerate it. The intravenous formulation is diluted with water and administered *via* a red rubber catheter into the rectum of a child lying prone. Once injected, the child has to be held down and the gluteal mounds held closed for a few minutes, so the medication is not pushed out [1]. The doses and onset times for different routes of administration of midazolam are shown in Table **3**.

Table 3. Dosage of Midazolam as a premedication [1, 2].

Route of Administration	Dose of Midazolam	Onset
Intravenous	0.1 mg/kg (max 2 mg)	Immediate
Oral (preferred)	0.5 mg/kg (max 10-20 mg)	5-10 mins
Nasal	0.2 - 0.3 mg/kg (split evenly between each nare, usually a highly concentrated form is used so that the volume is less than 1 mL per nare) * 0.1 mL extra is drawn up per nare in order to account for dead space in the nasal injector	10-12 min
Rectal	0.5 - 1 mg/kg (IV preparation diluted with water and injected *via* red rubber catheter)	fast onset, about 7-10 min

Ketamine

Ketamine is an NMDA receptor antagonist. Ketamine, like midazolam, has many routes of administration, including intravenous, intramuscular and oral. Ketamine has been used nasal trans-mucosally and rectally, but these routes are less utilized today. Oral ketamine and midazolam can be used together, the results of which are more satisfactory than either drug alone, and this combination is often used for premedication in infants with congenital cardiac malformations. The drawbacks of ketamine premedication include increased salivation, emergence delirium, postoperative nausea, and increased hospital discharge times (more common with the high dose intramuscular route). The advantages of ketamine include analgesia, decreased anesthetic requirements, and the ability to produce sedation without compromising respiration [1, 2, 7]. Ketamine is a reasonable and effective alternative for patients who have had a paradoxical reaction to midazolam in the past [1]. Intramuscular ketamine is usually reserved for patients who refuse to accept or can not swallow liquid medication. Often, it is used in patients who are combative or have some degree of developmental delay. The doses and onset of different ketamine routes of administration are shown in Table **4**.

Table 4. Dosage of Ketamine as a premedication [1, 2, 7].

Route of Administration	Dose of Ketamine	Onset
Intravenous	1-2 mg/kg	Immediate onset
Intramuscular	2-6 mg/kg	5-10 min
Oral	3-6 mg/kg	12-20 min
Nasal	5-6 mg/kg	20-40 min
Rectal	5 mg/kg	20-30 min

Dexmedetomidine

Dexmedetomidine is a potent, selective alpha-2 adrenergic agonist. There is adequate evidence to show that it can reduce preoperative anxiety as well as reduce opioid requirements postoperatively and potentiate analgesia. There is also the additional benefit of decreasing postoperative emergence delirium, and potentially decreasing postoperative nausea and shivering as well [7]. Different routes of administration have not been studied extensively within the pediatric population, and no consensus on dosing for pediatric premedication exists at this time. Intranasal administration requires a higher concentration to be used to decrease the administered medication volume. The negative effects of dexmedetomidine include longer onset time (with intranasal dosing) and the possibility of bradycardia and hypotension with larger doses [7]. Bioavailability of dexmedetomidine after oral, buccal and intramuscular administration has been studied, but not extensively and doses are not well established [2]. Dexmedeto-midone has been compared with midazolam as a premedication and they were both found to have little or no significant difference in recovery time and discharge from pacu, incidence of postoperative nausea and vomiting, and incidence of emergence agitation [8]. With dexmedetomidine, compared with midazolam, there was found to be a more satisfactory separation from parents preoperatively and reduced need for rescue analgesia postoperatively, according to a 2014 meta analysis [8]. The chart below provides suggested dosing for intravenous and intranasal dexmedetomidine. The suggested doses below are based on limited studies [2, 7 - 9] and are displayed in Table **5**.

Table 5. Dosage of Dexmedetomidine as a premedication [2, 7].

Route of Administration	Dose of Dexmedetomidine	Onset
Intravenous	0.5 mcg/kg (max 20 mcg) *administered slowly to avoid bradycardia *This dosing is for emergence agitation but can be extrapolated for premedication	Immediate onset
Intranasal	1-2 mcg/kg (split evenly between each nare, usually a highly concentrated form is used so that the volume is less than 1 mL per nare) * 0.1 mL extra is drawn up per nare in order to account for dead space in the nasal injector	45-60 min

Nonpharmacologic Preoperative Anxiety Reducing Strategies

Attempts at relieving preoperative anxiety without pharmacologic interventions have been attempted and studied. The theoretical benefits of nonpharmacologic interventions are many. They are usually a cheaper alternative, they are easily available, it saves the child any potential side effects from a pharmacologic alternative, and there are less preoperative or postoperative delays. Many studies have shown that alternative strategies are successful in reducing preoperative anxiety, with some studies claiming to show similar results when compared to oral midazolam. For example, one study from 2018 showed decreased preoperative anxiety in school aged children by bringing them into the operating room in a toy car, to a degree comparable with preoperative oral midazolam [10]. One study showed a statistically significant reduction in preoperative anxiety and pain in children who received relaxation guided imagery before induction of general anesthesia [11]. A number of studies have looked at the effects of music and music therapy to relieve anxiety in children prior to surgery, many of which cite success and the need for further testing [12 - 14]. Another article discussed the use of art therapy in combination with a preoperative clown visit as a useful adjunct to ease preoperative anxiety by enhancing the effects of oral midazolam in children. Decreased anxiety was noted at the time of parental separation, and parents and nursing staff were in agreement with the findings [15]. Some centers often offer children small toys or stuffed animals in the preoperative area which they can take with them to the operating room. Other facilities may offer a tablet computer to play cartoons and music videos of the child's choosing as they are separated from parents. There are many ways to distract a child in order to decrease their anxiety; not all of them will consistently be effective, more studies are needed, and they likely will not be as reliable as pharmacologic methods.

Developing a rapport with the patient and parents in the preoperative area by any means can be very effective in developing a trust between the provider and the patient and the patient's family, and aids with decreasing preoperative anxiety.

III. INDUCTION PRINCIPLES

In the pediatric population, there are two options for induction: inhalation and intravenous. Intravenous induction is the method of choice if the patient already has an intravenous catheter (IV). It is the method of choice for any patient deemed an aspiration risk, who requires an RSI [7]. Inhalation induction is often used in children coming from home for outpatient procedures who will not be amenable to IV placement. In the absence of any contraindications, inhalation induction is the method of choice in the younger pediatric population where there is no intravenous access. Contraindications include aspiration risk, potential for difficult ventilation (obesity, severe OSA, dysmorphic features), facial trauma, unknown NPO status and emergencies. In some situations in which there is potential for encountering a difficult airway (dysmorphic features, epiglottitis), inhalation induction is the preferred method for induction because it allows for a slow, steady onset, maintenance of spontaneous respiration and easy, quick reversibility [7]. However, in such situations, establishing intravenous access pre-induction is essential.

Monitors for induction should include all standard ASA monitors. Non-invasive blood pressure monitoring, pulse oximetry, end tidal carbon dioxide, electrocardiography and temperature. End tidal concentration of the volatile anesthetic should also be available for inhalation induction [16 - 18].

Inhalation Induction

Inhalation induction consists of sevoflurane (Sevo), oxygen, and nitrous oxide (optional). Sevo is the volatile anesthetic of choice since it is less irritating to the airways compared to desflurane or isoflurane. Halothane is no longer used due to its cardiac side effects and the availability of a much better alternative. Desflurane and isoflurane are not optimal agents for inhalation induction due to their unpleasant smell which can be irritating to the airways. Using a 2:1 mixture of nitrous oxide to oxygen allows the sevo to be taken up more quickly due to the 2nd gas effect, thereby speeding time from induction to loss of eyelash reflex and minimizing the time the patient is in stage 2. A slow induction consists of using the nitrous oxide/oxygen mixture, starting at a low dose sevo 1-2%, and increasing the sevo concentration every few breaths until the patient has loss of eyelash reflex. This method is only possible in compliant, calm children. Since nitrous oxide is an optional addition, used only to increase the speed of onset of the volatile anesthetic, some practitioners opt to start with a 1:1 mixture. As an optional adjunct, the dose can be adjusted based on provider's preference or experience, or patient conditions [7, 17].

A quicker induction can be accomplished by a similar nitrous oxide/oxygen mixture, and sevo at 8%, the circuit being primed with this mixture before applying the mask on the patient's face. Once the mask is applied, both the smell of sevo at 8%, and a well-sealed mask hold are both uncomfortable for the patients and they tend to struggle from the anesthesia providers' grasp. It is imperative to have help available during this time, in order to maintain hold of the patient in a safe manner. This technique produces a much faster induction to loss of eyelash reflex time, often under 60-90 seconds [7]. There is more likelihood of apnea with the faster induction method. It is during this time when the risk of obstruction is highest, therefore positive pressure and assisted ventilation should be provided if apnea occurs. It is during the stage 2 period when the risk of laryngospasm is also highest and therefore, emergency medications should always be available, including intramuscular and intravenous doses. Medications such as succinylcholine and atropine should be drawn up in intramuscular doses (with intramuscular needles ready for immediate administration) in case of an adverse event that may occur before intravenous access is established.

Once the patient is through stage 2, intravenous access should be obtained. If a single anesthesia provider is available, the operating room nurse should be asked to obtain intravenous access. If this is not possible, the anesthesiologist can place a laryngeal mask airway (LMA) in the patient, place the patient on the ventilator, and obtain intravenous access themselves. If a team-based approach is being utilized, the anesthesiologist can obtain intravenous access while the nurse anesthetist is mask ventilating the patient or vice versa. Any further necessary medications can then be given intravenously in order to facilitate obtaining a secure airway. If the plan is to continue with a sedation technique, such as is often utilized with pediatric gastroenterology procedures, once intravenous access is established, the patient is started on a propofol infusion and provided with supplemental oxygen once spontaneous ventilation has resumed.

During inhalation induction, when the patient is adequately anesthetized beyond stage two, the nitrous oxide can be turned off and the sevoflurane percentage can be reduced. Usually, a higher concentration than normal is required until a secure airway is obtained (around 3-4%). The patient should not be maintained on 8% sevo for longer than is necessary as they can have volatile anesthetic induced cardiac depression, which is concentration dependent. During induction, if at any point the patient becomes bradycardic, which often happens in the pediatric population on inhalation induction, the nitrous oxide should be turned off, FiO_2 should be 100%, and the sevo concentration should be reduced, if not completely turned off until heart rate recovers. Intramuscular atropine should be ready in the event that the initial maneuvers are not sufficient. Often the bradycardia occurs due to hypoventilation of the patient, and inappropriate assisted ventilation by the provider. Hypoxia leads to acute and immediate bradycardia, which if not immediately addressed, can lead to cardiac arrest. Adequate ventilation and avoidance of hypoxia is the priority. If ensuring adequate ventilation (with normal SpO_2) and turning off nitrous oxide and sevo does not immediately improve bradycardia, IM atropine should be administered. In patients with contraindications to nitrous oxide, it can be removed from the induction with only a small difference in induction to loss of eyelash reflex time.

Intravenous Induction

Intravenous induction is the safer method of induction because there is almost no stage 2 or excitement stage of anesthesia. There is a decreased incidence of respiratory complications in patients at risk when intravenous induction is completed *versus* inhalation induction, 10.7% *versus* 26% [18, 19]. If the patient already has intravenous access, any unanticipated events can be dealt with more quickly. There is no volatile anesthetic that could potentially irritate the airways. It is the preferred method for induction if the child already has an IV and it is the recommended method for patients with increased risk of perioperative respiratory complications, such as those with severe OSA, known history of asthma or reactive airway disease with recent and frequent wheezing, passive or active smoke exposure, recent upper respiratory symptoms (within the past two weeks), stridor or upper respiratory concerns, history of eczema, exercise induced wheezing, signs of atopy, two or more family members with atopy and presence of dry cough at night [7, 20]. In these children, it is likely safest to obtain a pre-induction IV. In a noncompliant or uncooperative patient, this can be done after administration of an oral premedication or even in the operating room under 1:1 inhaled nitrous oxide and oxygen.

In patients who require an RSI, such as in situations of unknown NPO status, traumas, full stomach, bleeding tonsils (potential blood in the stomach) or bowel obstruction, inhalation induction is not safe and a preoperative IV should be established and used for induction [17].

The most common medication used for induction is propofol. It is a short acting, widely available hypnotic medication that produces reliable and rapid sedation. It can be preceded with intravenous lidocaine to decrease the burning sensation on administration. Etomidate is a short acting imidazole derivative that also provides rapid and reliable induction, and is preferred in the context of hemodynamic instability. Ketamine is often used for intravenous induction of anesthesia in the setting of hemodynamic instability, and it has the added benefit of providing analgesia simultaneously. The doses for intravenous induction of different anesthetics are described in Table **6**.

Table 6. Intravenous induction agents and dosages [17].

Intravenous Induction Anesthetic	Pediatric weight based dosing
Propofol	2.5-3.5 mg/kg
Ketamine	1-2 mg/kg
Etomidate	0.2-0.3 mg/kg
Methohexital (barbiturate, less commonly used)	1-2.5 mg/kg

Parental Presence During Induction

The original intention for parental presence on induction was to alleviate parental and patient anxiety preoperatively and have a more cooperative patient. Current literature tends to support the notion that parental presence does not substantially allay anxiety in either the parent or patient [7, 21]. Some studies have shown that while the presence of a calm parent at the time of induction may help relieve anxiety in an anxious child, the presence of an anxious parent at induction can significantly increase preoperative anxiety in a child [22]. With the wide availability of reliable premedication options, decreasing patient and parent anxiety has become more easily accomplished. Under the circumstance where a child refuses all premedications or cannot receive them (*e.g.*, allergy) and is uncooperative, parental induction can be a useful technique. Such a situation is not common, but can sometimes be witnessed in patients with mild developmental delays, patients with anxiety/PTSD or patients with autism. The parents are brought to the operating room (OR) with the patient, they assist in allowing monitors to be placed on the patient (by playing or distraction) and remain with the patient as induction begins. Once the patient is anesthetized, but even before

IV or airway placement, the parents' role is complete and they are escorted out of the OR. The need for additional staff to act as an escort, as well as having the parents prepare themselves in appropriate attire to come to the OR can be disruptive to the normal workflow. Parental induction should be done on a case by case basis if the benefits of the parents' presence exceed the potential risk [21].

IV. PLANNING FOR PATIENTS WITH SPECIAL CONSIDERATIONS

Full Stomach / Need for RSI

There are many instances in which a child requires anesthesia and has a full stomach. Usually, these are trauma cases, emergency surgeries, or bowel/gastrointestinal tract surgeries where they have a risk of aspiration (ex. bowel obstruction, pyloromyotomy, gastroschisis/omphalocele, TE fistulas, foreign body aspiration or ingestion). For these surgeries, rapid sequence intubation is required to decrease the risk of aspiration. The operating room and anesthetic equipment should be prepared with the usual pediatric setup and machine check, as well as two sources of suction and suction catheters (in the event that one suction gets clogged with stomach content, the second source can be used immediately), two pulse oximetry monitors, two different laryngoscope blades, and styletted endotracheal tubes of an assortment of sizes [17].

A typical RSI involves careful preoxygenation, cricoid pressure applied to the neck in the approximate area of the cricoid cartilage, a rapid intravenous induction, fast-acting muscle relaxant administration, no ventilation prior to insertion of the endotracheal tube, and securing the airway with a cuffed endotracheal tube as quickly as possible. It is important to refrain from positive pressure ventilation in order to prevent introducing air into the potentially already distended stomach [17]. In infants and neonates, even a small amount of air in the stomach can make ventilation difficult by causing abdominal compression of the thorax. Unlike adults, infants and children have a lower functional residual capacity, higher metabolic demands, and can often not cooperate in optimal preoxygenation. It is not possible to ask an infant to take optimal tidal volume breaths prior to induction. Infants and children do not tolerate prolonged apnea time, and therefore become hypoxic quickly. Cricoid pressure is less reliable in children due to their airway anatomy and position of the esophagus with respect to the trachea. The amount of pressure to apply and where to apply it is not clear. Pressure placed down on a small, malleable airway can often interfere with obtaining an adequate view while intubating. Some studies suggest that cricoid pressure causes a decrease in tone of both esophageal sphincters [17].

There are studies that suggest avoiding cricoid pressure altogether. Instead, they advocate applying gentle positive pressure ventilation, using pressures that do not pose a risk of inserting air into the stomach until the patient is ready for intubation. This allows for the small airways to remain open during induction without inserting air into the belly. This technique avoids the fast onset hypoxia that is observed in infants and children due to their higher metabolic demands, lower functional residual capacity, and less than optimal preoxygenation. Succinylcholine (2 mg/kg IV) is the muscle relaxant of choice for an RSI, however, a modified RSI with rocuronium can also be used in patients in whom succinylcholine is contraindicated. The RSI dose of rocuronium is 1.2 mg/kg (same as adults).

Recent Illness or Upper Respiratory Tract Infection (URI)

Recent or current colds and URIs are commonly seen in the pediatric population, and may occur many times in one calendar year. For this reason, a patient may often show up for surgery with a current or recent URI. There is ample evidence to show that recent URIs in combination with anesthesia in the pediatric population put the patients at a higher risk of pulmonary complications intraoperatively and postoperatively due to increased airway hyperreactivity. The most common risks include bronchospasm, laryngospasm, decreased arterial blood pressures, hypoxia, stridor, difficult or prolonged intubation time, unanticipated admission, and increased length of hospital stay [23]. Often, the complications are quickly and easily managed with no long-term sequelae. In some instances, serious complications such as laryngospasm can cause respiratory induced cardiac arrest [24]. A URI within 2 weeks or on the day of surgery has been shown to increase the risk of pulmonary related adverse events by twofold [24]. Surgery on a patient currently sick with respiratory syncytial virus or flu has been shown not only to increase the risk of pulmonary adverse events, but also to increase the likelihood of intensive care unit (ICU) admission and increase the length of stay [24].

Other risk factors that contribute to pulmonary related adverse events include the history of reactive airway disease (RAD) or asthma, family history of asthma or atopy, passive smoke exposure, copious secretions, nasal congestion, ENT (ear, nose, and throat) procedures or procedures involving the airway, and young age, particularly age less than 1 year. All risk factors should be taken into account when deciding to proceed with a surgery in a patient with a recent or current URI [23, 24].

The decision whether to proceed with surgery in a patient with a recent or current URI should take into account the urgency of the procedure, degree of illness, timing of illness and any other risk factors the patient may have. Since children are so often sick, it is difficult to justify the cancellation of necessary procedures for a runny nose. However, the patient's risk should be evaluated thoroughly. In elective surgeries, if the child has an active illness, the surgery should be postponed. If the child had a mild illness within 2 weeks of presenting to surgery, with clear nasal secretions and an intermittent dry cough, but NO fevers, lethargy, wet cough or wheezing, and is otherwise healthy with no other risk factors, it is reasonable to proceed with the surgery, realizing that airway hyperreactivity can persist for up to six weeks post infection. In cases where the child has a moderate to severe illness or is recovering from a moderate to severe illness, it is best to postpone the elective surgery and avoid unnecessary risk.

Moderate and severe illness symptoms include fevers, lethargy, poor feeding, decreased urine output (if the parent says he or she has been using fewer diapers), wet cough, wheezing and purulent sputum. If the child has other risk factors for pulmonary complications such as a history of asthma, passive smoke exposure, personal or family history of atopy, bronchopulmonary dysplasia, need for airway manipulation, or airway surgery, it is best to postpone the surgery. For elective procedures that need to be delayed due to a current or recent URI, they should be delayed for 2-4 weeks after symptoms resolve. If the patient presents with a recent URI 2-4 weeks prior to surgery, and is no longer symptomatic, it is reasonable to proceed, again understanding the risk that hyperreactivity may still be present [23, 24].

For urgent procedures in patients with risk factors for pulmonary adverse events and a recent URI, a discussion should take place with the surgeon for optimal timing of the procedure, and all associated risks should be discussed with parents during the consent process. If a procedure is urgent or emergent, the child can still be optimized with premedications such as inhaled beta-2 agonists, antisialogogues, nasal decongestants, adequate suctioning, chest physiotherapy, use of incentive spirometry, or glucocorticoids as needed depending on the severity of the illness. Adjuncts for optimization can be utilized at all times during the perioperative process, before, during and after the anesthetic [24].

Autism

Autism occurs in about 2-5 patients per 10,000, with a gender ratio of 4:1 male: female. Children with autism spectrum disorder require special care during their entire perioperative experience. Autistic patients have a lifelong social disability and may often find it hard even to leave their homes. They rely on a daily, familiar routine; even coming into a hospital or healthcare setting can start to increase their anxiety and discomfort. Autistic children have difficulty with social communication, interactions, and social understanding. They often display repetitive patterns of behavior, prefer the familiar, and may be reluctant to make eye contact or be touched, especially by an unfamiliar person. They often process language literally because of a decreased ability to imagine or understand something metaphorical. Metaphors and magic, techniques often utilized in pediatrics to make children feel more comfortable, do not work with autistic children because they can not make metaphoric connections. When talking with parents, it is important to learn about the comforts and discomforts of the child and to speak quietly and gently. No jargon or metaphors should be used; the plan should be explained simply and clearly. If physical contact is necessary, permission from the child and parents should always be obtained before approaching and making contact [25, 26].

If possible, learning about the patient before the day of surgery is helpful so as to encourage the family to bring a comfort object with them (*e.g.* a favorite toy, blanket, or pillow). Early communication with the family is key to planning a smooth perioperative experience. With that in mind, an individualized but flexible treatment plan should be in place to accommodate the changing needs of the child. On the day of surgery, the patient should be given a private room, if possible, in a quiet environment with dim lighting. The minimum number of staff involved in the care should be assigned so as not to introduce too many new faces to the patient. These patients often need premedication, and it may be easier to allow the patient to self administer (depending on age and ability) or to allow the parents to administer the premedication rather than a preoperative nurse. Sometimes the premedication may have to be given mixed in a preferred food or drink such as juice or jello. Oral midazolam has great efficacy. Oral ketamine may be a better option in moderate to severe cases of autism spectrum. Oral midazolam-ketamine combination also is an effective combination for moderate to severe autism. A familiar face should always be allowed to be nearby for patient comfort (parent, caretaker). Parental presence at inductions are beneficial in the autistic patient population. Most autistic patients will not tolerate IV placement preoperatively, even with a premedication, so inhalation induction and IV placement post induction is usually the optimal technique. Intraoperative management should include multimodal analgesia and prophylactic antiemetics to facilitate a smooth postoperative course. The IV should be wrapped or covered so as to not distress the child on wakeup, and removed as quickly as the recovery allows. In the recovery area, parents should be brought to accompany the child as soon as possible. Emergence agitation is always a possibility and prophylactic treatment should always be considered. The postoperative care environment should be similar to the preoperative environment, including limited new faces, dim lights, quiet environment, and parents at the bedside. The goal of care for these patients is to do everything possible to decrease the stress of change that the patient experiences being out of their normal routine [25, 26].

Special Needs: Mental Disability, Developmental Delay

Children with special needs include those with cognitive disabilities, perceptive delays, motor disabilities, or a combination thereof. They can have cognitive deficits, speech or communication problems, associated physical disabilities, learning impairments, or social impairments. The most common physical disability in early childhood is cerebral palsy (CP). CP is a nonprogressive, common intellectual disorder caused by injury to the developing brain. CP presents with varying degrees of severity and various associated impairments. For example, about 43% of CP patients have dysphagia or dysfunctional swallowing and 50% have gastroesophageal reflux, both of which increase the risk of aspiration. Epilepsy, hypotonia, muscle spasms and limb contractures, scoliosis, temporomandibular disorder, visual and hearing deficits, and behavioral and communications problems are also commonly seen in this population. All of these associations can present a challenge to the anesthesiologist in the perioperative environment [27 - 30].

These children are at a higher risk of developing complications from anesthesia as compared to non-special needs pediatric patients. For example, they have higher risk of hypothermia (a compromised central nervous system can lead to impaired thermoregulatory mechanisms), hypotension, delayed emergence, seizures, airway obstruction, secretions, aspiration and pneumonia, postoperative stridor, laryngospasm, and bronchospasm. The severity of CP correlates with the postoperative complication incidence [27]. Each patient has to be taken care of with an individualized plan specific for their needs, and with sensitivity. The information from the parent or caregiver is essential since they know the patient best and they are able to communicate with the patient best. A review of the patient's home medications and what was taken the morning of the planned procedure is important to identify any risks that may present. Many patients are on chronic antispasmodic medications and antiepileptic medications which should be continued on the day of surgery. It is helpful to have the caregiver with the patient for as long as possible preoperatively and at induction if necessary, as well as postoperatively. Premedications are often very helpful. Oral midazolam is a great choice since many patients have seizures as comorbidity and midazolam can increase the seizure threshold. Since many patients have swallowing difficulties, intramuscular premedications can be a better option. Antisialogogues as a premedication (adding atropine to an intramuscular premedication) is often ideal to help with uncontrolled secretions. If clonidine is available, a preoperative clonidine patch may help with decreasing tone and improving spasticity in patients.

Vascular access in these patients may present a challenge, especially if the child has multiple chronic contractures. Also, some patients may have difficult airways due to comorbidities such as severe scoliosis or malocclusion of the jaw. In the event where an RSI is necessary or a difficult airway is suspected, every effort should be made to obtain a preoperative IV. Positioning can be a challenge in these patients due to spasms and contractures. Appropriate padding and pressure point checks should be done through the procedure. Antiemetics and multimodal analgesia should be employed to avoid postoperative stress from nausea, vomiting, and pain, and also to avoid opioid-related hypoventilation. The minimal alveolar concentration required for patients with CP or neurological deficits is less than that of healthy patients. Using a bispectral index monitoring device is helpful to titrate the amount of volatile anesthetic required. Any and all epileptogenic medications should be avoided in this patient population. Chronic antiepileptic use can decrease sensitivity toward nondepolarizing muscle relaxants, although how clinically relevant the effect is questionable. A twitch monitor should be utilized prior to redosing muscle relaxants. In the event that a regional technique can be utilized for anesthesia or even for postoperative pain, it is highly recommended and encouraged in this population given the respiratory risks of general anesthesia, airway manipulation, risk of emergence agitation, and postoperative nausea and vomiting (PONV). Postoperatively, the caregiver should be at the patients' bedside as soon as possible and all attempts to decrease postoperative anxiety in the patient and support symptomatically (*i.e.*, for secretions, hypothermia, pain, spasticity, agitation, PONV) should be undertaken [27, 28, 30, 31].

The Premature Infant / Bronchopulmonary Dysplasia

The premature infant is defined as a viable infant born after the 20th week of gestation and before full term (37 weeks gestation), weighing usually 500-2,499 grams at birth. Low birth weight is defined as less than 2500 grams at birth. Very low birth weight is defined as less than 1500 grams at birth. Extremely low birth weight is defined as less than 1000 grams at birth [32].

Apnea is common in premature infants, and is more common after anesthesia. As gestational age increases, risk of apnea decreases. With apneic episodes, infants can also develop bradycardia requiring treatment. Acute apnea is treated first with stimulation and then with simple airway maneuvers (chin lift, jaw thrust). If hypoxemia or apnea persists, positive pressure ventilation should be applied with a bag-mask. Some infants may be on stimulant therapy such as caffeine to stimulate spontaneous respirations. Nasal CPAP and mechanical ventilation are the last resort for life-threatening, persistent apnea or apneic episodes that are not responsive to simple maneuvers or stimulants. Apnea of prematurity usually resolves by 52-55 weeks post conceptual age. For this reason, most institutions have an admission policy for all premature infants having surgery that are less than 60 weeks post conceptual age. They are admitted postoperatively for at least 24 hours for apnea monitoring and pulse oximetry. Full term infants that are less than 44 weeks post conceptual age AND preterm infants (any infant born earlier than 37 weeks gestation) that are less than 60 weeks post conceptual age must be monitored for at least 23 hours after discharge from Phase I recovery [32].

Anemia in premature infants is more severe than anemia of infancy that is seen in all infants. Up to 75% of extremely low birth weight infants will receive a transfusion during their hospital stay. Anemia of prematurity is associated with poor weight gain, poor feeding, persistent tachycardia, and even persistent metabolic acidosis. Treatment options include blood transfusion, close monitoring, and administration of recombinant erythropoietin. There is no consensus on the adequate hemoglobin range. Most neonatologists favor hemoglobin levels within the 7-10 g/dL range, favoring higher or lower depending on the infants' other comorbidities and severity of illness. Pre-surgical hemoglobin of at least 10 g/dL at a minimum is recommended by many institutions [32].

Premature infants are at risk of developing hypoglycemia. This risk is seen with history of intrauterine growth restriction, hypothermia, respiratory distress, polycythemia, or maternal diabetes. Most neonatologists consider hypoglycemia requiring treatment to be less than 50 mg/dL or higher if the infant is symptomatic (tremors, eye-rolls, apnea, convulsions, cyanosis, weak/high pitched cry, poor feeding). Hypoglycemia should be monitored closely and treated aggressively to avoid acquired neurodevelopmental deficits. Treatment is with enteral feeds. If that alone is not sufficient, dextrose is bolused and infused. Often neonates require a dextrose infusion of D10 due to the high risk of rebound hypoglycemia following boluses. In a surgical setting, most infants present to the operative room already on a dextrose infusion. The stress of surgery causes an increase in blood glucose, so intraoperative glucose infusions are often reduced from the maintenance dose. Intraoperative glucose should be checked hourly and infusion titrated as needed [32].

Premature infants are deficient in the alveolar cells (type 2 pneumocytes) that produce surfactant and decrease surface tension in the alveoli, which is necessary for preventing alveolar collapse. Surfactant production is at 50% by 28 weeks gestation, and is complete by 36 weeks gestation. The risk of respiratory distress syndrome (RDS) and surfactant deficiency increases with decreasing gestational age, and is rarely seen in infants over 35 weeks gestational age. Risk factors that increase the risk of RDS include perinatal asphyxia, maternal diabetes, birth by cesarean section, cold stress, maternal history of multiple pregnancies, and history of affected siblings. Antenatal administration of corticosteroids is beneficial in any parturient with risk of preterm labor to increase surfactant production. Surfactant deficiency leads to decreased lung compliance, atelectasis, and decreased functional residual capacity. Clinically, infants present with tachypnea and show signs of respiratory distress, accessory muscle use, nasal flaring, sternal retractions, and grunting. Cyanosis or respiratory failure require mechanical ventilation. An arterial blood gas will show acidosis and hypoxemia. A chest x-ray classically shows a diffuse ground-glass appearance and air bronchograms. Treatment includes supplemental O_2 with a goal arterial oxygen partial pressure (PaO_2) of 55-70 mmHg, nasal cpap, or even mechanical ventilation. Some indications for mechanical ventilation include low PaO_2 less than 50 mmHg despite FiO_2 of 100%, persistent pH less than 7.2, or central apnea unresponsive to pharmacologic treatments. These infants are at risk for developing chronic lung disease; therefore the goal is to wean FiO_2 and ventilation aggressively and to minimize volutrauma and barotrauma. Goals are normoxia and permissive hypercapnia ($paCO_2$ 40-65). Each premature infant at risk of developing RDS receives artificial surfactant introduced into the lungs *via* the trachea shortly after birth to decrease the risk of pulmonary air leak and long term chronic lung disease, also known as bronchopulmonary dysplasia or BPD [32, 33].

In 2018, one in every ten infants born in the United States was born preterm. The rate of preterm birth is rising, largely in part due to assisted reproduction, older maternal age at first delivery, and less prenatal care in certain populations. As more of these babies are born, and mature into childhood and adulthood, more instances of long term sequelae of preterm birth will be seen. In the past, mostly the respiratory and neurologic complications have been discussed as these are the most common systems that are affected in development. BPD of prematurity often develops into a chronic obstructive lung disease [34, 35]. BPD can persist in varying severities of persistent pulmonary dysfunction. Symptoms are similar to those often seen in asthmatics, such as decreased exercise tolerance in young adulthood, abnormal ventilatory responses, abnormal pulmonary function tests, microaspiration, and reflux and associated aspiration pneumonia and chronic lung inflammation, and even development of pulmonary hypertension [36]. History of prematurity in infants, toddlers, and even young adults should prompt a review of systems of exercise tolerance, respiratory infections, and signs and symptoms of the presence of potential chronic lung disease. A pediatric pulmonologist is often involved in their care, and if not, it is not unreasonable to consider consultation with a pediatric pulmonary specialist. Treatment of infants with a history of bronchopulmonary dysplasia associated with prematurity have a higher incidence of pulmonary adverse events, and care should be taken to optimize their respiratory status preoperatively. If they are presenting for an elective surgery, all risk factors should be taken into consideration. For this reason, any signs of recent illness should prompt rescheduling. Discussion with parents about the potential need for oxygen therapy postoperatively, whether in the form of invasive ventilation or noninvasive supplemental oxygen should be complete and thorough. A plan for admission postoperatively should be in place. All efforts at avoiding airway irritation should be prioritized. The patient should receive a preoperative anxiolytic (depending on age and need), intubation should be avoided if possible, and the risks and benefits of a deep extubation technique to avoid bronchospasm on extubation should be weighed [33].

Sickle Cell Disease

Patients with sickle cell disease have abnormal hemoglobin (Hb) S which have sickle red blood cells that cause vessel occlusion leading to infarct in the lungs (acute chest syndrome), bones, brain, and spleen. These patients have anemia, decreased erythrocyte lifespan, increased bilirubin, and increased hemolysis. All infants with homozygous Hb SS should receive the pneumococcal vaccine and penicillin prophylaxis up to 6 years of age. The severity of the disease depends on the percentage of the abnormal Hb S and the presence of any other abnormal hemoglobin types. In sickle cell trait (SCT), sickling is unlikely to occur unless the patient is profoundly hypoxic, and patients usually do not have a history of crises. They often do not require special sickle cell treatment. Patients with the homozygous Hb SS have sickle cell disease (SCD). Sickling is much more likely in this patient population. Many patients may have evidence of sickling crises in the past, such as splenomegaly, splenic infarct, avascular necrosis of the bone, *etc.* Serious perioperative complications are possible such as stroke, acute chest syndrome, and pulmonary complications. Other abnormal hemoglobins such as Hb C and Hb D, when combined with Hb S, can also result in sickling. Neonates with fetal hemoglobin (Hb F) are less at risk for sickling. Hb F is replaced completely by 6 months of age [37]. Sickling can be precipitated by hypoxemia. The potential for sickling increases with acidosis, anemia, hypothermia, dehydration, sepsis, hypotension, and hypercarbia. Previous occlusive episodes can lead to impaired liver, heart, and renal function. Decreased serum cholinesterase activity is possible with impaired liver disease [37].

The patient's hematologist should be involved in the perioperative management of a patient with sickle cell disease. The patient should be optimized by the hematologist and cleared for all procedures. The hematologist should provide instructions for the management of fluid and pain while the patient is admitted, and they should give guidance on transfusion thresholds. All pediatric outpatients scheduled for surgery should be admitted to the hospital the day before for fluid management in the setting of NPO status. Any necessary lab work or preoperative transfusion can be completed at this time. These patients usually have a type, screened, and crossmatched available blood products ready before any procedures.

All children of African American or Mediterranean descent should be screened for sickle cell disease. If a child has known sickle cell trait, preoperative dehydration should be avoided with the encouragement of clear fluid intake until 2 hours prior to surgery, or by using maintenance intravenous fluids during the fasting period. Preoperative sedation should be avoided, as most preoperative sedatives are respiratory depressants. If a child has known sickle cell disease, a careful assessment should be done to identify any sequelae from previous crises. Previous pain management strategies should be ascertained. A minimum Hb level of 10 should be obtained with blood transfusion if necessary. The patient should be hydrated with a balanced salt solution at 1-1.5x maintenance while NPO. In an emergency, exchange transfusion should be performed [37].

During induction, all efforts to avoid complications such as laryngospasm and breath holding should be maintained. Intubation is undertaken after muscle relaxant administration. Many anesthetics have been used successfully; no specific anesthetic has been shown to increase or decrease morbidity related to SCD. Intraoperative goals of care include avoiding hypoxemia, hypothermia, hypercarbia, hypovolemia, and acidosis. High FiO_2 should be used to maintain 100% saturation, and ventilation should be controlled to avoid hypercarbia. Careful positioning is needed to minimize venous stasis and avoid regional ischemia. Techniques for careful positioning include padding all pressure points, positioning the child carefully, and rotating the blood pressure cuff position during a long procedure. Tourniquets should only be used if necessary and for a minimal amount of time. Careful fluid balance should be calculated to avoid under or over resuscitation. The benefit of general anesthesia *versus* regional anesthesia is unclear [37, 38].

Once the procedure is complete, the patient should be extubated fully awake, with continued oxygenation post extubation. Pulse oximetry should be maintained in the recovery area so as to prevent any unanticipated hypoxemia and incentive spirometry should be encouraged. Some studies indicate that the use of incentive spirometry decreases the risk of acute chest syndrome in SCD patients. In recovery, temperature control and fluid management should continue to be carefully managed, as these patients can develop crises at any time. Pulmonary complications are common in SCD and the patients should be frequently assessed for signs of pulmonary compromise. Adequate preoperative and postoperative pain management is a critical step to help prevent a sickle cell crisis. Usually the patient's hematologist has recommendations for postoperative pain control, but the patient or patient's family also has insight into their pain regimen. The patient and their family can be a great resource for learning about the child's normal pain requirements and can give insight into a pain regimen that has worked in the past. Early mobilization is encouraged [37, 38].

Obstructive Sleep Apnea (OSA)

OSA usually occurs in children due to chronic obstruction from hyperplasia of lymphoid tissue. Symptoms of OSA include loud snoring, difficult arousal, daytime somnolence, behavioral problems (attention deficit disorder, short attention), nocturnal enuresis, nocturnal gasps, or apnea. The majority of children with OSA are overweight or obese, but it is not a diagnostic requirement. OSA is diagnosed ideally with polysomnography (sleep study), which measures the amount of times the patient becomes apneic or hypopneic during the night. The AHI (apnea-hypopnea index) is then calculated and is defined as the average number of apnea to hypopnea episodes per hour. Table **7** depicts the range of AHI and associated severity of OSA [39].

Table 7. AHI scoring in the Pediatric Population.

Severity of Pediatric OSA	AHI score (average events per hour of sleep)
Mild	1-5
Moderate	5.1-10
Severe	>10

If no polysomnography is available, a nighttime oxygen saturation trend can help elucidate the severity of OSA combined with the patient's review of symptoms. A baseline O_2 saturation of less than 90% and a sleeping oxygen saturation dropping below 80% is strongly suggestive of severe OSA. An abnormal sleep study in a patient with OSA symptoms warrants a tonsillectomy and adenoidectomy (T&A), which is the most commonly completed pediatric surgery. Many T&As can be done in ambulatory surgery centers; however, a T&A for the indication of OSA often requires intensive monitoring and admission postoperatively. Indications for admission following T&A are described in Table **8**. Sleep study criteria for admission of a patient with known OSA following T&A are shown in Table **9** [39].

Table 8. Indications for admission following T&A.

Indications for admission following T&A
1. Age < 3 years
2. Significant OSA
3. Presence of craniofacial abnormalities such as patients with Down syndrome
4. Peritonsillar abscess history
5. Abnormal coagulation history or increased risk of bleeding
6. Systemic disease such as obesity, congenital heart disease, neuromuscular disorders, SCD, or those who don't have access to a medical facility near their homes.

Table 9. Sleep study criteria for admission of a patient with OSA following a T&A.

Indication for Admission Post T&A in OSA patients
1. Baseline $PaCO_2$ of 50 mmHg or greater
2. Baseline awake O_2 saturation less than 92%
3. Desaturation episodes to O_2 saturation less than 80%
4. AHI of greater than or equal to 10 (considered severe OSA in pediatric patients)

Children with OSA have a decreased response to rebreathing carbon dioxide and may be very sensitive to narcotics. A reduction of opioid doses is required, especially if their night time desaturations drop to below 85%. Mild OSA has not been shown to have an increased risk of complications following T&A. Moderate to severe OSA patients require more intensive monitoring postoperatively. A multimodal approach to pain management is recommended in an attempt to limit opioids. Preoperative oral acetaminophen or intraoperative intravenous acetaminophen can be given, and intraoperative ketamine 0.5 mg/kg can be given to decrease opioid use. Pre- or postoperative oral ibuprofen can also be given unless there is a contraindication for NSAIDs or surgeon preference to avoid NSAIDs. Ketorolac is usually not administered for fear of increased postoperative bleeding risk. Codeine should never be used due to incidences of postoperative deaths that led to a black box warning from the Food and Drug Administration (FDA). Up to 90% of mild-moderate OSA patients show improvement of symptoms after 6 months post T&A. Only about 30% of patients who are obese or who have severe OSA show similar improvement. Some patients may require nighttime oxygen, intranasal steroids or even evaluation for uvulopalatopharyngoplasty [39].

In any child with a history of OSA coming to the operative room, preoperative IV placement should be seriously considered, especially in obese children, as these children will obstruct easily during induction and emergence. For that reason, such patients should always be extubated awake, with evidence of the return of airway reflexes. Supplemental oxygen and a pulse oximeter for transport to the recovery area are always recommended. In patients with severe OSA, intensive monitoring in an intensive care setting should be considered depending on the severity of OSA and the type of surgery the patient is recovering from. Restlessness in the child may be a symptom of hypoxia or hypercarbia and may indicate obstruction or impaired ventilation. Nasal CPAP should be considered as ventilatory aid in obese patients, as many younger children do not tolerate larger mask positive pressure devices. Less severe OSA patients should at the very least be monitored closely in the recovery area for 4-6 hours postoperatively. Different institutions have different requirements [39].

Congenital Cardiac Anomalies

Patients with congenital heart disease (CHD) are at high risk for adverse events during anesthesia and surgery. They comprise a vulnerable population that should be taken care of by the appropriate providers at an institution with adequate and necessary resources for their care. The anesthesiologist and all care teams that the patient will encounter (surgeon, intensivist, pediatrician) must possess the skill and expertise needed for these patients, which differs based on their specific heart disease. There are several risk assessment tools in the literature to try to classify congenital heart disease patients, but ultimately it is up to the providers to determine the appropriate needs for these high risk patients [40 - 42].

The American College of Surgeons National Surgical Quality Improvement Program published a classification of congenital heart disease. The classification system breaks down CHD into minor, major, and severe categories based on the lesion burden and the patient's functional status. Minor lesions include minor cardiac conditions that may or may not need medication. Examples include small atrial septal defects, small-to-moderate asymptomatic ventral septal defects, or a completely repaired congenital lesion in which cardiac function is essentially normal. Major lesions include repaired congenital heart lesions that have residual abnormal function and may require medication. Severe lesions include pulmonary hypertension, cardiac dysfunction requiring a heart transplant, ventricular dysfunction requiring medications, or an uncorrected cyanotic heart defect. The ACS-NSQIP classification system is a great tool to utilize for the allocation of resources for a patient with congenital heart disease. Should the patient present to an institution with limited resources, it is a useful tool to assess whether they can be safely taken care of at that institution. A provider can decide based on the risk of an individual patient (taking into account their heart disease, age, other comorbidities and risk of surgical procedure) whether or not the available resources are adequate, or if they need to be transferred to another hospital or institution [41 - 43].

As mentioned in the section, "Triaging the Patient" earlier in this chapter, a study by Seattele *et al.* classified pediatric cardiac patients as low, moderate or high risk. The breakdown of the risk categories by Seattele *et al.* is a good summary of cardiac defects that an anesthesia provider may encounter. The study indicated that the "low risk" patients were safely taken care of at an outpatient facility, therefore not requiring special preoperative or postoperative monitoring or hospital admission. A moderate or high risk patient, according to their criteria, was safely taken care of at a pediatric facility with cardiac pediatric anesthesia providers [6]. To utilize their risk stratification to create inclusion/exclusion criteria for a non-pediatric anesthesia provider at a non-pediatric facility would be reasonable (refer to Table **2**). The intention of the study was to effectively allocate appropriate anesthesia resources at the institution using the risk assessment tool, which appeared to be successful based on their adverse outcome rates. If a pediatric patient with congenital heart disease falls into the low risk category, and a non-pediatric anesthesia provider feels it is within their scope of practice, and the hospital is well-equipped, it is reasonable to proceed with that patient's care.

CONCLUSION

Thorough preoperative evaluation is essential prior to administering anesthesia in all children. A detailed history, examination of various organ systems, identification of various risk factors, optimization of organ function and careful planning prior to administration of anesthesia is essential for a good postoperative outcome.

CONSENT FOR PUBLICATION

Not applicable.

CONFLICT OF INTEREST

The author declares no conflict of interest, financial or otherwise.

ACKNOWLEDGEMENTS

Declared none.

REFERENCES

[1]   Dodson G, Litman R. Preanesthetic preparation of the pediatric patient Basics of Pediatric Anesthesia. 2nd ed. Philadelphia: Ronald S. Litman 2017; pp. 71-84.

[2]   Krane EJ, Davis PJ, Kain ZN. Preoperative Preparation. In: Davis PJ, Cladis FP, Eds. Smith's Anesthesia for Infants and Children 9th Edition. location: Elsevier . 2017.

[3]   Basel A, Bajic D. Preoperative Evaluation of the Pediatric Patient 2018.https://www.anesthesiology .theclinics.com/article/S1932-2275(18)30083-1/fulltext [PMID: 30390788]

[http://dx.doi.org/10.1016/j.anclin.2018.07.016]

[4]   English A, Bass L, Boyle AD, Eshragh F. State Minor Consent Laws: A Summary 2010.https://www.freelists.org/archives/hilac/02-2014/pdftRo8tw89mb.pdf

[5]   Winiarski D, Klatt E, Kazerouninia A. Risks and Legal Issues in Caring for Minor Jehovah's Witness Patients 2018. https://forum.ashrm.org/2018/03/29/risks-and-legal-issues-in-caring-fo--minor-jeho vahs-witn-ss-patients/#:~:text=Risks%20and%20Legal%20Issues %20in%20Caring%20for%20Minor %20Jehovah's

[6]   Saettele AK, Christensen JL, Chilson KL, Murray DJ. Children with heart disease: Risk stratification for non-cardiac surgery. J Clin Anesth 2016; 35: 479-84.
        [http://dx.doi.org/10.1016/j.jclinane.2016.09.016] [PMID: 27871578]

[7]   Dave NM. Premedication and Induction of Anaesthesia in paediatric patients. Indian J Anaesth 2019; 63(9): 713-20.
        [http://dx.doi.org/10.4103/ija.IJA_491_19] [PMID: 31571684]

[8]   Peng K, Wu SR, Ji FH, Li J. Premedication with dexmedetomidine in pediatric patients: a systematic review and meta-analysis. Clinics (São Paulo) 2014; 69(11): 777-86.
        [http://dx.doi.org/10.6061/clinics/2014(11)12] [PMID: 25518037]

[9]   Plambech MZ, Afshari A. Dexmedetomidine in the pediatric population: a review. Minerva Anestesiol 2015; 81(3): 320-32.
        [PMID: 24824958]

[10]   Liu PP, Sun Y, Wu C, *et al.* The effectiveness of transport in a toy car for reducing preoperative anxiety in preschool children: a randomised controlled prospective trial. Br J Anaesth 2018; 121(2): 438-44.
        [http://dx.doi.org/10.1016/j.bja.2018.02.067] [PMID: 30032883]

[11]   Vagnoli L, Bettini A, Amore E, De Masi S, Messeri A. Relaxation-guided imagery reduces perioperative anxiety and pain in children: a randomized study. Eur J Pediatr 2019; 178(6): 913-21.
        [http://dx.doi.org/10.1007/s00431-019-03376-x] [PMID: 30944985]

[12]   Franzoi MA, Goulart CB, Lara EO, Martins G. Music listening for anxiety relief in children in the preoperative period: a randomized clinical trial. Rev Lat Am Enfermagem 2016; 24: e2841.
        [http://dx.doi.org/10.1590/1518-8345.1121.2841] [PMID: 27992027]

[13]   Ni CH, Tsai WH, Lee LM, Kao CC, Chen YC. Minimising preoperative anxiety with music for day surgery patients - a randomised clinical trial. J Clin Nurs 2012; 21(5-6): 620-5.
        [http://dx.doi.org/10.1111/j.1365-2702.2010.03466.x] [PMID: 21332853]

[14]   Millett CR, Gooding LF. Comparing Active and Passive Distraction-Based Music Therapy Interventions on Preoperative Anxiety in Pediatric Patients and Their Caregivers. J Music Ther 2018; 54(4): 460-78.
        [http://dx.doi.org/10.1093/jmt/thx014] [PMID: 29253180]

[15]   Dionigi A, Gremigni P. A combined intervention of art therapy and clown visits to reduce preoperative anxiety in children. J Clin Nurs 2017; 26(5-6): 632-40.
        [http://dx.doi.org/10.1111/jocn.13578] [PMID: 27627730]

[16]   Cote CJ, Lerman J, Anderson BJ. The practice of pediatric anesthesiaA practice of anesthesia for infants and children. 5th ed. Philadelphia: Elsevier Saunders 2013; pp. 1-6.

[17]   Ghazal EA, Mason LJ, Cote CJ. Preoperative evaluation, premedication, and induction of anesthesiaA practice of anesthesia for infants and children. 5th ed. Philadelphia: Elsevier Saunders 2013; pp. 31-63.

[18]   Simpao A, Litman R. Monitoring in pediatric anesthesia.Basics of Pediatric Anesthesia. 2nd ed. Philadelphia: Ronald S. Litman. 2017; pp. 71-84.

[19]   Ramgolam A, Hall GL, Zhang G, Hegarty M, von Ungern-Sternberg BS. Inhalational *versus* Intravenous Induction of Anesthesia in Children with a High Risk of Perioperative Respiratory

Adverse Events: A Randomized Controlled Trial. Anesthesiology 2018; 128(6): 1065-74.
[http://dx.doi.org/10.1097/ALN.0000000000002152] [PMID: 29498948]

[20] von Ungern-Sternberg BS, Boda K, Chambers NA, *et al.* Risk assessment for respiratory complications in paediatric anaesthesia: a prospective cohort study. Lancet 2010; 376(9743): 773-83.
[http://dx.doi.org/10.1016/S0140-6736(10)61193-2] [PMID: 20816545]

[21] Chundamala J, Wright JG, Kemp SM. An evidence-based review of parental presence during anesthesia induction and parent/child anxiety. Can J Anaesth 2009; 56(1): 57-70.
[http://dx.doi.org/10.1007/s12630-008-9008-3] [PMID: 19247779]

[22] Kain ZN, Caldwell-Andrews AA, Maranets I, Nelson W, Mayes LC. Predicting which child-parent pair will benefit from parental presence during induction of anesthesia: a decision-making approach. Anesth Analg 2006; 102(1): 81-4.
[http://dx.doi.org/10.1213/01.ANE.0000181100.27931.A1] [PMID: 16368808]

[23] Becke K. Anesthesia in children with a cold. Curr Opin Anaesthesiol 2012; 25(3): 333-9.
[http://dx.doi.org/10.1097/ACO.0b013e3283534e80] [PMID: 22499163]

[24] Houck P. Anesthesia for the child with a recent upper respiratory infection. 2019. UpToDate. Waltham, MA: UpToDate;

[25] Short JA, Calder A. Anaesthesia for children with special needs, including autistic spectrum disorder. Contin Educ Anaesth Crit Care Pain 2013; 13(4): 107-12.
[http://dx.doi.org/10.1093/bjaceaccp/mks065]

[26] van der Walt JH, Moran C. An audit of perioperative management of autistic children. Paediatr Anaesth 2001; 11(4): 401-8.
[http://dx.doi.org/10.1046/j.1460-9592.2001.00688.x] [PMID: 11442855]

[27] Wass CT, Warner ME, Worrell GA, *et al.* Effect of general anesthesia in patients with cerebral palsy at the turn of the new millennium: a population-based study evaluating perioperative outcome and brief overview of anesthetic implications of this coexisting disease. J Child Neurol 2012; 27(7): 859-66.
[http://dx.doi.org/10.1177/0883073811428378] [PMID: 22190505]

[28] Erasmus CE, Van Hulst K, Rotteveel JJ, Willemsen MAAP, Jongerius PH. Swallowing problems in cerebral palsy. Clinical practice. Eur J Pediatr 2012; 171: 409-14.
[http://dx.doi.org/10.1007/s00431-011-1570-y] [PMID: 21932013]

[29] Miamoto CB, Pereira LJ, Paiva SM, Pordeus IA, Ramos-Jorge ML, Marques LS. Prevalence and risk indicators of temporomandibular disorder signs and symptoms in a pediatric population with spastic cerebral palsy. J Clin Pediatr Dent 2011; 35(3): 259-63.
[http://dx.doi.org/10.17796/jcpd.35.3.738t75v74l1m1p22] [PMID: 21678667]

[30] Nolan J, Chalkiadis GA, Low J, Olesch CA, Brown TCK. Anaesthesia and pain management in cerebral palsy. Anaesthesia 2000; 55(1): 32-41.
[http://dx.doi.org/10.1046/j.1365-2044.2000.01065.x] [PMID: 10594431]

[31] Graham RJ, Wachendorf MT, Burns JP, Mancuso TJ. Successful and safe delivery of anesthesia and perioperative care for children with complex special health care needs. J Clin Anesth 2009; 21(3): 165-72.
[http://dx.doi.org/10.1016/j.jclinane.2008.06.033] [PMID: 19464608]

[32] Pukenas E, Dodson G, Griggs S, Litman R. The Premature Infant.Basics of Pediatric Anesthesia. 2nd ed. Philadelphia: Ronald S. Litman 2017; pp. 59-65.

[33] Muhly T, Litman R. The Formerly Premature Infant.In: Litman R, Ed Basics of Pediatric Anesthesia 2nd Edition Philadelphia: Ronald S Litman. 2017; pp. 67-70.

[34] Centers for Disease Control and Prevention. Reproductive Health, Maternal and Infants Health. [cited 2020 May 13]. https://www.cdc.gov/reproductivehealth/maternalinfanthealth/ pretermbirth.htm

[35]   Landry JS, Chan T, Lands L, Menzies D. Long-term impact of bronchopulmonary dysplasia on pulmonary function. Can Respir J 2011; 18(5): 265-70.
[http://dx.doi.org/10.1155/2011/547948] [PMID: 21969927]

[36]   Davidson LM, Berkelhamer SK. Bronchopulmonary Dysplasia: Chronic Lung Disease of Infancy and Long-Term Pulmonary Outcomes. J Clin Med 2017; 6(1): 4.
[http://dx.doi.org/10.3390/jcm6010004] [PMID: 28067830]

[37]   Lerman J, Cote CJ, Steward DJ. Medical Conditions Influencing Anesthetic ManagementManual of Pediatric Anesthesia. 7th ed. New York: Springer International Publishing AG Switzerland 2016; pp. 167-210.
[http://dx.doi.org/10.1007/978-3-319-30684-1_6]

[38]   Adjepong KO, Otegbeye F, Adjepong YA. Perioperative Management of Sickle Cell Disease. Mediterr J Hematol Infect Dis 2018; 10(1): e2018032.
[http://dx.doi.org/10.4084/mjhid.2018.032] [PMID: 29755709]

[39]   Lerman J, Cote CJ, Steward DJ. OtorhinolaryngologyManual of Pediatric Anesthesia. 7th ed. New York: Springer International Publishing AG Switzerland 2016; pp. 271-80.
[http://dx.doi.org/10.1007/978-3-319-30684-1_10]

[40]   Brown ML, DiNardo JA, Nasr VG. Anesthesia in Pediatric Patients With Congenital Heart Disease Undergoing Noncardiac Surgery: Defining the Risk. J Cardiothorac Vasc Anesth 2020; 34(2): 470-8.
[http://dx.doi.org/10.1053/j.jvca.2019.06.015] [PMID: 31345716]

[41]   Gottlieb EA, Andropoulos DB. Anesthesia for the patient with congenital heart disease presenting for noncardiac surgery. Curr Opin Anaesthesiol 2013; 26(3): 318-26.
[http://dx.doi.org/10.1097/ACO.0b013e328360c50b] [PMID: 23614956]

[42]   Brown ML, DiNardo JA, Odegard KC. Patients with single ventricle physiology undergoing noncardiac surgery are at high risk for adverse events. Paediatr Anaesth 2015; 25(8): 846-51.
[http://dx.doi.org/10.1111/pan.12685] [PMID: 25970232]

[43]   Faraoni D, Zurakowski D, Vo D, *et al.* Post-Operative Outcomes in Children With and Without Congenital Heart Disease Undergoing Noncardiac Surgery. J Am Coll Cardiol 2016; 67(7): 793-801.
[http://dx.doi.org/10.1016/j.jacc.2015.11.057] [PMID: 26892415]

CHAPTER 5

Induction, Maintenance, and Emergence

Aysha Hasan[1], Andrea Gomez-Morad[2] and Arvind Chandrankantan[3]

[1] *Department of Anesthesiology, St. Christopher's Hospital for Children, Philadelphia, PA, USA*

[2] *Department of Anesthesiology, Boston Children's Hospital, Boston, MA, USA*

[3] *Department of Anesthesiology, Texas Children's Hospital, Houston, TX, USA*

Abstract: Induction of anesthesia in the pediatric population differs significantly compared to adult care. Many pediatric inductions are performed with a mask-only technique. Intravenous access is rapidly obtained prior to securing the airway in the majority of cases. Maintenance of anesthesia can be achieved *via* an inhalational agent, intravenous agent, or a combination of both. Fluid should be administered judiciously. Multimodal pain management is superior to an opioid-only technique. Premature or sick infants and neonates require added glucose to their fluids and frequent glucose checks. Additional intravenous access, arterial access, or foley should be obtained once the patient's airway is secure and the patient is under a surgical plane of anesthesia. Emergence includes reversal agents if muscle relaxant was administered. Regardless of deep *versus* awake extubation, preparations for significant emergence delirium should be made for children aged 2-12 years. Common postoperative sequelae such as laryngospasm and emergence delirium are discussed.

Keywords: Bronchospasm, Emergence delirium, Fluid management, Inhalational induction, Intravenous induction, Laryngospasm, Maintenance of anesthesia, Oxygen desaturation, Pain, Parental presence induction, Postintubation stridor, Postoperative nausea and vomiting, Pulmonary edema, Respiratory insufficiency, Temperature instability, Temperature regulation.

INTRODUCTION

Induction, maintenance, and emergence of anesthesia are core principles that require an in-depth understanding to provide optimal anesthetic care. The anesthesiologist must devise an anesthetic plan that incorporates all aspects of the perioperative care of a pediatric patient. This chapter will go into further detail regarding each step in this process.

[8] **Corresponding author Bharathi Gourkanti MD:** Department of Anesthesiology, Cooper Medical School of Rowan University, Cooper University Health Care, Camden, NJ, United States; E-mail: gourkanti-bharathi@cooperhealth.edu

Bharathi Gourkanti, Irwin Gratz, Grace Dippo, Nathalie Peiris and Dinesh K. Choudhry (Eds.)
All rights reserved-© 2022 Bentham Science Publishers

INDUCTION

Planning an anesthetic induction for a pediatric patient often requires more flexibility and finesse than it would for an adult patient. In addition to preoperative evaluation of the patient's medical conditions and ensuring appropriate preoperative fasting (please see Chapter 4 for further description), one must consider other factors such as the patient's fears and parental concerns. Induction of anesthesia for a pediatric patient often starts prior to arrival into the operating room with anxiolysis in the preoperative holding area or at bedside. For further details on preoperative medications and anxiety-relieving techniques, please see Chapter 4.

Methods of Induction: Inhalational *vs* Intravenous

In comparison to anesthetic induction of adult patients, inhalational anesthetic inductions are often conducted in children due to intolerance of preoperative placement of intravenous (IV) access. The pediatric patient can differ vastly from the adult patient in terms of cooperation with the placement of vital monitors. Pediatric patients cannot rationalize unfamiliar situations and it can be very challenging to place all monitors on a patient upon arrival to the operating room. Even with premedication, children may still display emotional outbursts, become combative, scream, or cry when entering the unfamiliar operating room. Particularly combative patients may require initiation of inhalational anesthetic prior to monitor placement. A common inhalational induction technique for uncooperative patients consists of first priming the anesthesia circuit with 70% nitrous oxide, 30% oxygen and 8% sevoflurane, and placing the mask on the child. The child will inhale the combination and enter Guedel's stage 1 of anesthesia relatively quickly [2]. If the care team is only able to place a single monitor on the patient, the monitor of choice is the pulse oximeter. Pulse oximetry provides valuable information regarding oxygenation (and therefore ventilation) and perfusion (waveform, heart rate and regular rhythm) and is the most critical monitor to observe through the induction process [1]. In the interim, the anesthesiologist should monitor the patient visually for signs of perfusion and ventilatory obstruction. Once all standard ASA monitors are placed on the patient and the child has passed Guedel's stage 2 of anesthesia, a member of the care team should assist with intravenous access while keeping the patient in a deep state of anesthesia *via* mask ventilation. If the anesthesiologist does not have any assistance, a laryngeal mask airway (LMA) can be inserted to help stabilize the airway and continue ventilation and volatile anesthetic administration during IV placement attempts. After IV insertion, the anesthesiologist can then proceed with endotracheal intubation (if required). Common complications during inhalational induction include laryngospasm, bradycardia (especially in syndromic children or those with cardiac abnormalities), difficulty obtaining IV access, prolonged induction, and ventilatory obstruction (see Table **1**). Quick diagnosis and immediate correction of the underlying problem is important, especially if obstruction, bradycardia, or laryngospasm occur. Gradual slowing of the heart rate can often be managed with dialing down the concentration of sevoflurane from 8% as needed after the child passes through stage 2. Severe bradycardia should be treated immediately with intramuscular atropine (0.02 mg/kg) if no IV access has been established. Intramuscular injection of atropine and succinylcholine (4 mg/kg) should be used to relieve laryngospasm if it is not immediately relieved by positive pressure. Intramuscular weight-specific doses of these emergency medications should be drawn up and ready for administration with a small bore needle attached prior to induction. If IV access cannot be obtained after inhalational induction and after exhaustive measures have been undertaken by multiple providers, an elective case should be canceled.

In a cooperative child, ASA standard monitors should be placed prior to induction. Inhalational induction can be administered in a slow and stepwise fashion if the patient will tolerate a mask. One can often facilitate mask tolerance by adding artificial sweet flavoring to the mask (using flavored lip balm or scents) to disguise the anesthetic gas odor or creating games such as "blowing up" the anesthetic bag on the anesthesia machine *via* the mask. Induction of anesthesia can begin with a 50:50 mixture of nitrous oxide (which is odorless) and oxygen until the patient appears sedated. Sevoflurane is titrated in a stepwise approach beginning at 2% and incrementally increasing to 8% [3]. At this point, nitrous oxide can be discontinued and the child is maintained on 100% oxygen and sevoflurane while IV access is obtained. This will ensure that in an adverse event (*i.e.*, laryngospasm, bronchospasm, bradycardia, cardiac arrest), the child will maintain oxygenation for a greater period of time while the adverse reaction is being remedied. Once the child has intravenous access, intravenous induction agents can then be administered to deepen the plane of anesthesia prior to insertion of the endotracheal tube. If an LMA is the airway of choice, then intravenous access can safely be achieved after placement of the LMA as long as a deep plane of anesthesia has been achieved with inhalational agents.

A variety of medications can be used for the pediatric population when performing an intravenous induction (please see chapter 2 and chapter 4 for a detailed discussion of induction agents and dosing). Commonly known induction medications such as propofol and ketamine can be used in addition to using opioids or dexmedetomidine as adjuncts. Etomidate is rarely used as an induction medication in children due to concerns for adrenal suppression. If ketamine is the induction agent of choice, midazolam and glycopyrrolate can also be given to help avoid hallucinations and excessive salivation. Intravenous induction may be indicated in the presence of a full stomach, for pediatric trauma patients, in patients with suspected or known difficult airway, or for otherwise critically ill pediatric patients. The choice of an induction agent should be made based on the child's comorbidities and past medical history (as it is done in the adult population). Preoperative IV access enhances the safety of anesthetic induction due to the ability to "rescue" if the patient were to have laryngospasm or bronchospasm on induction, and for increased speed of anesthetic induction. Please see Table **1** for a further description of the advantages and disadvantages of an inhalational *versus* intravenous induction.

A combination of both inhalational induction and intravenous induction can also be used. If the anesthesiologist feels it may be unsafe to do a full inhalational induction and intravenous access is not available, a nitrous oxide: oxygen ratio can be used to help improve tolerance of IV insertion. This technique is useful in larger children that may be uncooperative with preoperative IV placement, but difficult to control during the excitatory phase of a purely inhalational induction. Alternatively, ketamine and midazolam given intramuscularly can induce a dissociative state, which may improve patient cooperation with obtaining IV access. Combination inductions are common and help the anesthesiologist facilitate the initiation of general anesthesia in a safe and comfortable manner. Table **1** provides a comparison of inhalational *vs.* intravenous induction advantages and disadvantages [4].

Table 1. Advantages and disadvantages of inhalation *vs.* intravenous induction.

Route of Administration	Advantages	Disadvantages
Inhalational	• IV not required • Spontaneous breathing is easier to maintain • Rapid return to recovery • Quick elimination from lungs • Painless • Volatile agents help dilate vasculature for intravenous access	• No IV access • Laryngospasm • Bradycardia • Requires help with IV placement or mask ventilation • Slow and variable speed to Guedel stages of anesthesia • Prolonged induction (especially in older children) • Pungent smell • Mask phobia • Cannot perform RSI

(Table 1) cont.....

Route of Administration	Advantages	Disadvantages
Intravenous	• Quicker onset of anesthesia • Intravenous access for medication delivery • Fluids can be given in advance • Premedication is given *via* IV for quicker onset • Children at risk for malignant hyperthermia (must avoid all volatile anesthetics aside from nitrous oxide) • RSI can be performed • Emergency medications faster onset	• Pain during IV placement • Pain during injection of induction agents • Fear of the IV even with a local anesthetic application at site • Bradycardia

Parental Presence Induction

One technique for maintaining a calm patient during the induction process is to invite the parent to be present for induction in the operating room. The parent should be given a detailed explanation of what to expect when they enter the operating room, and the induction technique and monitoring processes should be described. The parent should have a member of the team escorting them at all times. A chair should be given to the parent so they may sit with their child as he or she is anesthetized. Once the child is unconscious, the parent should be immediately escorted back to the waiting room.

Parental presence with induction can decrease patient anxiety and increase parental satisfaction, but it does not decrease the anxiety of the parent [5, 6]. Parental presence has been shown to not be superior to the use of a preoperative anxiolytic. However, for patients that refuse premedication or have comorbidities that would render premedication unsafe, a parental presence induction can be a useful technique.

Rapid Sequence Intubation

Considerations and management of rapid sequence induction and intubation are thoroughly discussed in Chapter 4.

Maintenance

After securing the airway, maintenance of anesthesia includes a plan for balancing patient amnesia and analgesia, surgical optimization, and maintenance of patient's hemodynamic stability throughout the surgical procedure. The choice of anesthetic agents and technique for maintenance will depend on the type and length of the surgery, patient comorbidities and discharge disposition from the recovery room. Similar to adults, there are three main techniques for maintenance of anesthesia: inhalational, IV, and regional anesthesia. These three techniques are frequently combined in the pediatric population to provide a balanced anesthetic.

During the maintenance phase, the anesthesia provider must take into consideration the oral and IV premedication given preoperatively. Absorption and effects of oral premedication are variable and have prolonged clearance compared to IV premedication. It is important to take this into consideration when planning a maintenance anesthetic to avoid excessive postoperative sedation. The goals of the anesthetic technique chosen for maintenance are to provide good surgical conditions, hemodynamic stability, and adequate intraoperative and postoperative pain management. During maintenance of anesthesia, it is important to recognize the differences in pharmacokinetics, fluid management and temperature control between age groups. In general, there is a lack of strong evidence in pediatric anesthesia to recommend one maintenance technique over the other and data from adults can't be extrapolated in children, and this is especially true in newborns and infants. As previously explained in chapter 2, there are many differences in pharmacokinetics in pediatric patients that affect the choice of anesthesia during maintenance.

Volatile anesthetic maintenance is the preferred technique for neonates and small infants because of its reliable clearance in the setting of variable organ maturity [9]. Volatile anesthetics are absorbed and eliminated by the lungs. The hydrophobic characteristics of the gasses allows them to be transferred quickly to the different compartments and be stored on the fat. The uptake, distribution and elimination of anesthetic gasses depend on cardiac output and clearance. The MAC of isoflurane is lower in preterm babies than in babies at term. The MAC of most common volatile agents (isoflurane and sevoflurane) increases with age until the first year of life and then decreases over time. Very high doses of volatile anesthetics are not recommended during the maintenance of anesthesia. Concentrations greater than 1.5 MAC produce epileptic activity. MAC requirements for isoflurane are highest between 1-6 months (1.87%) [24], for sevoflurane the MAC is the highest in neonates and decreases with age. Desflurane use in pediatrics is limited. In children, inhaled anesthetics have a faster washout compared to adults, for this reason, the cost/benefit of desflurane is not clear in pediatrics, the only potential benefit of desflurane over sevoflurane or isoflurane is the faster wake up, desflurane has also been associated with emergence agitation, and its irritative effects in the airway could potentially cause more laryngospasm and desaturations in children who are more susceptible to respiratory adverse events than adults [15].

A total intravenous anesthetic (TIVA) offers similar advantages as it does with the adult population. TIVA offers a quiet awakening, and a decreased incidence of postoperative agitation and postoperative nausea and vomiting (PONV), but can suffer from the unreliable emergence caused by context-sensitive half-times [10, 11].

Propofol infusions for maintenance of anesthesia should be carefully used and adjusted in neonates and small children. Propofol infusion is not contraindicated, but they are not frequently used in this population. One of the reasons is that there is enormous variability in response to propofol in neonates. The main elimination pathways of the propofol are by the liver during glucuronidation (53%) and hydroxylation (38%), very small amounts are excreted unchanged in the urine, and there are some theories about some degree of lung metabolism. Glucuronidation activity is low at birth and this is gradually improved until the age of 2-4 years when it reaches the adult level. The ability to metabolize propofol *via* hydroxylation is only 10% of the adult level at 10 months of age and 50% at 1.3 years. In contrast to metabolism, infants have an increased volume of distribution for propofol during the first year of life. The clearance of propofol in an adult is 30 ml/kg/min; in a two-year-old could be as high as 41 ml/kg/min, and this remains high until puberty [12]. In older children, propofol infusions for maintenance of anesthesia offer the advantages of reducing the incidence of PONV and delirium. Propofol infusions combined with short acting opioids are used as the anesthetic of choice in patients with malignant hyperthermia and in surgeries where neuromonitoring is used. Total intravenous anesthesia in children is based on weight and pharmacokinetic models; this model counts on the variations in growth and body compartments that change with the age and the maturation of the systems that are involved in metabolic process and clearance. Some pharmacokinetic models have been studied in pediatric patients; based on these models, Target Controlled Infusion (TCI) systems were developed. The TCI systems deliver an automatized infusion that is adjusted based on the desired effect site concentration. TCI systems are widely used in Europe but are not approved to be used in the United States by the FDA. Currently, the pediatric TCI programs used for propofol infusions in children have multiple limitations; between these limitations are the patient's interindividual variabilities, differences in volumes of distribution and debated pharmacodynamic parameters. The main pediatric pharmacokinetic models are Marsh (1991), Short (1994), Kataria (1999), Schuttler (2000), Paedfusor (Absalom 1998) [13].

Opioids like fentanyl are commonly used for the maintenance of anesthesia in pediatric patients. Precautions should be taken in neonates and young infants because these medications cross the blood brain barrier more easily than in older patients. Respiratory centers in the central nervous system are more sensitive to the action of opioids, making them more susceptible to apneas. Older pediatric patients around 2-3 years of age have a higher hepatic blood flow making the rates of metabolism and elimination of opioids faster; this causes a shorter half-life and faster need for redosing.

Dexmedetomidine, an alpha-2-agonist that produces sedative effects, when used during maintenance of anesthesia, decreases the need for opioids and other anesthetics. This drug has a different PK in neonates compared to older children and adults, and it has been suggested that lower doses of dexmedetomidine are required to achieve similar levels of sedative effects in neonates when compared to older children. Safety of the use of dexmedetomidine in pediatric patients is still under investigation. Studies involving children have shown minimal side effects of dexmedetomidine in neonates and small infants and in general, showed a good safety profile. It is recommended to decrease the dose in neonates compared to older children to achieve the same degree of sedation and minimize the side effects. A prolonged effect and clearance were observed in ex-premature infants born at 28-35 weeks compared with those born at 36-44 weeks. Some described side effects of dexmedetomidine in neonates and infants are hypertension, hypotension, and agitation [14].

Regional anesthesia or infiltration of local anesthetics provide intraoperative or postoperative pain control. Regional anesthesia alone or combined with sedation requires patient cooperation, which is very unlikely to be achieved in the pediatric population (and can lead to a higher risk of block failure or complications), unless the patient is heavily sedated. Regional anesthesia is frequently performed under general anesthesia in pediatric patients and is considered to be a safe practice [7]. A multi-center analysis by the Pediatric Regional Anesthesia Network in 2018 showed that in over 100,000 pediatric regional cases done under general anesthesia, there were no cases of permanent neurologic deficit – thus demonstrating a level of safety comparable to that seen in the adult population [23]. In fact, due to the low risk of complications, the American Society of Regional Anesthesia and the European Society of Regional Anesthesia published guidelines which advise that the performance of regional anesthesia in pediatrics under general anesthesia is the standard of care [24].

Neurotoxicity Considerations with Anesthesia

One area of concern that has been brought to media attention is the anesthetic neurotoxicity risk in the developing pediatric brain. In animal studies, common anesthetic and sedating drugs have been linked to abnormal development of the central nervous system and can negatively affect behavior, learning and memory [21]. Thus, the need for surgery or anesthesia in patients younger than 3 years old should be considered carefully [8]. However, SmartTots, a collaborative partnership between the Food and Drug Administration and the International

Anesthesia Research Society funds current research into this topic and has released a consensus statement that states that there is not enough clinical evidence currently to state definite permanent harm to children undergoing anesthesia and that the potential neurotoxic risks of undergoing anesthesia must be weighed against the potential harm of delaying or canceling a surgical procedure [22].

Fluid Administration

Fluid homeostasis is the balance between the intracellular and extracellular water; this balance implies the interaction of multiple systems. Total body water and water distribution in pediatric patients has been previously discussed in chapter 2. The goal of intraoperative intravenous fluid administration during maintenance of anesthesia is to preserve the physiologic balance between body intravascular and extravascular water volumes and electrolytes. Fluid and electrolytes therapy in hospitalized children include maintenance, replacement of fluid deficits and requirements. Intraoperative fluid administration traditionally has included the replacement of basal maintenance requirements (based on metabolic rates and demands), the fasting deficit, the replacement of surgical insensible losses secondary to surgical trauma and exposure and the replacement of intraoperative bleeding. The well-known formula of fluid administration created by Dr. Holliday and Segar published in 1957 [16], was based on measurements of caloric requirement of hospitalized children. Since then, this formula has remained as the method used to calculate maintenance of fluid required in pediatric patients. Fluid deficits due to fasting are usually replaced 50% in the first hour, 25% during the second hour and 25% during the third hour of surgery, it is also accepted to be replaced 50% in the first hour and the remaining 50% in the second hour.

For example as demonstrated below in Table **2**, for a 8-year-old 20 kg patient undergoing a 3 hour open umbilical hernia repair, with last fluid and meal at 12 hours ago. We can calculate the intraoperative fluid requirements as follows:

- Maintenance/basal rate (Holliday and Segar): 4,2,1 formula:
- (4x10) + (2x10) + 0 = 60ml/h
Fasting: 10h. 60ml/h x 10h = 600ml
Insensible losses or maintenance for surgical exposure: Minor surgery. 3 ml x Kg/h. = 60ml/h

Table 2. Example of traditional intraoperative fluid replacement in a 20 kg patient undergoing 3 hour umbilical hernia repair.

-	1h	2h	3h	total
Fasting	300ml	150ml	150ml	600ml
Basal maintenance	60ml	60ml	60ml	180ml
Surgical insensible losses	30 ml	60ml	60ml	150ml
Bleeding mlx3	0	10mlx3=30ml	5mlx3+15ml	45ml
Total	390ml	300ml	285ml	**975ml**

Recent tendencies for intraoperative fluid management imply the use of goal-directed fluid therapy. Several devices had been utilized to monitor intravascular volume, diagnose hypovolemia and predict fluid responsiveness [17]. These technologies are still under investigation in pediatric patients and until now, there is not a clear goal standard for intraoperative diagnosis of hypovolemia in the pediatric population due to the difficulty of standardization between the different ages and the maturation and physiology of the cardiovascular system. Glucose containing solutions should be considered in the pediatric population at higher risk for hypoglycemia. Patients at high risk for hypoglycemia are patients younger than 3 months, malnourished, children with parenteral nutrition, certain metabolic diseases and increased metabolic rate.

Temperature Control

Pediatric patients are more susceptible to changes in temperature than adults during surgery. Strict temperature control is important during maintenance of anesthesia in pediatric patients. Temperature regulation and management is discussed more in detail in Chapter 1.

Emergence

Neuromuscular Reversal

Similar to adults, there are a number of factors which can affect neuromuscular blocker metabolism in children. The most common is the use of antiepileptic agents, which accelerate neuromuscular blocker metabolism. In these children, regular twitch monitoring along with assessment of blockade needs is important for optimizing surgical conditions. The available data at this point suggests that sugammadex is safe for use in children who are 2 years of age or greater. Below the age of 2, it should be utilized with caution. A recent excellent review should be further reading for those commonly using sugammadex in young children [18].

Awake *Versus* Deep Extubation

The decision to perform awake *versus* deep extubation is practitioner, type of surgery, and institution dependent. In pure pediatric hospitals due to a predominance of shorter procedures, many children are extubated under the deep plane of anesthesia (deep extubation). What constitutes a deep extubation is a spontaneously breathing child, with approximately 2-3 cc/kg of tidal volume, with no response to noxious stimuli such as posterior pharyngeal suctioning or deflating the tracheal cuff of an endotracheal tube. Once the endotracheal tube is removed, masking with a good seal is maintained until the child emerges completely from anesthesia. This type of extubation is generally used for higher turnover cases where there has not been high rates of blood loss and children are not prone to aspiration. The latter point is especially important since the child will emerge from anesthesia with an unprotected airway. If there is concern for aspiration, then an awake extubation is preferred.

"Awake extubation" is when the patient has almost completely emerged from anesthesia prior to extubation. This is generally used for longer surgeries with higher fluid or blood transfusion rates, as well as those children who are aspiration prone, such as gastrointestinal surgery. The decision therefore depends on a number of factors, including the comfort of the provider with deep and awake extubation.

Emergence Delirium

Emergence delirium is on the spectrum of emergence disorders, spanning from emergence agitation (EA) all the way to emergence delirium (ED). There are 3 scales for EA/ED (Watcha scale, Cravero scale, PAED scale). The PAED scale is the only scale with a validated scoring system- however, a head to head comparison of the 3 shows that all can be reliably utilized. Risk factors for emergence agitation include the age of the child, anesthetic agents administered, surgical procedure and use of adjunct drugs [19]. EA/ED is viewed as a self-limited disorder, with the caveat that the child being agitated can be distressing for parents and caregivers in the post-anesthesia care unit. The use of purely intravenous techniques has been associated with a lower incidence of EA/ED. That being said, the self-limited nature of EA/ED requires the practitioner to do a risk: benefit ratio of utilizing TIVA purely for the purpose of EA/ED reduction. Identification of ED is done using the aforementioned scales. The PAED scale is the most granular and uses 5 distinct, non-overlapping criteria (seen in Fig. (**1**)) with a scoring system that determines the likelihood of ED.

Behavior	Not at all	Just a little	Quite a bit	Very much	Extremely
Make eye contact with caregiver	4	3	2	1	0
Actions are purposeful	4	3	2	1	0
Aware of surrounding	4	3	2	1	0
Restless	0	1	2	3	4
Inconsolable	0	1	2	3	4

1 – Calm; 2 – Not calm but could be easily consoled; 3 – Moderately agitated or restless and not easily calmed; 4 – Combative, excited, thrashing around

Fig. (1). PAED scale. Adapted from Sikich N, Lerman J. Development and psychometric evaluation of the pediatric anesthesia emergence delirium scale. Anesthesiology. 2004; 100: 1142.

The lower the score, the higher the likelihood that the symptomatology is from EA rather than ED. Several medications have been used for EA/ED successfully, including midazolam, propofol, and dexmedetomidine. Given that all medications have associated risks, prudence should be exercised with their administration. In order to distinguish pain from ED in the emergence period, which is often difficult, many providers administer a single dose of postoperative pain medication (fentanyl or morphine). A chart of commonly used medications for ED is provided in Table **3** below.

Table 3. Chart of medications helpful for EA/ED prevention and therapy.

Agent	EA/ED Prevention	EA/ED Therapy
Desflurane	-	N/A
Sevoflurane	-	N/A
Propofol bolus	-/+	+
Propofol infusion	+	N/A
Ondansetron	-/+	-/+
Dexmedetomidine/Clonidine	+	++
Fentanyl	+	+
Ketamine	+/-	-
Midazolam	+	+

Pain

Postoperative pediatric pain is quite common, and the symptoms of pain upon emergence are quite variable by age group. There are several validated scales to study pediatric pain (FACES, FLACC) which are validated by age group. Pediatric pharmacokinetics of commonly used anti-nociceptive medications, especially opioids, can vary significantly. For example, even in children with obstructive sleep apnea, doses of commonly used opioids can have a greater effect due to upregulation of opioid receptors. Furthermore, medications that are metabolized through the CYP2D6 mechanism are affected by a number of pharmacogenomic factors, such as being a poor metabolizer *versus* an ultra-rapid metabolizer. In brief, there is a very narrow therapeutic window of administration of medications for those who fall outside the range of normal for CYP2D6 metabolism. This dichotomy leads to problematic balances between adequate analgesia and risk of over-sedation, which affects several commonly used medications, including codeine, oxycodone, and tramadol [20].

Temperature Instability

Children with postoperative temperature issues are generally hypothermic. This is a function of the multiple exothermic heat loss sites in the operating room, where heat is lost through conduction, convection, and radiation. Given the high body surface area of pediatric patients, especially infants and neonates, it is very common for children to arrive at the PACU hypothermic. Generally, covering the children with warm blankets, including their heads, which have a high percentage of BSA in children, quickly reverses the hypothermia. Shivering can theoretically be treated with meperidine as is done in adults, although this is rarely done in practice. If the hypothermia is quickly corrected with blankets, warmed intravenous fluids and forced air warmers can be used to restore temperature homeostasis.

Other important perioperative complications and considerations include: laryngospasm, bronchospasm, postoperative nausea and vomiting, postoperative desaturations, post-intubation stridor and pulmonary edema. Please see Chapter 6 for further discussion on these important topics.

CONCLUSION

Administering general anesthesia to the pediatric patient has many nuances that are different from anesthetizing the adult patient. The large range of pediatric patients encountered, from a small neonate to an adult-sized teenager, requires that the anesthesia provider create a customized perioperative anesthetic plan for every patient. Understanding these considerations is essential to delivering safe and effective care to pediatric patients in the perioperative period.

CONSENT FOR PUBLICATION

Not applicable.

CONFLICT OF INTEREST

The author declares no conflict of interest, financial or otherwise.

ACKNOWLEDGEMENTS

Declared none.

REFERENCES

[1]   Siddiqui BA, Kim PY. Anesthesia Stages InStatPearls. StatPearls Publishing 2020.

[2]   Stages and Signs of General Anesthesia | Anesthesiology Core Review: Part One Basic Exam | AccessAnesthesiology | McGraw-Hill Medical Accessanesthesiologymhmedicalcom 2020 .https://accessanesthesiology.mhmedical.com/content.aspx?sectionid=61588520&bookid=974

[3]   Fassoulaki A, Staikou C. Pretreatment with nitrous oxide enhances induction of anesthesia with sevoflurane: A randomized controlled trial. J Anaesthesiol Clin Pharmacol 2015; 31(4): 511-6.
        [http://dx.doi.org/10.4103/0970-9185.169079] [PMID: 26702210]

[4]   Zielinska M, Holtby H, Wolf A. Pro-con debate: intravenous *vs* inhalation induction of anesthesia in children. Paediatr Anaesth 2011; 21(2): 159-68.
        [http://dx.doi.org/10.1111/j.1460-9592.2010.03488.x] [PMID: 21210885]

[5]   Sadeghi A, Khaleghnejad Tabari A, Mahdavi A, Salarian S, Razavi SS. Impact of parental presence during induction of anesthesia on anxiety level among pediatric patients and their parents: a randomized clinical trial. Neuropsychiatr Dis Treat 2017; 12: 3237-41.
        [http://dx.doi.org/10.2147/NDT.S119208] [PMID: 28260897]

[6]   Kain ZN, Mayes LC, Caramico LA, *et al.* Parental presence during induction of anesthesia. A randomized controlled trial. Anesthesiology 1996; 84(5): 1060-7.
        [http://dx.doi.org/10.1097/00000542-199605000-00007] [PMID: 8623999]

[7]   Lönnqvist PA, Ecoffey C, Bosenberg A, Suresh S, Ivani G. The European society of regional anesthesia and pain therapy and the American society of regional anesthesia and pain medicine joint committee practice advisory on controversial topics in pediatric regional anesthesia I and II: what do they tell us? Curr Opin Anaesthesiol 2017; 30(5): 613-20.
        [http://dx.doi.org/10.1097/ACO.0000000000000508] [PMID: 28786855]

[8]   Rappaport BA, Suresh S, Hertz S, Evers AS, Orser BA. Anesthetic neurotoxicity--clinical implications of animal models. N Engl J Med 2015; 372(9): 796-7.
        [http://dx.doi.org/10.1056/NEJMp1414786] [PMID: 25714157]

[9]   Brussee JM, Yu H, Krekels EHJ, *et al.* First-Pass CYP3A-Mediated Metabolism of Midazolam in the Gut Wall and Liver in Preterm Neonates. CPT Pharmacometrics Syst Pharmacol 2018; 7(6): 374-83.
        [http://dx.doi.org/10.1002/psp4.12295] [PMID: 29745466]

[10]   Costi D, Cyna AM, Ahmed S, *et al.* Effects of sevoflurane versus other general anaesthesia on emergence agitation in children. Cochrane Database of Systematic Reviews 2014; 9
        [http://dx.doi.org/10.1002/14651858.CD007084.pub2]

[11] Ortiz AC, Atallah ÁN, Matos D, da Silva EM. Intravenous versus inhalational anaesthesia for paediatric outpatient surgery. Cochrane Database of Systematic Reviews 2014; (2):
[http://dx.doi.org/10.1002/14651858.CD009015.pub2]

[12] Chidambaran V, Costandi A, D'Mello A. Propofol: a review of its role in pediatric anesthesia and sedation. CNS Drugs 2015; 29(7): 543-63.
[http://dx.doi.org/10.1007/s40263-015-0259-6]

[13] Constant I, Rigouzzo A. Which model for propofol TCI in children. Paediatr Anaesth 2010; 20(3): 233-9.
[http://dx.doi.org/10.1111/j.1460-9592.2010.03269.x] [PMID: 20470319]

[14] Anderson BJ, Allegaert K. The pharmacology of anaesthetics in the neonate. Baillieres Best Pract Res Clin Anaesthesiol 2010; 24(3): 419-31.
[http://dx.doi.org/10.1016/j.bpa.2010.02.019] [PMID: 21033017]

[15] Cameron CB, Robinson S, Gregory GA. The minimum anesthetic concentration of isoflurane in children. Anesth Analg 1984; 63(4): 418-20.
[http://dx.doi.org/10.1213/00000539-198404000-00007] [PMID: 6703367]

[16] Holliday MA, Segar WE. The maintenance need for water in parenteral fluid therapy. Pediatrics 1957; 19(5): 823-32.
[http://dx.doi.org/10.1542/peds.19.5.823] [PMID: 13431307]

[17] Coeckelenbergh S, Zaouter C, Alexander B, *et al.* Automated systems for perioperative goal-directed hemodynamic therapy. J Anesth 2020; 34(1): 104-14.
[http://dx.doi.org/10.1007/s00540-019-02683-9] [PMID: 31555916]

[18] Grigg E. Sugammadex and neuromuscular reversal: special focus on neonatal and infant populations. Curr Opin Anaesthesiol 2020; 33(3): 374-80.
[http://dx.doi.org/10.1097/ACO.0000000000000847] [PMID: 32324657]

[19] Dahmani S, Delivet H, Hilly J. Emergence delirium in children: an update. Curr Opin Anaesthesiol 2014; 27(3): 309-15.
[http://dx.doi.org/10.1097/ACO.0000000000000076] [PMID: 24784918]

[20] Patino M, Sadhasivam S, Mahmoud M. Obstructive sleep apnoea in children: perioperative considerations. Br J Anaesth 2013; 111 (Suppl. 1): i83-95.
[http://dx.doi.org/10.1093/bja/aet371] [PMID: 24335402]

[21] Jevtovic-Todorovic V. Exposure of developing brain to general anesthesia what is the animal evidence? Anesthesiology. Anesthesiology 2018; 128(4): 832-9.
[http://dx.doi.org/10.1097/ALN.0000000000002047] [PMID: 29271804]

[22] Consensus Statement on the Use of Anesthetic and Sedative Drugs in Infants and Toddlers http://smarttots.org/wp-content/uploads/2015/05/ConsensusStatementV10-10.2017.pdf

[23] Walker BJ, Long JB, Sathyamoorthy M, *et al.* Complications in Pediatric Regional Anesthesia: An Analysis of More than 100,000 Blocks from the Pediatric Regional Anesthesia Network. Anesthesiology 2018; 129(4): 721-32.
[http://dx.doi.org/10.1097/ALN.0000000000002372] [PMID: 30074928]

[24] Ivani G, Suresh S, Ecoffey C, *et al.* The European Society of Regional Anaesthesia and Pain Therapy and the American Society of Regional Anesthesia and Pain Medicine joint committee practice advisory on controversial topics in pediatric regional anesthesia. Reg Anesth Pain Med 2015; 40(5): 526-32.
[http://dx.doi.org/10.1097/AAP.0000000000000280] [PMID: 26192549]

CHAPTER 6

PACU Management and Emergence Delirium

Malgorzata Lutwin-Kawalec[1], Sheaba Varghese[1] and **Dinesh K. Choudhry, FRCA[2]**

[1] *Department of Anesthesia and Perioperative Medicine, Nemours Children's Health, Delaware Valley, Wilmington, DE, USA*

[2] *Department of Anesthesiology, Shriners Hospital for Children, Philadelphia, PA, USA*

Abstract: Recovery of children from anesthesia may be complicated by multiple unique issues encountered in the postanesthesia care unit (PACU). **Emergence delirium** is a dissociated state of consciousness, irritability, uncooperativeness, and inconsolability that may cause injury to the child or staff. **Malignant hyperthermia** is a rare genetic state of hypermetabolism that presents with hyperthermia, hypercarbia, acidosis, rhabdomyolysis, and arrhythmias. Timely treatment with dantrolene is lifesaving. Common postoperative respiratory events include stridor, laryngospasm, and bronchospasm. **Postextubation stridor** is noisy breathing during inspiration caused by airway mucosal injury or pressure from an endotracheal cuff, treated with humidified oxygen, racemic epinephrine, and dexamethasone. **Laryngospasm**, a partial or complete closure of the glottis, is an emergency that may lead to hypoxic cardiac arrest and requires timely recognition and treatment with positive pressure ventilation (PPV), medications, and possibly intubation. **Bronchospasm** is a clinical manifestation of exacerbated underlying airway hyperreactivity, treated with inhaled bronchodilators, intravenous epinephrine, and steroids. Cardiovascular events include arrhythmias and blood pressure abnormalities. **Bradycardia** is a common dysrhythmia in children usually caused by hypoxemia or vagal stimulation, treated with oxygen, PPV, and intravenous epinephrine, or anticholinergics. Narrow complex tachycardias—**sinus tachycardia** and **supraventricular tachycardia**—may be caused by pain, hypoxia, emergence agitation, or medications such as epinephrine or anticholinergics. Their management depends on etiology and consists of vagal maneuvers, adenosine, or synchronized cardioversion. Known risk factors for **postoperative nausea and vomiting (PONV)** in children include surgeries of longer than 30 minutes, age over 3 years, strabismus surgery, and previous history of PONV. Our standardized PACU handoff tool is discussed.

Keywords: Apnea of prematurity, Bradycardia, Bronchospasm, Cardiac arrest, Child Life, Discharge, Emergence delirium, Family-centered care, Guidelines,

---

** **Corresponding author Bharathi Gourkanti MD:** Department of Anesthesiology, Cooper Medical School of Rowan University, Cooper University Health Care, Camden, NJ, United States; E-mail: gourkanti-bharathi@cooperhealth.edu*

Bharathi Gourkanti, Irwin Gratz, Grace Dippo, Nathalie Peiris and Dinesh K. Choudhry (Eds.)
All rights reserved-© 2022 Bentham Science Publishers

Handoff, Hypotension, Laryngospasm, Malignant hyperthermia, Narrow complex, Non-triggering anesthetic, Postanesthesia care unit, Postextubation stridor, Postobstructive pulmonary edema, Postoperative nausea and vomiting, Premature atrial contractions, Premature ventricular contractions, Tachycardia.

PATIENT HANDOFF & RECOVERY ENVIRONMENT

Children recovering from anesthesia are at risk for serious physiologic compromise because of the proximity of the surgical procedure, residual effects of anesthetics, and underlying conditions. The American Society of Anesthesiologists' "Standards for Postanesthesia Care" provides a road map for patient recovery [1]. All patients who receive general anesthesia, regional anesthesia, or monitored anesthesia care should be admitted to the postanesthesia care unit (PACU) or its equivalent, such as the intensive care unit (ICU), unless otherwise specified by the anesthesiologist responsible for that patient. During transport, a patient should be accompanied by an anesthesia team member knowledgeable with the patient's condition, who should continually evaluate the patient and intervene if necessary. Upon arrival to the PACU, the patient should be reevaluated and a verbal report given to a PACU nurse. We use a thorough standardized handoff tool, which is hanging on the wall in each recovery space (Table **1**). Care should not be transferred to PACU staff until the patient's status is satisfactory and the nurse accepts the responsibility.

Table 1. PACU handoff tool.

OR Nursing: - Name, age, weight   - Isolation   - Surgery performed   - Local anesthetic usage by surgery (yes/no)   - Drains/tubes – location/number   - Special instructions – chest tube to suction/arm elevated   - Dressings, packings   - Special equipment – Iceman, sequential compression devices
Anesthesia: - Past medical history/past surgical history & anesthesia history   - Allergies   - Home & preoperative medications   - Patient & parental anxiety, special family considerations   - Anesthesia type (general & regional)   - Airway – instrumentation, difficulty of mask ventilation & intubation, extubation awake *vs.* deep   - Lines – location/type   -Intraoperative medications – muscle relaxants, analgesics including acetaminophen & ketorolac, antibiotics, infusion double checks

(Table 1) cont.....

- Fluids – urine output, blood loss, intravenous fluids & blood products
- Laboratory – last operating room (OR) checks, need for PACU draws
-Key OR events – respiratory events, hypoxemia, temperature abnormalities, hypotension, arrhythmias, vomiting
- OR documentation complete (yes/no)
- Disposition
- PACU orders for pain medications
-The thing I'm most concerned about is…
Credit: Leslie Jackson, CRNA (used with permission)

Each PACU patient location should be equipped with oxygen supply, a suction apparatus, a self-inflating resuscitation bag, and monitors including a pulse oximeter, thermometer, electrocardiogram (ECG), and automated blood pressure device (Fig. **1**). Emergency drugs as well as resuscitation carts should be readily available (Fig. **2**). The PACU should be located close to the operating rooms to allow for rapid response by the anesthesia team when immediate presence is required for complications. An alarm system for quick backup is of great value. At our institution, an overhead "Anesthesia now to PACU" is utilized. Our PACU staff is well trained and competent in recognizing and treating various complications that may occur in pediatric patients during recovery.

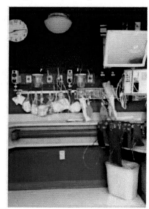

Fig. (1). Well-organized PACU patient location.

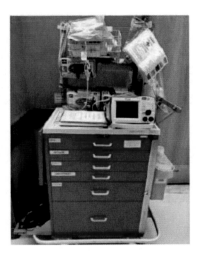

Fig. (2). Code cart with medications and airway equipment. Please notice the cognitive aid we use called Pedi Crisis hanging on the cart.

GUIDELINES FOR DISCHARGE

Prior to discharge:

- The patient should be reevaluated and a note documenting readiness for discharge placed in the chart.
- The patient should be alerted and oriented with mental status at baseline.
- Vital signs should be stable and within acceptable limits.
- A responsible adult should be available to accompany the patient home and be able to report any complications.
- Written discharge instructions should be provided to the responsible adult [2].

EMERGENCE DELIRIUM

Emergence delirium [ED] is one of the most common adverse reactions encountered in pediatric anesthesia and is defined as an abnormal mental state that develops as patients emerge from a general anesthetic. There are four stages of anesthesia: analgesia, delirium, surgical, and medullary depression. Stage two of anesthesia is considered to be the phase of "excitement and delirium" in which there can be an irregular breathing pattern or possibly breath-holding in an unconscious patient. Children can present with inconsolability, incoherence, thrashing, and lack of eye contact or purposeful movement [3]. The cause of ED is still uncertain, but it has been speculated that it is secondary to rapid redistribution of anesthetic. Inhalation anesthetics cause specific excitation of locus coeruleus neurons, and sevoflurane particularly plays an important role in paradoxical excitation [4]. ED is most commonly encountered with volatile anesthetics such as sevoflurane and desflurane and less likely in patients who have had total intravenous (IV) anesthesia.

ED can occur any time after extubation through the patient's stay in the recovery room. It is important to determine if a child is experiencing ED or having pain with purposeful movements and to distinguish these from behavioral issues. To assist with properly identifying ED, the Pediatric Anesthesia Emergence Delirium (PAED) scale can be used in patients 2 years of age and older (Table **2**) [5].

Table 2. Pediatric Anesthesia Emergence Delirium scale [5].

Points	Patient Description	Not at All	Slightly	Quite a Bit	Very Much	Extremely
1	Eye contact	4	3	2	1	0
2	Purposeful movement	4	3	2	1	0
3	Aware of surroundings	4	3	2	1	0
4	Restless	0	1	2	3	4
5	Inconsolable	0	1	2	3	4

There are many other scales that can be used to determine if a child is experiencing delirium in addition to the PAED scale. The Watcha scale (Table **3**), which grades the child from asleep to agitated and thrashing, appears to be more practical and simpler [6].

Table 3. The Watcha scale.

Behavior	Score
Asleep	0
Calm	1
Crying, but can be consoled	2
Crying, but cannot be consoled	3
Agitated and thrashing around	4

Risk factors for developing ED include the age of the patient, surgical procedure, use of sevoflurane or other volatile anesthetic, and poorly controlled pain [3]. Surgical procedures that have a higher incidence of ED include otolaryngologic procedures. Additionally, there has been discussion about if the actual surgical procedure makes a difference if the pain is adequately controlled at the time of emergence. The age group that is at the highest risk is 3 to 9 years, but it can occur at any age [7]. A shortened time to emergence was also found to be an independent risk factor [8]. Medications associated with ED are listed in Table **4** and other risk factors in Table **5**.

Table 4. Medications associated with emergence delirium.

Medications Associated with Emergence Delirium	Medications NOT Associated with Emergence Delirium
Volatile anesthetics	Propofol
Sevoflurane	Narcotics
Desflurane	Nitrous oxide
Isoflurane	Dexmedetomidine
Enflurane	Ketamine

Table 5. Risk factors for the development of emergence delirium [3].

Risk Factors for Development of Emergence Delirium
Age 2 to 5 years
Preoperative anxiety and behavior
Type of anesthesia
Pain
Type of surgery
Shortened time to emergence
Child temperament

Prevention of ED

Identifying children in the preoperative area who may be at risk of developing ED can help with prevention and management. A child's temperament should be noted preoperatively as children with underlying behavioral issues are more likely to behave similarly during emergence, when they awaken from an anesthetic. It is important to take measures to prevent recurrence in patients who have experienced ED previously, such as administering dexmedetomidine or administering a total IV anesthetic. The best prevention for ED is to avoid inhalational anesthetics and use propofol as the primary anesthetic. Ensuring appropriate pain control with regional blocks or appropriate narcotic use is also beneficial.

Treatment of ED

Common treatment options include dexmedetomidine or propofol. Patients can receive dexmedetomidine at 0.5 to 1 mcg/kg as a bolus or a continuous infusion of

0.1 mcg/kg/hr. Dexmedetomidine activates presynaptic alpha 2 receptors in the locus coeruleus and prevents ED [4]. Using a total IV anesthetic with propofol in addition to a narcotic is helpful in decreasing the incidence of ED. If total IV anesthesia is not being used, a bolus of propofol of 1 mg/kg at the end of the case may help decrease the incidence of ED [9], although not as reliably.

MALIGNANT HYPERTHERMIA

Malignant hyperthermia (MH) is a feared, life-threatening complication of general anesthesia inherited in an autosomal dominant pattern. The most common mutation is in the RYR1 gene for a sarcoplasmic reticulum ryanodine receptor, which is responsible for calcium regulation in skeletal muscle cells. Triggering agents, which include halogenated inhalational anesthetics and succinylcholine, induce prolonged opening of functionally altered ryanodine receptors leading to an unregulated calcium accumulation in muscle cell cytosol resulting in sustained muscle contraction. The sustained muscle contraction leads to a hypermetabolic state with an increase in oxygen consumption, carbon dioxide production, hyperthermia, and cellular acidosis [10].

Some of the genetic disorders associated with MH susceptibility include central core disease, multiminicore myopathy, King-Denborough syndrome, and Native American myopathy [11]. Children with other diseases such as Duchenne or Becker muscular dystrophy can develop rhabdomyolysis and hyperkalemia with exposure to volatile anesthetics and succinylcholine, but this does not represent true MH because of lack of the hypermetabolic state [11].

Signs and Symptoms

Clinical signs of MH include hypercapnia, masseter muscle rigidity or generalized muscle rigidity, acidosis, and peaked T waves indicating hyperkalemia and hyperthermia (Table 6) [11]. Masseter muscle rigidity [MMR] presents as an increase in jaw muscle tension that results in an inability to open the mouth after the administration of succinylcholine. MMR may be an early sign of MH; therefore, additional monitoring for other signs of MH is necessary. In the presence of MMR, urine should be checked for myoglobinuria and core temperature should be followed. Levels of Creatine kinase (CK) and electrolytes should be monitored to ensure that early detection occurs if the patient deteriorates. As MH presentation progresses, the patient will develop muscle rigidity and myoglobinuria secondary to rhabdomyolysis. The sustained muscle contraction and rhabdomyolysis lead to increased lactic acid production and a resultant metabolic acidosis.

Table 6. Signs of malignant hyperthermia.

Early Signs	Late Signs
Tachycardia	Rhabdomyolysis
Hyperthermia	Metabolic acidosis
Increase in end-tidal carbon dioxide	Myoglobinuria
Masseter muscle rigidity (possibly)	Acute kidney injury

Triggers

All volatile anesthetics and depolarizing muscle relaxants are considered triggers for MH (Table **7**). For a patient who is susceptible to MH, nitrous oxide, IV anesthetics, opioids, and nondepolarizing muscle relaxants are safe to use.

Table 7. Non-triggering and MH-triggering medications.

Medications Safe to Use in MH-Susceptible Patients	MH-Triggering Medications
Nitrous oxide	Sevoflurane
Propofol	Isoflurane
Ketamine	Desflurane
Fentanyl	Enflurane
Local anesthetics	Depolarizing muscle relaxant – succinylcholine

If a patient during prior anesthesia experienced signs and symptoms of MH, additional precautions must be taken to avoid another crisis. Children who are MH susceptible can have a misleading history of a prior anesthetic without issues, but it is important to remember that MH can present even after an uncomplicated prior anesthetic.

Preparing for a Non-triggering Anesthetic

Obtaining a detailed patient history is one of the most important aspects of preoperative evaluation. If a patient has a family history of MH susceptibility, has tested positive, or has had an MH episode in the past, certain measures should be taken prior to surgery to ensure a safe anesthetic. The anesthesia machine should be flushed with high flows of oxygen, and charcoal filters should be placed on the machine to prevent residual volatile anesthetic from reaching the patient. The vaporizers should ideally be removed from the machine or tape placed over dials so that the anesthesia gas is not accidentally turned on. The MH cart should be kept outside the operating room. A total IV anesthetic should be performed with medications that have been found to be safe in MH (refer to Table **7**). A common anesthetic technique is total intravenous anesthesia (TIVA) with propofol infusion and narcotic of choice.

Treatment of an MH Episode

Table **8** lists interventions recommended if an MH episode occurs [12, 13].

Table 8. Summary of management of an MH episode.

Turn off all triggering agents, notify the surgical team and get additional personnel for help → **contact the MH hotline (1-800-644-9737)**
Send additional personnel to obtain MH cart
Transition to total intravenous anesthetic
Disconnect patient from anesthesia machine and manually ventilate with self-inflating bag
Attach charcoal filters if available or flush anesthesia machine with 10 L oxygen
Obtain arterial blood gas and draw CK levels
Start dantrolene 2.5 mg/kg dose for a maximum dose of 10 mg
Continue dantrolene therapy at 1 mg/kg every 4-6 hours for 24 hours
Cool patient: • ice to axilla, groin, head • cold IV fluids • Nasogastric tube and open body cavity lavage with cold water • Stop cooling when temp < 38 °C
Monitor urine output
Trend CK levels and acid base balance
Correct metabolic acidosis with 1-2 mEq/kg sodium bicarbonate
Transfer patient to ICU to monitor CK and arterial blood gas trend, continue hydration and monitor urine output for 24 hours

Treatment of MH includes IV dantrolene administration, hyperventilation, hydration, and cooling of the patient. Dantrolene is a ryanodine receptor antagonist that inhibits the release of calcium from the sarcoplasmic reticulum by decreasing the activation of calcium-dependent RYR1 and is the definitive treatment but may also work through a sarcolemma channel [14]. Common side effects of dantrolene include nausea, muscle weakness, and diuresis. Hyperventilation is a quick and easy treatment to implement.

Active cooling should be discontinued once the patient's core temperature reaches 38 °C [13]. In addition to other treatment measures, an IV fluid bolus should be administered with an aggressive fluid replacement while monitoring urine output.

Administer dantrolene 2.5 mg/kg to a maximum dose of 10 mg every 5 minutes. Treatment should continue with a maintenance dose of 1 mg/kg/dose every 4 to 6 hours and should be continued for at least 24 hours. Dantrolene can be discontinued once the following criteria have been met: metabolic stability for 24 hours, core temperature less than 38 °C, declining CK level, no evidence of ongoing myoglobinuria, and resolution of muscle rigidity [13].

The patient should be monitored in the ICU for at least 24 hours. In the ICU, electrolyte disturbances should be monitored and treated, in particular hyperkalemia that can lead to arrhythmias. Standard treatment of hyperkalemia includes IV calcium gluconate or chloride, sodium bicarbonate, and regular insulin and dextrose [12]. Appropriate fluid replacement should be instituted while monitoring urine output. Rhabdomyolysis can lead to severe kidney damage if the patient is not properly hydrated. A CK level should be obtained at the initial time of insult and then monitored throughout the ICU stay to ensure declining levels.

Testing

The caffeine-halothane contracture test (CHCT) is the "gold standard" for MH diagnosis and is used to determine a patient's MH susceptibility [15, 16]. The CHCT can be performed only in patients weighing at least 20 kg or who are older than 10 years because of the amount of muscle that is needed for the test. The CHCT can be performed only at one of the designated testing centers and requires a fresh tissue sample from the vastus medialis or vastus lateralis muscle. Downfalls of the CHCT include age limitations, cost of testing, and a limited number of centers that are able to perform testing. MH is inherited in an autosomal dominant manner, which means that a person has a 50% chance of passing the condition to the next generation. If a patient has not inherited the altered gene, then that person is not at risk of passing on MH susceptibility. The Malignant Hyperthermia Association of the United States (MHAUS) has a complete list of additional recommendations and resources (www.mhaus.org).

PERIOPERATIVE ADVERSE RESPIRATORY EVENTS

Perioperative adverse respiratory events account for three-quarters of pediatric critical events [17] and one-third of all perioperative cardiac arrests in children [18]. It is estimated that 15% of pediatric PACU patients develop one or more respiratory complications, including hypoxemia, cough, airway obstruction, laryngospasm, bronchospasm and postoperative stridor [19].

Hypoxemia

Main causes of hypoxemia in the PACU include:

- atelectasis
- decreased respiratory drive due to residual anesthesia and opioid medications
- muscle relaxant-related and sedation-related low muscle tone [20]

Laryngospasm

Laryngospasm is a sustained closure of the vocal cords causing partial or complete airway obstruction. Transient laryngeal closure is a vagal reflex that protects against aspiration in an awake state, but it can also occur during light planes of general anesthesia, and, if sustained, it can rapidly result in hypoxemia and bradycardia and may lead to cardiac arrest. Laryngospasm has an overall incidence of 0.87% in the general population, 1.74% in children 1 to 9 years old, and 2.82% in infants [21]. Common risk factors related to the patient, procedure, and anesthesia are listed in Table **9** below [20 - 22].

A 2005 Australian laryngospasm case review study showed 61% incidence of hypoxemia, 6% incidence of bradycardia, 4% incidence of post-obstructive pulmonary edema, and 3% incidence of pulmonary aspiration [23].

Table 9. Risk factors for laryngospasm.

Anesthesia-Related Factors:
• Airway instrumentation in light planes of anesthesia
• Presence of airway blood or secretions
• Lack of pediatric experience of anesthesia provider
Patient-Related Factors:
• Age < 3 years
• Recent upper respiratory infection (URI)
• History of airway hyper-reactivity or asthma
• Gastroesophageal reflux disease
• Exposure to passive smoking
Surgery-Related Factors:
• Shared airway procedures
• Tonsillectomy and adenoidectomy (25% incidence of postoperative nausea and vomiting [PONV])
• Dental procedures
• Hypospadias repair
• Emergency surgeries

Prevention of Laryngospasm

Prevention of laryngospasm includes postponing a non-emergent surgery in a child with a history of a recent URI, avoidance of airway manipulation in light planes of anesthesia, and preventing laryngeal stimulation by airway secretions. The "No Touch" technique, which consists of suctioning and lateral position to drain blood or secretions while anesthetized, followed by avoidance of any stimulation until eye opening when extubation takes place, has been shown to decrease the incidence of post-extubation laryngospasm [22]. The results of studies on IV lidocaine for the prevention of laryngospasm are conflicting [21].

Treatment of Laryngospasm

Initial treatment of laryngospasm includes airway suctioning and **positive pressure ventilation with 100% oxygen** and the jaw firmly pulled forward. It is important to avoid vigorous ventilation as this will likely distend the stomach and may cause regurgitation. If these interventions do not resolve the laryngospasm, **IV anesthetic followed by a muscle relaxant** is necessary. Intravenous propofol in 0.5 mg/kg increments has been reported to relieve laryngospasm in more than 75% of cases [22].

Succinylcholine is the relaxant of choice, but one must keep in mind a rare possibility of undiagnosed myopathy in children, which may cause MH after succinylcholine is given. Nevertheless, laryngospasm is one of the indications for succinylcholine use [12]. While taking care of pediatric patients, it is useful to have pre-drawn syringes of "emergency drugs" such as propofol, atropine, and succinylcholine and carry them to the PACU with the patient. Succinylcholine 0.1-2 mg/kg IV will break the laryngospasm, which should be given in conjunction with 0.02 mg/kg of atropine to prevent bradycardia [22]. If there is no IV access, both **atropine and succinylcholine can be given intramuscularly (IM)** in 0.02 mg/kg and 4 mg/kg doses, respectively. With the IM route, either deltoid or the lateral quadriceps muscle can be used, and the time it takes to break laryngospasm is 45 to 60 seconds [22].

Intralingual (IL) succinylcholine 2 mg/kg injected with a small needle in the body of the tongue takes 75 seconds for full relaxation. This route is associated with arrhythmias and requires interrupting the ventilation attempts by removal of tight-fitting masks in this dire situation with low oxygen saturation. Also, bleeding from the injection site in the oral cavity may occur and can further complicate the issue. This technique, in our opinion, should preferably be avoided. **Intraosseous (IO) access** can also be used if present or readily available. When administered by IO access, 1 mg/kg of succinylcholine has a similar onset to the IV route [22]. Once laryngospasm is broken, supplemental oxygen should be continued and ventilation closely monitored. Further support of the airway may require tracheal intubation if gastric content aspiration or pulmonary edema is suspected.

Postobstructive Pulmonary Edema

One of the feared complications of laryngospasm is postobstructive pulmonary edema caused by high negative intrathoracic pressure secondary to forced inspiration attempts against closed vocal cords. It presents with rales, low oxygen saturation, and pink frothy oropharyngeal secretions. Treatment involves continuous positive airway pressure (CPAP) of 5-10 cm H_2O with supplemental oxygen, diuretics, and fluid restriction. The need for intubation and postoperative ventilation must be judged on a case-by-case basis.

Bronchospasm

Bronchospasm is a common cause of airway obstruction in children [24]. It presents with oxygen desaturation, decreased lung compliance, expiratory wheezing, or complete absence of breath sounds. Bronchospasm is usually a clinical manifestation of:

- acute asthma exacerbation
- viral bronchiolitis
- anaphylaxis [25]

Asthma is a chronic airway disease associated with inflammation, reversible smooth muscle constriction, and mucus production. Viral respiratory infection, exercise, tobacco exposure, weather fluctuations, and even air pollution may trigger excessive bronchoconstriction that is a hallmark of asthma exacerbation. Symptoms may include wheezing, coughing, shortness of breath, and chest tightness. According to 2018 data from the Centers for Disease Control (CDC), 5.53 million children have asthma in the United States. Compared with adults, children have higher asthma prevalence and a higher rate of visits to the primary care physician and emergency department [26].

Bronchiolitis, a viral lower respiratory tract infection affecting kids 2 years and younger, is another common cause of bronchospasm. This disease is most often caused by the respiratory syncytial virus and is frequent in the winter months. Factors associated with the severe disease include age less than 12 weeks, history of prematurity, underlying cardiopulmonary disease, and immunodeficiency [27].

Anaphylaxis is an acute systemic allergic reaction that is typically mediated by immunoglobulin E. Perioperative triggers include neuromuscular blocking agents, chlorhexidine skin prep solution, antibiotics, colloids, and latex. Acute onset rash, wheezing, bronchospasm, hypotension, or shock are common findings. Early recognition of anaphylaxis is challenging yet crucial, as severity and rate of progression in this complication are generally rapid and unpredictable, and prompt intervention is vital [25].

Treatment of Bronchospasm and Anaphylaxis

The most important intervention in both anaphylaxis and bronchospasm, in general, is epinephrine administration. In bronchospasm, 1-2 micrograms/kg IV (max 1 mg) or 10 micrograms/kg subcutaneously/IM (max 0.5 mg) are recommended as per Critical Event Checklist guidelines from the Society of Pediatric Anesthesia. Other recommendations include supplemental oxygen, inhaled albuterol, IV methylprednisolone 1 mg/kg (max 60 mg), or dexamethasone 0.15-0.25 mg/kg (max 16 mg) [12]. Ketamine, an N-methyl- D-aspartate receptor antagonist, also has bronchodilatory effects [28]. Treatment of anaphylaxis may require higher doses of IV epinephrine in the range of 1-10 micrograms/kg to increase blood pressure and reduce mediator release from mast cells. The IM route in the anterolateral surface of the mid-thigh can also be used. Other interventions involve removing suspected triggers if possible, giving oxygen for hypoxemia, IV crystalloid 10-30 ml/kg for hypotension, diphenhydramine 1 mg/kg IV/IO (max 50) and famotidine 0.25 mg/kg IV (max 20 mg) to reduce histamine-mediated effects, methylprednisolone 2 mg/kg IV/IO (max 100 mg) to reduce mediator release, and inhaled albuterol (4-10 puffs) to reduce bronchoconstriction [12]. Epinephrine may need to be repeated every 5 to 15 minutes. If the patient is hemodynamically unstable and not responding to repeat doses of epinephrine and fluids, an IV epinephrine infusion may need to be initiated. If severe airway compromise is present, the child should be intubated and mechanically ventilated [25]. Once the patient is stabilized, a chest radiograph should be considered, and, if anaphylaxis is suspected, a tryptase assay should be sent as elevated levels support this diagnosis.

Postextubation Stridor

Postextubation stridor is defined as high-pitched inspiratory wheezing in a patient who required intubation for the procedure. It usually occurs because of a tight-fitting endotracheal tube or repeated and traumatic intubation attempts. This inspiratory stridor is caused by turbulent air flow in the airway as a result of mucosa swelling in the extrathoracic airway, larynx, or trachea. Treatment includes cool humidified mist, nebulized 2.25% racemic epinephrine (0.25-0.5

ml+ 2 ml NS), and IV dexamethasone 0.5 mg/kg, if not given previously in the operating room. Racemic epinephrine results in vasoconstriction of blood vessels in the swollen mucosa. Clinicians need to be aware of a potential rebound effect after nebulized racemic epinephrine, which necessitates an observation for at least 4 hours after the treatment to avoid an unobserved worsening of the respiratory symptoms [20].

Postoperative Apnea

Neonates and young infants are at increased risk of developing apnea in the PACU, with the greatest risk being in premature babies. A strong inverse correlation exists between gestational age (GA) and postconceptual age (PCA) and apnea [29]. These children often have irregular breathing patterns, respiratory immaturity, and abnormal responses to hypoxia and hypercapnia. Apnea is defined as cessation of breathing for more than 15 seconds or more than 10 seconds if accompanied by hypoxia or bradycardia. This lack of breathing must be differentiated from periodic breathing, which involves repetitive pauses in respirations lasting 5 to 10 seconds. The normal response to hypercapnia in older children and adults leads to an increase in tidal volume and respiratory rate. In premature babies, hypoxia initially causes a brief increase in ventilation followed by a more sustained decrease in ventilation. Any residual anesthetic or muscle relaxant further complicates the response to hypoxia and hypercapnia [20, 30]. Anemia with hematocrit levels of less than 30, regardless of GA or PCA, is another known risk factor for apnea.

Preventive treatment with IV caffeine 10 mg/kg should be considered for patients at high risk. Treatment of apnea depends on the severity and involves tactile stimulation, supplemental oxygen, bag mask ventilation, and cardiopulmonary resuscitation (CPR) if cardiac arrest occurs. The General Anesthesia Compared to Spinal Anesthesia (GAS) study by Davidson *et al.* showed a reduction in early postoperative apnea (within the first 30 min in PACU) in infants undergoing inguinal hernia repair under a spinal anesthetic compared with those who had general anesthesia. There was no difference in late apnea occurring between 30 min and 12 hours postoperatively between the two groups [30]. Early apnea was found to be a strong predictor of late apnea. Even though spinal anesthesia did not reduce the risk of apnea in this trial, it decreased the severity of episodes and the need for significant interventions.

A classic study by Cote *et al.* describes the apnea risk for preterm infants to be more than 5% until PCA of 48 weeks when born at 35 weeks. For babies born at 32 weeks GA, the risk did not go below 5% until 50 weeks PCA. The risk of apnea did not go below 1% until PCA of 54 weeks and 56 weeks when born at

GA of 35 weeks and 32 weeks, respectively [29]. Each practitioner and institution must evaluate the risk of apnea in former premature infants and standardize their monitoring and admission criteria. At our institution, premature babies younger than 53 weeks PCA are admitted for overnight observation with continuous pulse oximetry monitoring and need to have a 12-hour apnea-free period prior to discharge home. Patients who receive preventive treatment with caffeine should still be admitted for observation.

CARDIOVASCULAR EVENTS

Cardiac arrhythmias and blood pressure fluctuations are rare in children recovering from anesthesia [24]. Sinus arrhythmia, defined as phasic heart rate (HR) increase during inspiration and decrease during expiration, is a common normal rhythm variation in children. Low HR may be a normal variant in a well-conditioned healthy athlete.

Bradycardia

Bradycardia is the most frequent perioperative dysrhythmia and is defined as:

- HR < 100 in neonates
- HR < 80 in infants
- HR< 60 in children > 1 year [12]

Hypoxia due to inadequate ventilation is the cause of bradycardia until proven otherwise. Other etiologies include medications such as opioids, neuromuscular blockers, reversal agents, and vagal stimulation. In infants, cardiac output is HR dependent, and bradycardia may result in hypotension. Treatment depends on the cause and involves positive pressure ventilation with supplemental oxygen when bradycardia is caused by inadequate ventilation or atropine 0.01-0.02 mg/kg IV when vagal etiology is suspected. If the patient becomes hypotensive with signs of poor perfusion, epinephrine 10 mcg/kg IV should be administered. If the child becomes pulseless, one needs to call for help and start chest compressions without delay. Epinephrine needs to be administered and the American Heart Association (AHA) algorithm for resuscitation followed. For persistent bradycardia unresponsive to oxygen and medications, cardiology consult and pacing should be considered [12].

Narrow Complex Tachycardia

Narrow complex tachycardia can be divided into sinus tachycardia (ST) and supraventricular tachycardia (SVT) (Table **10**).

Table 10. Sinus tachycardia *vs.* supraventricular tachycardia [31].

Sinus Tachycardia (ST)	Supraventricular Tachycardia (SVT)
HR infant < 220 HR child <180	HR infant >220 HR child >180
Gradual onset	Sudden onset
HR variability with respirations or stimulation	Minimal HR variability
ECG: P waves present	ECG: P waves absent on abnormal

Sinus tachycardia usually represents a compensatory mechanism to maintain cardiac output and oxygen delivery. It may be caused by a variety of factors, including hypoxia, hypercarbia, fever, hypovolemia, bleeding, pain, agitation, and emergence delirium, or medications such as epinephrine or anticholinergics.

SVT is common in the pediatric population, affecting as many as 1 in 250 children [32], and is usually related to a known or unrecognized disease such as conduction abnormality, structural heart defect, toxin ingestion, or infections [33]. It often involves a reentry mechanism through an accessory atrioventricular pathway. SVT treatment involves vagal maneuvers such as applying ice to the patient's face, IV "rapid push" adenosine of 0.1 mg/kg for the first dose (max 6 mg) and 0.2 mg/kg for the second dose (max 12 mg), and synchronized cardioversion, 0.5-1 J/kg, if SVT is accompanied by hypotension or altered mental status [12]. If no pulse can be detected, one needs to call for help, start chest compressions, and follow the AHA Pediatric Advanced Life Support (PALS) algorithm for cardiac arrest.

Premature Atrial Contractions

Premature atrial contractions (PACs) are usually a benign finding in the postoperative period and require no treatment. Premature ventricular contractions (PVCs) are less common than PACs and can be divided into uniform and multiform based on morphology (the terms unifocal and multifocal are no longer used). Isolated PVCs can occur in children with a structurally and functionally normal heart and may be caused by electrolyte abnormalities or drug toxicities [34]. More worrisome etiologies include myocarditis, cardiomyopathies, conduction abnormalities, congenital heart defects, rhabdomyolysis, and malignant hyperthermia. Personal and family cardiac history should be gathered, 12-lead ECG obtained, electrolytes checked, and cardiac consult requested in case of positive history or prolonged QT interval [35].

Hypotension

Hypotension is defined as sustained low blood pressure with potential for end-organ hypoperfusion, typically more than 20% below baseline [12]. Systolic blood pressure (SBP) of less than 70 mmHg + (age x 2) should be considered hypotension. For example, for a 4-year-old, SBP of less than 78 mmHg, which is below the 5th percentile for age, is considered hypotension. For a term baby, hypotension is considered as SBP of less than 60 mmHg, and, for an infant, it is less than 70 mmHg. These numbers are only a guide and vary for individual patients and situations. Hypotension is most commonly related to preload abnormalities and treatment depends on etiology: hypovolemia caused by dehydration is treated with IV crystalloid and bleeding is treated with blood products and source control. Contractility and afterload issues are rare in otherwise healthy children and are treated with inotropic agents and vasopressors, respectively. Although rare, it is important to rule out an undiagnosed cardiac disease, sepsis, thyroid or adrenal crisis, and anaphylaxis as possible causes of hypotension in the PACU.

Cardiac Arrest

Cardiac arrest in pediatric patients undergoing non-cardiac surgery is rare (< 1 per 10,000) [24, 36], but, when it occurs, nearly 20% of anesthesia-related pediatric cardiac arrests present during emergence, transport to PACU, or recovery from anesthesia. According to the Wake Up Safe database analysis [37] published in 2017, 69% of these events were judged by institutional review to have been preventable. Individual provider factors such as decision making, inexperience, failure to call for assistance, and distraction were most commonly identified as the primary root cause. Other factors included inadequate supervision of trainees, competing priorities, inadequate monitoring during transport to the PACU, verbal miscommunication, lack of leadership, and underlying patient's disease. All preventable events were respiratory in nature. The outcomes of these early postoperative arrests were good, with 3.8% mortality, which is significantly better than previously reported mortality rates for pediatric PACU cardiac arrests and pediatric cardiac arrests in general. This likely reflects confounding factors such as sicker patients transported directly from the OR to the PACU for a planned admission and data only from pediatric hospitals with the advantage of staff with pediatric expertise. Identified modifiable measures include adequate monitoring during transport to the PACU, adequate supervision of trainees, transition of care from anesthesia providers to PACU nursing after emergence from anesthesia, and frequent reassessment by the anesthesiologist during recovery.

POSTOPERATIVE NAUSEA AND VOMITING (PONV)

The **P**ostoperative **Vo**miting in **C**hildren (**POVOC**) score has been validated and used for many years to evaluate a patient's risk for PONV.

The POVOC score includes:

- duration of surgery > 30 min
- age > 3 years
- strabismus surgery
- personal history of postoperative vomiting (POV) or history of PONV in parents or siblings

Risk Assessment

Postoperative nausea and vomiting (PONV) is a common PACU problem with emesis rates twice as high in children as in adults [38]. PONV can increase patient discomfort, prolong PACU length of stay, and result in unplanned admission or readmission to the hospital with increased health care cost [39]. PONV prophylaxis is an important component of Enhanced Recovery After Surgery (ERAS) programs. Proactive risk stratification is important to lower baseline risk and decide what approach to prophylaxis is likely to be most effective.

Depending on the presence of none, 1, 2, 3, or 4 risk factors, the estimated incidence of POV is 9%, 10%, 30%, 55%, and 70%, respectively [39]. Use of caudal and peripheral nerve blocks was found to decrease the risk in the same study, but the difference was not statistically significant. It is possible that regional anesthesia reduces the need for large doses of volatile anesthetics and postoperative opioids which were shown to contribute to POV [39, 40].

Stepwise Approach to PONV Prophylaxis

A stepwise approach to PONV prophylaxis includes:

1. Assessment of risk (low, moderate, high) using a validated risk score
2. Baseline risk reduction strategies [41]:
    - use of regional anesthesia
    - use of propofol for induction and maintenance
    - avoidance of nitrous oxide and volatile anesthetics
    - minimal use of perioperative opioids
    - adequate hydration

3. Pharmacologic prophylaxis

Since antiemetics (Table **11** & **12**) carry the risk of adverse effects ranging from headache to potentially significant QT prolongation and malignant arrhythmias, each patient should be evaluated separately and prophylaxis tailored to an individual patient's risk.

Table 11. Antiemetic doses for POV prophylaxis in children [41].

Drug	Dose
Dexamethasone*	150 mcg/kg up to 5 mg
Dimenhydrinate	0.5 mg/kg up to 25 mg
Dolasetron**	350 mcg/kg up to 12.5 mg
Droperidol***	10-15 mcg/kg up to 1.25 mg
Granisetron	40 mcg/kg up to 4 mg
Ondansetron****	50-100 mcg/kg up to 4 mg
Tropisetron	0.1 mg/kg up to 2 mg

*Dexamethasone may cause tumor lysis syndrome in children with leukemia **Dolasetron has an FDA Black Box Warning because of the risk of QT prolongation and torsade de pointes ***Droperidol has an FDA Black Box Warning because of risk of QT prolongation ****Ondansetron may cause ventricular tachycardia in children with prolonged QT syndrome

- For low-risk patients, a "wait and see" approach may be considered.
- Patients at moderate-to-high risk should receive prophylaxis with a combination pharmacologic therapy or a multimodal approach that includes two or more non-pharmacologic/pharmacologic interventions.

Table 12. Pharmacologic POV combination therapy [41].

Pharmacologic Combination Therapy for Children
Ondansetron 0.05 mg/kg + dexamethasone 0.015 mg/kg
Ondansetron 0.1 mg/kg + droperidol 0.015 mg/kg
Tropisetron 0.1 mg/kg + dexamethasone 0.5 mg/kg

One example of this multimodal PONV risk reduction approach in high-risk patients is the recent study by Muhly *et al.*, which combined inhalational general anesthesia with regional anesthesia (a femoral and sciatic nerve block), dexamethasone, ondansetron, intraoperative low-dose propofol infusion, and ketorolac for an outpatient anterior cruciate ligament (ACL) reconstruction. The authors reported a significant decrease in postoperative emesis rate from baseline 17% to 5% following this guideline implementation, as well as an increase in the percentage of patients managed without postoperative opioids from 16% to 38% [42].

Non-pharmacologic Prophylaxis

Non-pharmacologic interventions include P6 acupuncture point stimulation and IV hydration. Acupuncture is increasingly being integrated into pediatric care. The precise mechanism has been debated with the dominant explanation being stimulation and release of beta-endorphins, enkephalins and serotonin, as well as regulation of the autonomic nervous system (Moffet, 2006). P6 is located on the inner forearm above the transverse crease of the wrist, between the tendons of palmaris longus and flexor radialis. One of the ways to find it is to place three fingers of the patient's other hand across the wrist and then place your thumb above the patient's three fingers (Fig. **3**). P6 can be stimulated by needle insertion and manipulation (acupuncture), electrical stimulation of the inserted need (electroacupuncture), electrical stimulation of the skin without a needle (noninvasive electroacupuncture), applying pressure (acupressure), or directing a laser beam to the point (laser stimulation). A meta-analysis by Jindal *et al.* of 23 studies including both adult and pediatric patients showed that P6 acupuncture and acustimulation were effective in reducing POV in children [44]. A 2006 meta-analysis by Dune *et al.* focused on children aged 4 to 18 years. Twelve trails examined vomiting and two trials looked at nausea for 24-hour outcomes. Use of acupressure and acupuncture was associated with a significant reduction in both nausea and vomiting in children. No difference was found between antiemetic and acupuncture groups in the incidence of vomiting, suggesting equivalent effectiveness of both techniques [43].

P6 stimulation can be used before or after induction of anesthesia and stimulation over the median nerve has been used for PONV prophylaxis in PACU. One difficulty in using acupuncture in children is fear of needles, which may sometimes be mitigated by distraction with toys and pictures. Noninvasive electrical or laser stimulation, as well as acupressure, may represent better options for pediatric patients in whom these mitigation strategies fail to reduce anxiety and improve needle acceptance.

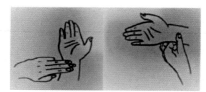

Fig. (3). Place three fingers of the patient's other hand across the wrist and then place your thumb above the patient's three fingers to find the P6 location. Illustration prepared by the author (Malgorzata Lutwin-Kawalec).

Failed Prophylaxis

In case of failed prophylaxis, the following treatment approach is recommended:

- use an antiemetic from a different class than the prophylactic drug(s) administered
- re-administer the same drug only if > 6 hours after PACU
- do not re-administer dexamethasone or transdermal scopolamine

CHILD LIFE SERVICES AND TEAM APPROACH TO PERIOPERATIVE CARE

At our hospital, we strongly emphasize and provide family-centered care. Child Life services are an important component of this team approach. The perioperative period is full of stress-generating factors such as fear of the unknown, separation from parents, loss of control, fear of body damage, or pain [45].

Each child is unique and has different coping mechanisms that depend on age, developmental level, and previous experiences in health care environments. Use of psychological preparation, age-appropriate therapeutic play, and encouragement provided by Child Life specialists help minimize adverse behavioral effects of hospitalization and surgery. It has been shown that these interventions decrease emotional distress, increase a child's understanding of planned procedures, act as non-pharmacological pain control modalities, and shorten recovery time. They also increase overall parental satisfaction with the care their child receives, which is an important component in the age of quality-based care. There is also emerging evidence that providing Child Life services decreases the overall cost of care by shortening the length of stay and needs for sedation and pain medications. Our Child Life specialists meet patients in a preoperative holding area, where they initiate a therapeutic relationship with the child and family and then accompany the patient to the operating room, provide guidance and distraction during induction of anesthesia allowing the anesthesia team to concentrate on safe and efficient patient care, and resume the child's management in the recovery room.

CONCLUSION

Children recovering from anesthesia can present with a multitude of challenging complications. Safe and efficient pediatric postanesthesia care requires a team approach, well-trained and dedicated nursing staff, a family-centered environment, and immediate availability of expert help, emergency drugs, and airway equipment.

CONSENT FOR PUBLICATION

Not applicable.

CONFLICT OF INTEREST

The author declares no conflict of interest, financial or otherwise.

ACKNOWLEDGEMENTS

Declared none.

REFERENCES

[1] American Society of Anesthesiologists. Standards for Postanesthesia Care 2019. https://www.asahq.org/standards -and-guidelines/standards-for-postanesthesia-care

[2] Practice guidelines for postanesthetic care: a report by the American Society of Anesthesiologists Task Force on Postanesthetic Care. Anesthesiology 2002; 96(3): 742-52. [http://dx.doi.org/10.1097/00000542-200203000-00033] [PMID: 11873052]

[3] Vlajkovic GP, Sindjelic RP. Emergence delirium in children: many questions, few answers. Anesth Analg 2007; 104(1): 84-91. [http://dx.doi.org/10.1213/01.ane.0000250914.91881.a8] [PMID: 17179249]

[4] Yasui Y, Masaki E, Kato F. Sevoflurane directly excites locus coeruleus neurons of rats. Anesthesiology 2007; 107(6): 992-1002. [http://dx.doi.org/10.1097/01.anes.0000291453.78823.f4] [PMID: 18043068]

[5] Sikich N, Lerman J. Development and psychometric evaluation of the pediatric anesthesia emergence delirium scale. Anesthesiology 2004; 100(5): 1138-45. [http://dx.doi.org/10.1097/00000542-200405000-00015]

[6] Bajwa SA, Costi D, Cyna AM. A comparison of emergence delirium scales following general anesthesia in children. Paediatr Anaesth 2010; 20(8): 704-11. [http://dx.doi.org/10.1111/j.1460-9592.2010.03328.x] [PMID: 20497353]

[7] Lee CA. Paediatric emergence delirium: an approach to diagnosis and management in the postanaesthesia care unit. J Perioper Crit Intensiv Care Nurs 2017; 3: 140.

[8] Voepel-Lewis T, Malviya S, Tait AR. A prospective cohort study of emergence agitation in the pediatric postanesthesia care unit. Anesth Analg 2003; 96(6): 1625-30. [http://dx.doi.org/10.1213/01.ANE.0000062522.21048.61] [PMID: 12760985]

[9] Moore AD, Anghelescu DL. Emergence delirium in pediatric anesthesia. Paediatr Drugs 2017; 19(1): 11-20. [http://dx.doi.org/10.1007/s40272-016-0201-5] [PMID: 27798810]

[10] Schneiderbanger D, Johannsen S, Roewer N, Schuster F. Management of malignant hyperthermia: diagnosis and treatment. Ther Clin Risk Manag 2014; 10: 355-62. [PMID: 24868161]

[11] Litman RS, Griggs SM, Dowling JJ, Riazi S. Malignant hyperthermia susceptibility and related diseases. Anesthesiology 2018; 128(1): 159-67. [http://dx.doi.org/10.1097/ALN.0000000000001877] [PMID: 28902673]

[12]   Critical Event Checklist https://www.pedsanesthesia.org/critical-events-checklist/

[13]   Litman RS, Smith VI, Larach MG, *et al.* Consensus Statement of the Malignant Hyperthermia Association of the United States on Unresolved Clinical Questions Concerning the Management of Patients With Malignant Hyperthermia. Anesth Analg 2019; 128(4): 652-9.
         [http://dx.doi.org/10.1213/ANE.0000000000004039] [PMID: 30768455]

[14]   Stowell KM. DNA testing for malignant hyperthermia: the reality and the dream. Anesth Analg 2014; 118(2): 397-406.
         [http://dx.doi.org/10.1213/ANE.0000000000000063] [PMID: 24445638]

[15]   Allen GC, Larach MG, Kunselman AR. The sensitivity and specificity of the caffeine-halothane contracture test: a report from the North American Malignant Hyperthermia Registry. Anesthesiology 1998; 88(3): 579-88.
         [http://dx.doi.org/10.1097/00000542-199803000-00006] [PMID: 9523799]

[16]   www.mhaus.org

[17]   Tay CL, Tan GM, Ng SB. Critical incidents in paediatric anaesthesia: an audit of 10 000 anaesthetics in Singapore. Paediatr Anaesth 2001; 11(6): 711-8.
         [http://dx.doi.org/10.1046/j.1460-9592.2001.00767.x] [PMID: 11696149]

[18]   Bhananker SM, Ramamoorthy C, Geiduschek JM, *et al.* Anesthesia-related cardiac arrest in children: update from the Pediatric Perioperative Cardiac Arrest Registry. Anesth Analg 2007; 105(2): 344-50.
         [http://dx.doi.org/10.1213/01.ane.0000268712.00756.dd] [PMID: 17646488]

[19]   von Ungern-Sternberg BS, Boda K, Chambers NA, *et al.* Risk assessment for respiratory complications in paediatric anaesthesia: a prospective cohort study. Lancet 2010; 376(9743): 773-83.
         [http://dx.doi.org/10.1016/S0140-6736(10)61193-2] [PMID: 20816545]

[20]   von Ungern-Sternberg BS. Respiratory complications in the pediatric postanesthesia care unit. Anesthesiol Clin 2014; 32(1): 45-61.
         [http://dx.doi.org/10.1016/j.anclin.2013.10.004] [PMID: 24491649]

[21]   Alalami AA, Ayoub CM, Baraka AS. Laryngospasm: review of different prevention and treatment modalities. Paediatr Anaesth 2008; 18(4): 281-8.
         [http://dx.doi.org/10.1111/j.1460-9592.2008.02448.x] [PMID: 18315632]

[22]   Gavel G, Walker RWM. Laryngospasm in anaesthesia Contin Educ Anaesth Crit Care Pain 2014; 14: 47-51.
         [http://dx.doi.org/10.1093/bjaceaccp/mkt031]

[23]   Visvanathan T, Kluger MT, Webb RK, Westhorpe RN. Crisis management during anaesthesia: laryngospasm. Qual Saf Health Care 2005; 14(3): e3.
         [http://dx.doi.org/10.1136/qshc.2002.004275] [PMID: 15933300]

[24]   Murat I, Constant I, Maud'huy H. Perioperative anaesthetic morbidity in children: a database of 24,165 anaesthetics over a 30-month period. Paediatr Anaesth 2004; 14(2): 158-66.
         [http://dx.doi.org/10.1111/j.1460-9592.2004.01167.x] [PMID: 14962332]

[25]   Edwards LR, Borger J. Pediatric Bronchospasm StatPearls. Treasure Island, FL: StatPearls Publishing 2020.

[26]   Akinbami LJ, Moorman JE, Bailey C, *et al.* Trends in asthma prevalence, health care use, and mortality in the United States, 2001-2010. NCHS Data Brief 2012; (94): 1-8.
         [PMID: 22617340]

[27]   Ralston SL, Lieberthal AS, Meissner HC, *et al.* Clinical practice guideline: the diagnosis, management, and prevention of bronchiolitis. Pediatrics 2014; 134(5): e1474-502.
         [http://dx.doi.org/10.1542/peds.2014-2742] [PMID: 25349312]

[28]   Nievas IF, Anand KJ. Severe acute asthma exacerbation in children: a stepwise approach for escalating therapy in a pediatric intensive care unit. J Pediatr Pharmacol Ther 2013; 18(2): 88-104.

[http://dx.doi.org/10.5863/1551-6776-18.2.88] [PMID: 23798903]

[29]   Coté CJ, Zaslavsky A, Downes JJ, *et al.* Postoperative apnea in former preterm infants after inguinal herniorrhaphy. A combined analysis. Anesthesiology 1995; 82(4): 809-22.
[http://dx.doi.org/10.1097/00000542-199504000-00002] [PMID: 7717551]

[30]   Davidson AJ, Morton NS, Arnup SJ, *et al.* Apnea after awake regional and general anesthesia in infants: The General Anesthesia Compared to Spinal Anesthesia Study--comparing apnea and neurodevelopmental outcomes, a randomized controlled trial. Anesthesiology 2015; 123(1): 38-54.
[http://dx.doi.org/10.1097/ALN.0000000000000709] [PMID: 26001033]

[31]   Manole MD, Saladino RA. Emergency department management of the pediatric patient with supraventricular tachycardia. Pediatr Emerg Care 2007; 23(3): 176-85.
[http://dx.doi.org/10.1097/PEC.0b013e318032904c] [PMID: 17413437]

[32]   Perry JC, Garson A Jr. Supraventricular tachycardia due to Wolff-Parkinson-White syndrome in children: early disappearance and late recurrence. J Am Coll Cardiol 1990; 16(5): 1215-20.
[http://dx.doi.org/10.1016/0735-1097(90)90555-4] [PMID: 2229769]

[33]   Bhat SR, Miyake C, Wang NE. Considerations in the diagnosis and emergency management of pediatric tachycardias. Pediatric Emergency Medicine Reports 2012.

[34]   Alexander ME, Berul CI. Ventricular arrhythmias: when to worry. Pediatr Cardiol 2000; 21(6): 532-41.
[http://dx.doi.org/10.1007/s002460010131] [PMID: 11050277]

[35]   McInerny TK, Adam HM, Campbell DE, DeWitt TG, Foy JM, Kamat DM, Eds. American Academy of Pediatrics Textbook of Pediatric Care. Washington, DC: American Academy of Pediatrics 2016.
[http://dx.doi.org/10.1542/9781610020473]

[36]   Flick RP, Sprung J, Harrison TE, *et al.* Perioperative cardiac arrests in children between 1988 and 2005 at a tertiary referral center: a study of 92,881 patients. Anesthesiology 2007; 106(2): 226-37.
[http://dx.doi.org/10.1097/00000542-200702000-00009] [PMID: 17264715]

[37]   Christensen RE, Haydar B, Voepel-Lewis TD. Pediatric cardiopulmonary arrest in the postanesthesia care unit, rare but preventable: analysis of data from Wake Up Safe, The Pediatric Anesthesia Quality Improvement Initiative. Anesth Analg 2017; 124(4): 1231-6.
[http://dx.doi.org/10.1213/ANE.0000000000001744]

[38]   Lerman J. Surgical and patient factors involved in postoperative nausea and vomiting. Br J Anaesth 1992; 69(7) (Suppl. 1): 24S-32S.
[http://dx.doi.org/10.1093/bja/69.supplement_1.24S] [PMID: 1486011]

[39]   Eberhart LHJ, Geldner G, Kranke P, *et al.* The development and validation of a risk score to predict the probability of postoperative vomiting in pediatric patients. Anesth Analg 2004; 99(6): 1630-7.
[http://dx.doi.org/10.1213/01.ANE.0000135639.57715.6C] [PMID: 15562045]

[40]   Apfel CC, Philip BK, Cakmakkaya OS, *et al.* Who is at risk for postdischarge nausea and vomiting after ambulatory surgery? Anesthesiology 2012; 117(3): 475-86.
[http://dx.doi.org/10.1097/ALN.0b013e318267ef31] [PMID: 22846680]

[41]   Gan TJ, Diemunsch P, Habib AS, *et al.* Consensus guidelines for the management of postoperative nausea and vomiting. Anesth Analg 2014; 118(1): 85-113.
[http://dx.doi.org/10.1213/ANE.0000000000000002] [PMID: 24356162]

[42]   Muhly WT, Ganley T, Jantzen E, *et al.* Reducing postoperative nausea and vomiting in pediatric patients undergoing anterior cruciate ligament reconstruction: A quality report. Paediatr Anaesth 2020; 30(4): 446-54.
[http://dx.doi.org/10.1111/pan.13813] [PMID: 31894609]

[43]   Dune LS, Shiao SY. Metaanalysis of acustimulation effects on postoperative nausea and vomiting in children. Explore (NY) 2006; 2(4): 314-20.
[http://dx.doi.org/10.1016/j.explore.2006.04.004] [PMID: 16846819]

[44]   Jindal V, Ge A, Mansky PJ. Safety and efficacy of acupuncture in children: a review of the evidence. J
         Pediatr Hematol Oncol 2008; 30(6): 431-42.
         [http://dx.doi.org/10.1097/MPH.0b013e318165b2cc] [PMID: 18525459]

[45]   Brewer S, Gleditsch SL, Syblik D, Tietjens ME, Vacik HW. Pediatric anxiety: child life intervention
         in day surgery. J Pediatr Nurs 2006; 21(1): 13-22.
         [http://dx.doi.org/10.1016/j.pedn.2005.06.004] [PMID: 16428010]

CHAPTER 7

Emergency Intubation and Difficult Airway Management

Nathalie Peiris¹ and Pravin Taneja²

¹ Department of Anesthesiology and Perioperative Medicine, Nemours Children's Health, Delaware Valley, Wilmington, DE, USA

² Department of Anesthesiology, St. Christopher's Hospital for Children, Philadelphia, PA, USA

Abstract: Knowing how to manage a difficult airway in a pediatric patient is important. Physical characteristics that are indicators for a difficult airway and difficult ventilation will be discussed. Management of an anticipated difficult airway using different intubating techniques and intubating devices will be described. Unlike the adult patient, an awake intubation is often not possible and methods for anesthetizing the patient will also be explained. In the case of an unanticipated difficult airway where intubation and ventilation are not possible, front of neck access is the next step. Certain airway emergency situations such as stridor in a pediatric patient and mask ventilation of a neonate causing abdominal distension will also be described and its management. Emergent intubations in an unfamiliar setting outside of the operating room can prove to be difficult for the anesthesia provider. This chapter will also describe the difficulties encountered and methods of management.

Keywords: Anesthesia induction of difficult airway patient, Difficult mask ventilation in the neonate, Emergency intubation outside of operating room, Fiberoptic intubation through supraglottic airway, Needle cricothyrotomy, Pediatric difficult airway, Predictors of difficult intubation, Predictors of difficult mask ventilation, Stridor, Supraglottic airway, Video laryngoscopy.

INTRODUCTION

As discussed in previous chapters, the anatomical and physiological differences of the pediatric patient make the act of securing the airway more difficult compared to the adult patient. With the addition of the difficult airway in a pediatric patient, the anesthesia provider is faced with many clinical challenges.

* **Corresponding author Bharathi Gourkanti MD:** Department of Anesthesiology, Cooper Medical School of Rowan University, Cooper University Health Care, Camden, NJ, United States; E-mail: gourkantibharathi@cooperhealth.edu

Bharathi Gourkanti, Irwin Gratz, Grace Dippo, Nathalie Peiris and Dinesh K. Choudhry (Eds.)
All rights reserved-© 2022 Bentham Science Publishers

The Pediatric Difficult Intubation (PeDI) registry has defined the criteria for pediatric difficult airway as:

1. Failure to visualize vocal cords on direct laryngoscopy by an experienced provider.
2. Impossible direct laryngoscopy because of abnormal anatomy.
3. Failed direct laryngoscopy within last 6 months.
4. Direct laryngoscopy felt to be harmful in a patient with suspected difficult laryngoscopy [14, 15].

The closed claims database of the American Society of Anesthesiologists and the Perioperative Cardiac Arrest Registry have shown that respiratory complications are one of the most common causes for perioperative morbidity and mortality in children [12,13].

Preoperative Evaluation and Predictors of Difficult Airway

Often, a pediatric difficult airway can be identified upon preoperative physical examination of the patient. History of a congenital dysmorphic syndrome (which may be obvious upon observation of the patient) should increase concern for abnormal and potentially difficult airway anatomy. The pediatric difficult airway can be divided into two components: difficult mask ventilation and difficult intubation. Ability to perform effective mask ventilation despite difficult intubation significantly reduces the dangers associated with airway management. The PeDI registry found that patient weight less than 10 kilograms, micrognathia, greater than 2 tracheal intubation attempts and 3 direct laryngoscopy attempts before an indirect technique were independent factors that increased risks of patient complications during airway management [15].

Risk factors for difficulty with mask ventilation include any comorbidities that cause upper airway obstruction. These include:

- Obesity
- Macroglossia
- Masses in the mouth (such as oropharyngeal airway tumors)
- Neck masses (such as cystic hygromas)

Physical risk factors for difficult intubation include:

- Micrognathia, Short thyromental distance (< 3 of patient's finger breadths)
- Small mouth opening (< 2 of patient's finger breadths), Mallampati score 3 or 4
- Midface hypoplasia
- Facial asymmetry (in particular, ear deformities)
- Temporomandibular joint immobility
- Shortened and increased circumference of neck, history of neck radiation,

extrinsic neck masses causing compression
• Limited head and neck range of motion

In addition to a physical exam, one must also conduct a thorough history of the patient. If there is a concern for a syndromic child, identifying the syndrome is important in order to determine where the difficulty lies in managing the airway. A list of syndromes associated with a difficult airway is shown in Table **1**. Inquiring about a history of subglottic or tracheal stenosis is also important to determine if a smaller size tube may be needed. Finally, obtaining previous anesthetic/airway records for the patient (in terms of ease of mask ventilation/intubation and what airway devices and endotracheal size tubes were used) is also vital because often one can follow the same airway technique to secure the airway.

Table 1.

Syndrome	Airway Concerns
Beckwith-Wiedemann Syndrome	Macroglossia
Pierre Robin Sequence	Micrognathia; airway obstruction secondary to tongue falling back (improves with age)
Goldenhar Syndrome	Micrognathia; Facial asymmetry; Limited mouth opening; fusion of cervical vertebrae
Treacher Collins	Micrognathia; Airway obstruction due to maxillary and mandibular hypoplasia (worsens with age); Limited mouth opening
Trisomy 21 (Down Syndrome)	Macroglossia; Atlantoaxial instability; Subglottic Stenosis
Mucopolysaccharidosis (Hunter's and Hurler's syndrome)	Accumulation of mucopolysaccharides in airway soft tissue (poor laryngeal and pharyngeal tissue compliance); Short and thickened neck; Atlantoaxial instability; Airway obstruction (worsens with age); difficulty with mask ventilation and intubation
Apert Syndrome, Crouzon Syndrome, Pfeiffer Syndrome	Midface hypoplasia; Cervical vertebrae fusion (associated with Apert)
Klippel-Feil Syndrome	Cervical vertebrae fusion

The goal of preoperative evaluation of a potentially difficult airway is to make an airway plan and backup plans should the initial attempt fail. With any concern for

a difficult airway, a pediatric otorhinolaryngology surgeon should be consulted in case the need for a surgical airway arises.

Advanced Tools for Difficult Airway

Video Laryngoscopes

Indirect laryngoscopy *via* video laryngoscopy has only been around since 2001; however, it has revolutionized airway management. Direct laryngoscopy with a Miller or Macintosh blade requires a skilled operator and one experienced in tracheal intubations. Video laryngoscopy offers the advantage of better visualization of the glottic opening without alignment of the 3 airway axes required for direct laryngoscopy. This can be helpful for intubating patients with concerns for cervical spine injury.

Studies have shown that video laryngoscopy results in higher successful intubations compared to direct laryngoscopy by novices in the adult population and has become standard of care when conventional direct laryngoscope fails or there is an anticipated difficult airway in the adult population [4].

On the other hand, for the pediatric population, studies have not shown video laryngoscopy to be superior to direct laryngoscopy in patients with normal airways [5]. One reason is that the blades for the video laryngoscope often are difficult or too large to use in pediatric patients. Studies have shown that the use of video laryngoscopy improved laryngeal views; however, time for intubation is prolonged in comparison to conventional direct laryngoscopy. Even with its challenges, video laryngoscopy still serves as a rescue device after failed conventional laryngoscopy and for patients with difficult airway anatomy and thus has been incorporated into pediatric difficult airway guidelines and clinical reviews [6]. Expertise with video laryngoscopy in pediatric patients is an important tool for airway management.

The two most popular pediatric video laryngoscopes used include the Glidescope®, which uses an angulated blade and the Storz CMAC® laryngoscope, which uses a nonangulated blade (although recently has come out with an angulated blade called the "D-blade").

One significant complication that may occur during indirect laryngoscopy intubation is oropharyngeal or dental trauma due to focusing on the image on the screen. This can be mitigated by inserting the video laryngoscope blade and endotracheal tube into the oral cavity under direct visualization before looking at the monitor. Removal of the video laryngoscope blade from the oral cavity should also be done under direct visualization.

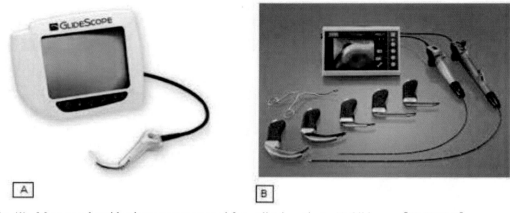

Fig. (1). Most popular video laryngoscopes used for pediatric patients **A)** Glidescope®**B)** CMAC®.

Circumstances where video laryngoscopy would be difficult include situations where there is a lack of space for the equipment in the mouth, such as patients with small mouth opening, macroglossia or large oropharyngeal masses.

Another drawback for indirect video laryngoscopy is its lack of functionality in the trauma airway – where blood and secretions obscure the camera.

Glidescope®

Glidescope® is created with a hyper-acute curved blade and is thus most effective for patients with severe airway abnormalities (*i.e.*, patients with "anterior" airways). However, in order to have successful intubation using the Glidescope®, one requires a stylet that is shaped to the same curvature as the blade. Glidescope® does create its own rigid stylets that can be used. Due to the varying size array of blades required for pediatric patients, one can take a standard disposable malleable stylet and mold it to mimic the curve of the blade in use. With a camera located at the distal end of the blade, the tongue does not need to be swept to the left (unlike with direct laryngoscopy). The ideal placement of the blade in the patient's mouth is midline or slightly left of the midline in order to accommodate passage of the endotracheal tube on the right.

Unlike with direct laryngoscopy (where the difficulty is with visualization of the glottic opening), the largest disadvantage of Glidescope® video laryngoscopy in the pediatric population is the difficulty in directing the endotracheal tube to and through the cords. A recent observational study of 200 children who underwent Glidescope® intubations showed an 80% first pass success rate and the most trouble experienced was passing the endotracheal tube in the area from the arytenoids to just below the vocal cords [3]. This is believed to be due to the hyperacute angle of the styletted endotracheal tube in comparison to the relatively straight airway [3].

Methods to correct for this include clockwise or counterclockwise rotation of the endotracheal tube and external manipulation of laryngeal structures. Other methods suggested to reduce the acute angle of the endotracheal tube include withdrawal of the stylet, "downgrading" the view (making a grade 1 Lehane Cormack view a grade 2 view Lehane Cormack view), and "reverse loading" the stylet into the endotracheal tube (forming a concave curve rather than the preformed convex curve to follow the posterior tracheal wall) [3].

CMAC®

The traditional CMAC® blades are designed similarly to the traditional Miller and Macintosh blades with a camera and light source at the distal tip. Thus, in "normal" pediatric airways, CMAC® may be more beneficial to use rather than the Glidescope®. Due to the less acute angle of the blade, intubation is successful without the need for a hyper-curved endotracheal tube. The blade design allows for the use of either direct or indirect laryngoscopy during intubation attempts. This is beneficial because one can convert from direct laryngoscopy to indirect laryngoscopy in the same attempt and thus minimize complications with multiple attempts. This can also be helpful in teaching airway trainees direct laryngoscopy skills while the anesthesiologist is able to visualize and confirm relevant anatomy seen on the monitor.

If using the CMAC® for direct laryngoscopy, one must use the same techniques used for direct laryngoscopy such as positioning the patient in the appropriate "sniffing" position for airway axis alignment and inserting the blade on the right side and sweeping the tongue to the left. If using the C-mac for video indirect laryngoscopy, one would employ similar techniques as used for Glidescope intubations.

Supraglottic Airways

Supraglottic airways (SGAs) have gained popularity in difficult airway management in both adult and pediatric populations. First created in the 1980s, SGAs are advantageous due to improving difficult ventilation, aiding as an airway adjunct after failed intubation, and relative ease of placement. SGAs have been incorporated into difficult airway management algorithms created by the American Society of Anesthesiologists and Difficult Airway Society and serve as a rescue device in the "can't ventilate, can't intubate" scenario.

In the pediatric population, SGAs have a lower failure rate (0.86%) than in the adult population (1.1%) [1]. Similar to adults, benefits in the pediatric population include the ability to bypass upper airway obstruction to allow for adequate ventilation, act as a rescue device in the "can't intubate, can't ventilate" scenario and serve as a conduit for difficult intubation.

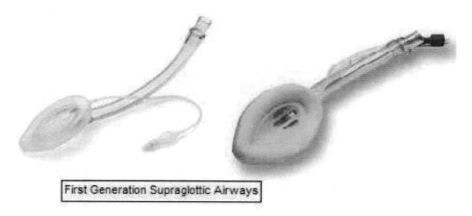

Fig. (2). First generation supraglottic airways include: LMA Unique® and LMA Classic®

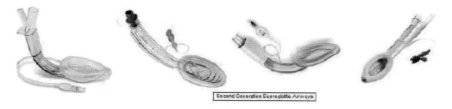

Fig. (3). Second generation supraglottic airways include: LMA supreme®, air-Q®, Ambu Aura-I®, LMA proseal®

Second generation SGAs differ from first generation SGAs by having a better design to decrease tip malposition, poor mask seal, risk of aspiration and increase the ease of intubation with an endotracheal tube. In particular, the air-Q® laryngeal mask airway has been shown to be the ideal conduit for successful tracheal intubation in pediatric patients due to its widened and shortened shaft, which allows passage of an endotracheal tube with its pilot balloon [2].

Flexible Fiberoptic Bronchoscope

The use of a flexible fiberoptic bronchoscope is considered gold standard for difficult airway management of adult and pediatric patients. The fiberoptic scope can be used to intubate both nasally and orally – which is beneficial when there is limited mouth opening. Similar to video laryngoscopy, head and neck manipulation is not required for successful intubation and thus, fiberoptic intubations can be used when there is a known or suspected unstable cervical spine. In addition, the fiberoptic scope can be used to intubate through an SGA and in combination with video laryngoscopy – which shall be discussed more in detail in a later section.

Similar to video laryngoscopy, airways filled with blood or secretions will obscure the lens of the scope and limit its use. Set-up for fiberoptic intubation is often time consuming and, in an acute unanticipated difficult airway, may be more difficult to attempt than video laryngoscopy. Proficiency in pediatric fiberoptic intubation may not be as common due to the increased popularity of video laryngoscopy. In addition, proficiency at adult fiberoptic intubations may not translate to pediatric fiberoptic intubations due to the technical challenges of navigating a smaller scope through a small airway.

One significant limitation of pediatric fiberoptic intubation is the inability to perform awake fiberoptic intubation. Unlike in the adult population, pediatric patients are often unable to tolerate awake fiberoptic intubation due to lack of cooperation and may cause significant distress and discomfort.

Role of Passive Oxygenation

Due to increased oxygen consumption and lower oxygen reserve in pediatric patients, desaturation and subsequent bradycardia occur more quickly. Passive oxygenation is a method to help prolong time to desaturation and increase the time during intubation attempts. Studies have shown that passive oxygenation/apneic oxygenation *via* nasal cannula (at least 0.2 L/kg/min, ideally 1-2L/kg min with max 15 L), oral rae tube placed in the corner of the pharynx, SGA, high flow nasal cannula, or intubating mask has extended time to hypoxemia during laryngoscopy [10, 11].

Anesthetizing Techniques for Difficult Airway

As mentioned previously, pediatric fiberoptic intubations often need to take place while the patient is sedated or under general anesthesia.

If a patient's airway appears favorable for mask ventilation, one can induce general anesthesia by administering an inhalational induction with sevoflurane while maintaining spontaneous respirations. Then an IV can be started, and intravenous anesthetics can deepen the anesthetic for an intubation attempt.

If there is concern for difficulty with mask ventilation, an IV should be placed while the patient is awake. One can consider oral, intramuscular or intranasal premedication options for anxiolysis prior to IV attempt (premedication options are detailed in a separate chapter). One can also consider placing IV with administration of 50:50 nitrous: oxygen mixture in OR.

Administration of an antisialogogue (such as glycopyrrolate) can help to eliminate airway secretions. Preoxygenation with 100% FiO_2 and place a nasal cannula or oral rae in the oral cavity for passive oxygenation.

A slow intravenous induction can then be started and titrated to the patient's spontaneous respirations. One can consider intravenous anesthetics such as a propofol infusion (for older children, starting at 50-100mcg/kg min, for infants, starting at 150-200 mcg/kg/min and increasing by 25mcg/kg/min to effect), a dexmedetomidine infusion (1 mcg/kg bolus over 10 minutes followed by 0.5-1mcg/kg/hr-can re-bolus up to 4 mcg/kg) or a remifentanil infusion (0.05mcg/kg/min). The combination of dexmedetomidine and propofol, or dexmedetomidine and remifentanil, have proven to be successful infusions to keep patients sedated. One can also consider low dose propofol infusion with a low dose of sevoflurane to keep the child anesthetized but breathing spontaneously. Otherwise, ketamine (0.5-1mg/kg at a time) and midazolam (0.05-0.1mg/kg at a time) boluses have also been shown to help sedate while not affecting respirations.

Unlike in adults, local anesthetic topicalization needs to be more carefully administered due to volume limitations to keep under local anesthetic toxicity levels. Oftentimes, one can eliminate the need for topicalization if the patient is deeply anesthetized enough to suppress some airway reflexes. However, if performing a sedated intubation in an older child who is more awake, one should draw up the maximum amount of local anesthetic that can be used to prevent accidental local anesthetic toxicity, and stick to that dosage. If doing nasal intubation, one can consider only anesthetizing one nostril rather than both to help decrease the amount of local anesthetic given. Wait 30 seconds to 1 minute after administration of local anesthetic for the full numbing effect prior to continuing.

The key to anesthetizing a difficult airway in a pediatric patient is patience. One must up-titrate anesthetics slowly and continuously assess the patient to determine if the child is "deep enough" to tolerate airway manipulation while breathing spontaneously. Suggested methods to detect this include a Larson maneuver (laryngospasm notch pressure), or a jaw thrust for 5 seconds with evaluation for patient reactivity (such as an increase in heart rate, increase in respirations, or patient movement) [8].

To Paralyze or not to Paralyze

Traditionally, muscle relaxants have been avoided in difficult airway intubations. However, a recent observational study described ventilation complications (hypoxemia and laryngospasm) in spontaneously breathing patients who were "too light" *versus* those with controlled ventilation [9]. Thus, consideration could be given to administering muscle relaxants when there is airway reactivity (particularly if it causes laryngospasm and complete inability to ventilate). Contraindications to muscle relaxation include patients with mucopolysaccharidosis, history of head and neck radiation or airway masses (where relaxation can cause a further obstruction) [5].

Flexible Fiberoptic Bronchoscope Intubation Through SGA Technique

A successful innovative intubation technique in a pediatric difficult airway is the flexible fiberoptic intubation through a supraglottic airway. The benefit of this technique is that oxygenation and ventilation can be maintained *via* the SGA *via* bronchoscope adapter while the endotracheal tube can be navigated *via* the flexible fiberoptic, using the SGA as a conduit, and into the trachea. This can be beneficial to "buy time" in the emergent unanticipated difficult airway. In an analysis from the Pediatric Difficult Intubation registry, an observational study showed that first-attempt success rate was similar for video laryngoscopy *versus* fiberoptic intubation through a supraglottic airway [7].

As mentioned previously, certain SGAs (such as the air-q®) are designed to have an endotracheal tube fit through them. However, if one does not have access to the air-q® or other intubating SGAs, one can use a traditional SGA and cut the aperture bars located in the mask bowl of the SGA. This helps to prevent the fiberoptic scope and endotracheal tube from getting caught as it exits the SGA shaft.

Steps to Intubation Through SGA

1. Ensure endotracheal tube and fiberoptic scope fits through the SGA. Lubricate SGA, tube and scope.
2. Preoxygenate the patient *via* SGA and ensure the patient is adequately anesthetized and sedated. Use passive oxygenation *via* nasal cannula to help prolong the time before needing to reoxygenate the patient between tracheal intubation attempts.
3. Load endotracheal tube onto the scope and have an assistant stabilize SGA. Navigate scope through SGA (SGA may need to be adjusted to allow scope to slide through) and then slide endotracheal tube over scope.
4. Once the endotracheal tube is confirmed to be in the correct position through

the cords, remove the scope and hold the tube and SGA in the same place. Can oxygenate and ventilate through the endotracheal tube if needed.

5. Remove endotracheal tube connecting port and set aside. Deflate SGA cuff.
6. Use a second endotracheal tube to "plug" the end of the correctly placed tube to prevent it from sliding out as you remove SGA. Provide counter pressure on the tube as you remove SGA to decrease the risk of unintended extubation.
7. Once the SGA cuff is seen in the mouth, stabilize the endotracheal tube at the proximal end and remove SGA and second endotracheal tube.
8. Reconnect endotracheal tube connecting port and to circuit and confirm tracheal placement.

Glidescope® with Flexible Fiberoptic Technique

As previously mentioned, navigating the endotracheal tube into the trachea is often the most difficult portion of Glidescope® intubation due to its hyperangulated blade. One method to circumvent this problem is to intubate using a combination of Glidescope® and flexible fiberoptic. This technique leverages the advantages of both tools. The Glidescope® is used to provide an improved view of the glottis and to help displace the soft tissue and create space for the navigation of the fiberoptic and preloaded endotracheal tube. The fiberoptic functions as a flexible stylet and allows for improved mobility of the endotracheal tube to be maneuvered past any obstruction and into the trachea.

This technique would require a second practitioner since both the fiberoptic and Glidescope® would be used simultaneously.

Similar to intubating *via* SGA, one needs to make sure the patient is adequately anesthetized and passive oxygenation is implemented prior to attempt.

Anticipated Difficult Airway

Any pediatric patient that is identified to have a known difficult airway during preoperative history and physical examination should have his or her surgery conducted in a setting that has the staff, expertise, and tools in managing the pediatric difficult airway.

Other questions and considerations in planning for an anticipated difficult airway include (adapted from 16]:

1. Is the procedure elective, urgent, or emergent?
2. In the event that the airway is unable to be secured, can the patient be awakened and can an alternative airway plan be planned for a later time?
3. Are any further studies needed to evaluate the airway?

4. Can the airway be optimized prior to sedation/anesthesia?
5. What is the level of sedation (awake-rare in pediatric patients, sedated, or anesthetized) required to secure the airway?
6. If sedation or anesthesia is attempted, can a patent airway and spontaneous ventilation be preserved?
7. Should a surgical airway be electively performed?
8. What is the preferred intubation route (oral or nasal)?
9. What is the method of securing the airway (fiberoptic, video laryngoscopy, or supraglottic airway)?
10. Is the difficult airway cart available, and what equipment will be used from it?
11. If there is a loss of airway, what is the rescue route?
12. Is there a need for emergency surgical airway access, and will an ENT surgeon need to be present in the room?
13. Is there a need to prepare for emergent complex advanced rescue procedures (*i.e.*, emergent tracheostomy, sternotomy, vascular access for extracorporeal membrane oxygenation)?

If any of these considerations can be optimized for the patient at a pediatric tertiary care hospital – then the recommendation should be made to transfer to such a hospital for a higher level of care.

Fig. (**4**) depicts a flowchart with suggestions on how to manage a difficult airway in a pediatric non-tertiary hospital setting.

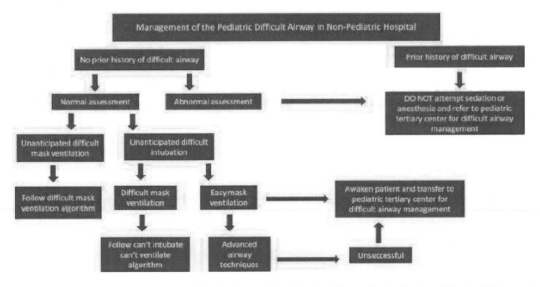

Fig. (4). Management of Pediatric Difficult Airway Outside of a Nonpediatric Tertiary Hospital (adapted from 16).

Unanticipated Difficult Airway

However, the more common emergent scenario that anesthesiologists may encounter is the unanticipated difficult airway. As previously described, the difficult pediatric airway can be subdivided into difficult mask ventilation and difficult intubation. See Fig. (5) for the difficult mask ventilation algorithm.

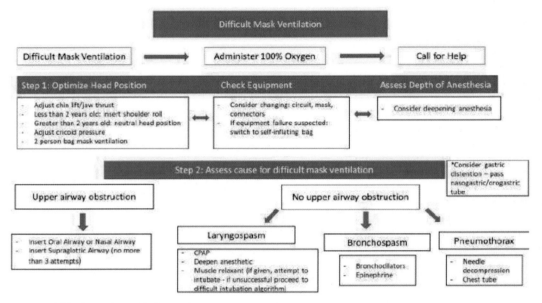

Fig. (5). Difficult mask ventilation pathway.

The most common cause of difficulty with mask ventilation is obstruction of the upper airway, this can be remedied by adjusting the head position (*i.e.*, extension) and performing a jaw thrust or chin lift. If the patient is less than 2 years old, the head may be larger in proportion to the rest of the body and cause flexion and obstruction of the airway. Thus, a shoulder roll is beneficial to relieve obstruction and open up the airway. Other methods to help with ventilation include a 2-person masking technique or inserting an oral or nasal airway or supraglottic airway.

If difficulty with mask ventilation is not due to upper airway obstruction, the two most common causes are laryngospasm or bronchospasm. Laryngospasm is due to a laryngeal reflex causing vocal cord closure (which in awake patients, protects against aspiration). In an anesthetized patient, laryngospasm can be prolonged and cause difficulty with mask ventilation and hypoxia. Treatment includes: continuous positive pressure, deepening the anesthetic with intravenous anesthetics (such as propofol 1-2mg/kg) or inhaled anesthetics (using volatile anesthetics, however, may not be effective if truly impaired ventilation), and mainstay of treatment: muscle relaxants such as succinylcholine (intravenous: 0.5 mg/kg; intramuscular: 4 mg/kg) or rocuronium (intravenous: 1.2 mg/kg) [16]. Bronchospasm is the spasm of the smooth muscles of the lower airway (bronchi) and is a vagally mediated reflex caused by histamine release or noxious stimuli and is commonly seen in patients with reactive airway disease. The mainstay of treatment includes intravenous or subcutaneously administered epinephrine and bronchodilators (although not effective in true bronchospasm where there is no gas exchange). One consideration during difficult mask ventilation that is specific to younger pediatric patients is the development of gastric distension during mask ventilation. Gastric distension may impede lung expansion and make mask ventilation impossible. If gastric distension is noted, decompression with an oral or nasal gastric tube may be needed to increase respiratory compliance.

The options for pediatric difficult intubation vary depending on whether mask ventilation is possible. As long as one is able to mask ventilate a patient, there are a variety of options available for securing the airway including, intubating through a supraglottic airway, trying different airway techniques, or awakening the child. Fig. (**6**) shows the pathway for a difficult intubation.

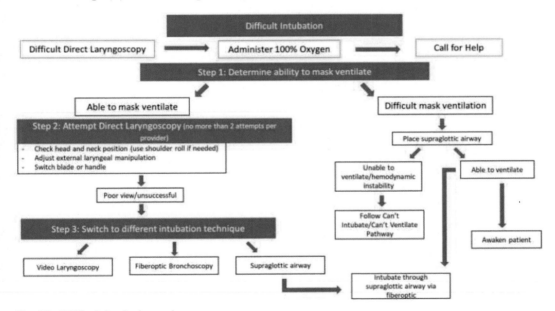

Fig. (6). Difficult intubation pathway.

Intubation attempts should be limited to a maximum of two direct laryngoscopy attempts prior to switching to a different intubating technique due to airway trauma that occurs with each attempt. It is also important during this process to continuously oxygenate the patient with either nasal cannula or supraglottic airway to help increase time to desaturation. The primary goal is to avoid entering the "cannot intubate, cannot ventilate" situation.

The "cannot intubate, cannot ventilate" scenario is a rare true emergency where mortality is high. Fig. (**7**) depicts management in this emergent situation.

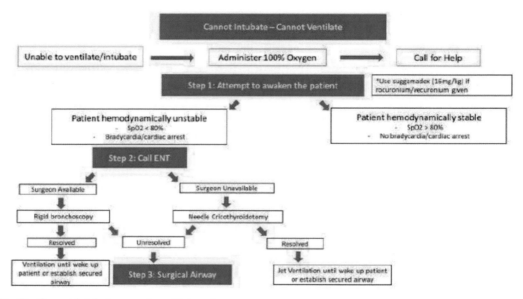

Fig. (7). Cannot intubate-cannot ventilate pathway.

When faced with a "cannot intubate – cannot ventilate" scenario, the odds of a successful outcome decrease as the age of the child decreases. The first step would be to attempt to wake the patient so that the patient could resume his or her own respirations – neuromuscular blockade reversal should be used as needed. A pediatric otolaryngologist should also be called immediately once initiation of this pathway occurs. Ideally, the surgeon would be the operator to perform a rigid bronchoscopy, or surgical airway access as necessary. However, if there is hemodynamic instability and a surgeon is not available, the anesthesiologist must perform emergent front of neck access. Front of neck access is defined as the creation of a surgical airway *via* accessing the cricothyroid membrane or anterior tracheal wall. The goal in this emergent scenario is oxygenation and not ventilation in order to prevent end organ damage or death. This is typically accomplished by an anesthesiologist *via* an emergent needle/cannula cricothyroidotomy in order to perform jet ventilation. There is a 60% success rate [17], and risks of complications, including posterior tracheal wall perforation, increase as the age of the child decreases. In addition, risks with jet ventilation include barotrauma, pneumothorax, and subcutaneous emphysema. Steps to perform emergent front of neck access: [18]

1. Place the patient in extension (shoulder roll under patient, head in extension).
2. Identify the cricothyroid membrane *via* landmarks or with the help of ultrasound.
3. Stabilize the larynx using the nondominant hand. With the dominant hand, use a 14-16 gauge angiocath and attach a 5 cc syringe filled with saline and air. Aim at a 45 degree angle caudad and aspirate until bubbles confirm in the trachea.
4. Thread angiocath over the needle and connect to an oxygen source with flows at 10-15 L/min. Cautiously inflate and allow for full expiration prior to the next inflation.
5. Maintain upper airway patency *via* oral airway or supraglottic airway (to help with expiration).

A successful cannula cricothyroidotomy is not a secured airway. It needs to be held securely at all times to avoid dislodgement or kinking of the cannula. It is also prone to blockage due to secretions and blood. Transition to a formal tracheostomy should be conducted as soon as possible by a surgeon.

If one attempts to do jet ventilation, there are jet ventilation devices on the market such as Enk Oxygen Flow Modulator® or Rapid O$_2$ insufflator®. However, if one is in an emergent situation and do not have those supplies available, one can attach the barrel of a 3 cc syringe to the end of the cannula (with the plunger removed) and fit an endotracheal tube adaptor into it which can then connect to a self-inflating bag to supply manual ventilation [19].

For younger patients (particularly neonates), cannula cricothyroidotomy becomes particularly challenging due to anatomical differences, inability to identify landmarks and higher risk of posterior wall perforation. If successful cricothyroidotomy cannot be performed, the "scalpel-finger-bougie" technique can be used as a last-ditch effort for airway access. This involves a vertical incision from the base of thyroid cartilage to top of manubrium, blunt dissection down to trachea with fingers, small horizontal incision at the identified landmark on the trachea, direct bougie insertion followed by endotracheal tube insertion [20]. This technique should only be used in the most dire situations and with impending patient demise.

Emergency Intubations Outside the Operating Room

Pediatric emergency intubations that occur outside of the operating room can be a stressful situation. Unlike in the operating room, where intubations typically occur in a controlled and selective fashion, the emergent intubation thrusts the anesthesia provider into unknown circumstances. In this environment, lack of supplies, drugs, monitoring, and skilled airway staff members in non-ideal conditions add stress and difficulty in a situation that carries a high risk of morbidity and mortality. One review of pediatric emergent intubations reported that it was three times more likely for complications to occur during the emergent intubation rather than the planned intubation and twice as likely for complications to occur during off-hours [21]. The emergency or "stat" intubation can happen in any part of the hospital, from the emergency room, to the hospital floor, to the intensive care unit. Lack of familiarity with the environment and not knowing where supplies or help arecan be very disorienting. In addition, due to the cardiopulmonary physiology of the pediatric patient and unsuccessful attempts at airway prior, one may arrive at emergent intubation to find the patient in extremis – causing increased stress and risk for error.

When an anesthesia provider is called for pediatric emergency intubation, the provider must first assess the patient's hemodynamics and "ABCs" (airway, breathing, circulation). Obtain pertinent health information from the bedside healthcare provider such as the reason for hospitalization and important cardiac and pulmonary medical history, age and weight of child, allergies, NPO status, and any known airway history. Upon assessment of the child, determine if there are concerns about a difficult airway and, if so, whether the patient's respiratory status can allow for transport to the operating room setting for controlled intubation and surgical assistance. If the child is in need of emergent intubation at bedside, one can follow the mnemonic SOAP ME as seen in Table **2** to ensure that the provider has everything for rapid sequence intubation. Ideally, another anesthesia provider should be called to assist, however during off-hours, that may not be possible. If this is to be done at bedside, the provider must clearly delineate roles and assign tasks to bedside healthcare providers to help with the management of the acute patient. Clear communication with all providers in the room is paramount to the successful intubation of a decompensating child in an unfamiliar arena.

Table 2. SOAP ME mnemonic for rapid sequence intubation.

S – Suction	- Yankauer or Soft Tip Suction
O – Oxygen	- Self-inflating bag or Mapleson with appropriate sized mask connected to oxygen source - Preoxygenate patient (keep child on noninvasive ventilation if has it with FiO_2 100%)
A – Airways	- Appropriate size cuffed endotracheal tubes (1 size below and above, consider uncuffed endotracheal tube if neonate) with stylet - Appropriate size direct laryngoscopy blade - Appropriate size oral and nasal airway, tongue depressor and lubricant for ease of placement - Appropriate size supraglottic airway and lubricant for ease of placement
P – Positioning	- Sniffing position (Place shoulder roll if appropriate)

M – Monitors and Meds	- Blood pressure (cycling every 3-5 minutes), Pulse oximetry, EKG
	- Determine working intravenous access (in emergent situation, can consider intramuscular muscle relaxant)
	- Rapid sequence induction medications dosed appropriately to weight
	  - IV induction agent (ketamine, propofol, etomidate)
	  -Muscle relaxant (succinylcholine, rocuronium)
	- Sedation infusion post-intubation

E – $EtCO_2$ and other Equipment	- Quantitative capnography or color change $EtCO_2$ cap - Back up direct laryngoscopy blade and video laryngoscopy

CONCLUSION

Difficult airways in children are a major factor in anesthesia-related morbidity and mortality. Understanding the various pathological states and syndromes that are associated with airway abnormalities is critically important. A thorough preoperative evaluation, familiarity with the newer devices for airway management, and prior preparation and planning are essential for safe anesthetic management of these children.

CONSENT FOR PUBLICATION

Not applicable.

CONFLICT OF INTEREST

The author declares no conflict of interest, financial or otherwise.

ACKNOWLEDGEMENTS

Declared none.

REFERENCES

[1]   Jagannathan N, Sohn L, Fiadjoe JE. Paediatric difficult airway management: what every anaesthetist should know! Br J Anaesth 2016; 117(S1) (Suppl. 1): i3-5.https://bjanaesthesia.org/article/S0007-0912(17)33760-1/pdf
        [http://dx.doi.org/10.1093/bja/aew054] [PMID: 27095241]

[2]   El-Emam EM, El Motlb EAA. Blind tracheal intubation through the Air-Q intubating laryngeal airway in pediatric patients: Reevaluation–A randomized controlled trial. Anesth Essays Res 2019; 13(2): 269-73.
        [http://dx.doi.org/10.4103/aer.AER_42_19] [PMID: 31198243]

[3]   Zhang B, Gurnaney HG, Stricker PA, Galvez JA, Isserman RS, Fiadjoe JE. A prospective observational study of technical difficulty with GlideScope-guided tracheal intubation in children. Anesth Analg 2018; 127(2): 467-71.
        [http://dx.doi.org/10.1213/ANE.0000000000003412] [PMID: 29750689]

[4]   Channa AB. Video laryngoscopes. Saudi J Anaesth 2011; 5(4): 357-9.
        [http://dx.doi.org/10.4103/1658-354X.87262] [PMID: 22144919]

[5]   Fiadjoe J, Nishisaki A. Normal and difficult airways in children: "What's New"-Current evidence. Paediatr Anaesth 2020; 30(3): 257-63.
        [http://dx.doi.org/10.1111/pan.13798] [PMID: 31869488]

[6]   Xue FS, Liu YY, Li HX, Yang GZ. Paediatric video laryngoscopy and airway management: What's the clinical evidence? Anaesth Crit Care Pain Med 2018; 37(5): 459-66.
        [http://dx.doi.org/10.1016/j.accpm.2017.11.018] [PMID: 29331616]

[7]   Burjek NE, Nishisaki A, Fiadjoe JE, et al. Videolaryngoscopy versus Fiber-optic Intubation through a Supraglottic Airway in Children with a Difficult AirwayAn Analysis from the Multicenter Pediatric Difficult Intubation Registry. Anesthesiology. Anesthesiology 2017; 127(3): 432-40.
        [http://dx.doi.org/10.1097/ALN.0000000000001758] [PMID: 28650415]

[8]   Abelson D. Laryngospasm notch pressure ('Larson's maneuver') may have a role in laryngospasm management in children: highlighting a so far unproven technique. Paediatr Anaesth 2015; 25(11): 1175-6.
        [http://dx.doi.org/10.1111/pan.12731] [PMID: 26426878]

[9]   Garcia-Marcinkiewicz AG, Adams HD, Gurnaney H, et al. A Retrospective Analysis of Neuromuscular Blocking Drug Use and Ventilation Technique on Complications in the Pediatric Difficult Intubation Registry Using Propensity Score Matching. Anesth Analg 2019.
        [PMID: 31567318]

[10]   Riva T, Pedersen TH, Seiler S, et al. Transnasal humidified rapid insufflation ventilatory exchange for oxygenation of children during apnoea: a prospective randomised controlled trial. Br J Anaesth 2018; 120(3): 592-9.
        [http://dx.doi.org/10.1016/j.bja.2017.12.017] [PMID: 29452816]

[11]   Stein ML, Park RS, Kovatsis PG. Emerging trends, techniques, and equipment for airway management in pediatric patients. Paediatr Anaesth 2020; 30(3): 269-79.
        [http://dx.doi.org/10.1111/pan.13814] [PMID: 32022437]

[12]   Jimenez N, Posner KL, Cheney FW, Caplan RA, Lee LA, Domino KB. An update on pediatric anesthesia liability: a closed claims analysis. Anesth Analg 2007; 104(1): 147-53.
        [http://dx.doi.org/10.1213/01.ane.0000246813.04771.03] [PMID: 17179260]

[13]   Ramamoorthy C, Haberkern CM, Bhananker SM, et al. Anesthesia-related cardiac arrest in children with heart disease: data from the Pediatric Perioperative Cardiac Arrest (POCA) registry. Anesth Analg 2010; 110(5): 1376-82.
        [http://dx.doi.org/10.1213/ANE.0b013e3181c9f927] [PMID: 20103543]

[14]   Huang AS, Hajduk J, Rim C, Coffield S, Jagannathan N. Focused review on management of the

difficult paediatric airway. Indian J Anaesth 2019; 63(6): 428-36.
[http://dx.doi.org/10.4103/ija.IJA_250_19] [PMID: 31263293]

[15]   Fiadjoe JE, Nishisaki A, Jagannathan N, *et al.* Airway management complications in children with difficult tracheal intubation from the Pediatric Difficult Intubation (PeDI) registry: a prospective cohort analysis. Lancet Respir Med 2016; 4(1): 37-48.
[http://dx.doi.org/10.1016/S2213-2600(15)00508-1] [PMID: 26705976]

[16]   Krishna SG, Bryant JF, Tobias JD. Management of the difficult airway in the pediatric patient. J Pediatr Intensive Care 2018; 7(3): 115-25.
[http://dx.doi.org/10.1055/s-0038-1624576] [PMID: 31073483]

[17]   Stacey J, Heard AM, Chapman G, *et al.* The 'Can't Intubate Can't Oxygenate' scenario in Pediatric Anesthesia: a comparison of different devices for needle cricothyroidotomy. Paediatr Anaesth 2012; 22(12): 1155-8.
[http://dx.doi.org/10.1111/pan.12048] [PMID: 23066666]

[18]   Henderson JJ, Popat MT, Latto IP, Pearce AC. Difficult Airway Society guidelines for management of the unanticipated difficult intubation. Anaesthesia 2004; 59(7): 675-94.
[http://dx.doi.org/10.1111/j.1365-2044.2004.03831.x] [PMID: 15200543]

[19]   Chong CF, Wang TL, Chang H. Percutaneous transtracheal ventilation without a jet ventilator. Am J Emerg Med 2003; 21(6): 507-8.
[http://dx.doi.org/10.1016/S0735-6757(03)00166-9] [PMID: 14574664]

[20]   Sabato SC, Long E. An institutional approach to the management of the 'Can't Intubate, Can't Oxygenate' emergency in children. Paediatr Anaesth 2016; 26(8): 784-93.
[http://dx.doi.org/10.1111/pan.12926] [PMID: 27277897]

[21]   Carroll CL, Spinella PC, Corsi JM, Stoltz P, Zucker AR. Emergent endotracheal intubations in children: be careful if it's late when you intubate. Pediatr Crit Care Med 2010; 11(3): 343-8.
[PMID: 20464775]

CHAPTER 8

Pediatric Trauma Patient

Kathleen Kwiatt[1] and **Fatimah Habib[1]**

[1] Department of Anesthesiology, Cooper Medical School of Rowan University, Cooper University Health Care, Camden NJ, USA

Abstract: Every day in the United States, 33 children on average will die from an injury, and another 25 thousand will suffer a nonfatal injury. Given this tragically high incidence, anesthesiologists must prepare for the management of traumatic events, regardless of whether one's routine practice includes pediatrics. The anesthesiologist has the opportunity to add value at multiple points of care: initial assessment and airway management; intraoperative and resuscitative efforts; providing sedation to facilitate diagnostics and procedures; pain management. Advanced trauma life support (ATLS) has devised algorithms and guidelines to simplify and standardize the initial assessment and treatment of the trauma patient. Familiarity with and adherence to these guidelines improves morbidity and mortality outcomes. This chapter will explore the common risks that children face and how to respond when trauma occurs.

Keywords: Abdominal trauma, Burns, Cervical spine clearance, Epinephrine, Full stomach, GCS, Massive transfusion, Missed injuries, Pediatric airway characteristics, Pediatric trauma, Pediatric vital signs, Primary survey, SAMPLE, Secondary survey, Shock, Sugammadex, Tension pneumothorax, Thoracic trauma, Thromboembolism, Tranexamic acid, Traumatic brain injury, Traumatic airway, Whole blood.

INTRODUCTION

Pediatric trauma is the leading cause of morbidity and mortality for children under the age of 19 and results in more deaths than all other causes combined for this age group. An average of 12,000 children die annually in the United States from an injury. An additional 9.2 million present to an emergency department with a nonfatal injury. Pediatric trauma patients are not just miniature adults; both the mechanisms of injury and causes of mortality differ from those observed in adults. The leading cause of injury-related mortality varies by age. Children under 1 year old are most likely to suffocate, ages 1-4 are most likely to drown, and ages 5-19

* **Corresponding author Bharathi Gourkanti:** Department of Anesthesiology, Cooper Medical School of Rowan University, Cooper University Health Care, Camden NJ, USA; E-mail: gourkantibharathi@ cooperhealth.edu

Bharathi Gourkanti, Irwin Gratz, Grace Dippo, Nathalie Peiris and Dinesh K. Choudhry (Eds.)
All rights reserved-© 2022 Bentham Science Publishers

are most likely to die from a motor vehicle collision. Over 80% of deaths result from a head injury. Gunshot victims die as a result of their injuries at the highest rate [1].

For each death, another 40 children are hospitalized, and over 1100 require emergency treatment for their injuries. Males and females are at equal risk until age 1 when the incidence becomes higher in males. Falls are the leading cause of nonfatal injury, and other common causes include animal bites, poisoning, blunt force trauma, burns, drowning, and motor vehicle collisions. Blunt force trauma occurs 9 times for every 1 episode of penetrating trauma, and children are less likely to suffer penetrating trauma compared to adults [1].

Each childhood injury impacts the future of the child, their family, and their community. Trauma creates physical, emotional, temporal, and financial burdens. Understanding these statistics creates an impetus to identify and reduce risks with preventative measures, and to prepare to manage the events when they cannot be prevented. The anesthesiologist plays an important role in the effort to reduce morbidity and mortality through pre-hospital planning, airway management and resuscitative efforts, intraoperative care, and pain management, and contributes to a reduction of the burdens to patients, families, and society.

PRE-HOSPITAL PLANNING

Whenever possible, young and seriously injured children should be transported to pediatric trauma facilities, as in-hospital mortality outcomes are improved at pediatric centers. However, every facility that provides emergency care must prepare to resuscitate and stabilize a child because an injured child can present to any emergency department. Time is critical, so to promote efficiency, roles and responsibilities should be delineated prior to patient arrival. The following roles and responsibilities should be appointed: team leader, primary and secondary survey, airway management (often an anesthesia provider), establishing IV access and obtaining laboratory samples (sometimes an anesthesia provider), and monitoring vital signs. It is important to perform these tasks simultaneously and not sequentially [2].

After assigning roles, ensure that equipment is available and prepared for use. At a minimum, suction, oxygen, bag-valve mask, intubation equipment, anesthetics and neuromuscular agents, resuscitation medications, defibrillator, code cart, warming devices, and trauma shears should be immediately accessible and in working order. Obtain blood and a CPR board when clinically warranted. Personnel should don protective equipment. All teams that will be involved in the care of the trauma patient should be notified of the impending arrival, including the operating room, radiology, and the intensive care unit. While trauma centers often coordinate the supply of equipment, the responsibility of airway equipment and medications is often delegated to the anesthesia team, especially in community hospitals. A summary of prehospital planning is presented in Table **1**.

Table 1. Prehospital Planning.

Equipment	Medications*	Identify Roles	Notify Teams
- Ambu Bag - Mask - Oxygen - Suction - Monitors - IV/ IO access equipment - Intubation cart - Defibrillator/ code cart - Warming devices - Trauma shears - Broselow tape - CPR board	**Induction** - Propofol - Etomidate - Ketamine **Muscle Relaxants** - Succinylcholine - Rocuronium **Reversal** - Sugammadex - Naloxone - Flumazenil **Resuscitation** - Atropine - Epinephrine **Blood**	- Team leader - Airway (often an anesthesiology provider) - IV/ IO access + labs - Vitals - Primary survey - Record keeper	- OR - Radiology - ICU

* selection should be appropriate for the clinical scenario

Prior to patient arrival, the team should be briefed on the expected patient, with as much information as possible: name, age, mechanism of injury, current condition, allergies, and past medical history. An estimated weight should be determined. Commonly used techniques to estimate patient weight include the Broselow tape, the Leffler formula, and the Theron formula [3] (Table **2**). The Broselow tape is a color-coded tape that estimates a patient's weight based on height and provides recommended medication doses and equipment sizes based on that measurement. The Broselow tape is accurate for children <143 cm in height and outperforms mathematical formulas for children ≤25 kg. The Leffler formula estimates weight based on age and performs similarly to the Broselow tape for patients 25.1 − 40 kg. The Theron formula also estimates weight based on age and is more accurate than the Broselow tape in patients > 40 kg, as the Broselow tape underestimates weight in the setting of obesity [6].

Table 2. Leffler and Theron formulas to estimate weight.

	Leffler Formula	Theron Formula
Age < 1	$m = 1/2 \cdot a_m + 4$	
Ages 1 - 10	$m = 2a_y + 10$	$m = e^{0.175571x\ a_y\ +\ 2.197099}$

KEY
m = weight in kilograms
a_m = age (months)
a_y = age (years)

PRIMARY SURVEY

Systematic assessment of the pediatric trauma patient according to Advanced Trauma Life Support (ATLS) protocols begins with the primary survey, as summarized in Table **8** [4, 5]. The majority of trauma-related deaths are the direct result of hemorrhagic shock, respiratory failure, or brain injuries. The primary survey facilitates a sequential patient evaluation to identify the most life-threatening processes first so that they can be addressed before progressing through the algorithm. Utilizing the **ABCDE** mnemonic, the primary survey should be applied universally to each trauma patient to avoid overlooking a mortal injury. Resuscitation is initiated at any time it is needed during this assessment.

A: Airway. Evaluate the airway for patency. Talking or crying provides reassurance that the airway is patent. Suction blood and vomit and remove foreign bodies (dislodged teeth). The tongue is the most common cause of obstruction in unconscious patients. Maneuvers to open the airway include performing a chin lift or jaw thrust and insertion of an oral or nasal airway. Advanced airway management, including considerations for difficult traumatic airways and cervical spine management, is detailed later in this chapter.

B: Breathing. Evaluate breathing by inspection, palpation, percussion, and auscultation. Determine the respiratory rate, the normal respiratory rate per age is presented in Table **3**. Tachypnea is compensatory for respiratory distress and is also seen with pain and agitation. Bradypnea is an ominous sign and suggests that the patient's compensatory mechanisms have been exhausted or that the patient suffers from a toxic exposure (drugs, alcohol, organophosphates, carbon monoxide), and respiratory arrest is imminent. Inspect for tracheal deviation, flail chest, and penetrating injuries. Palpate for subcutaneous emphysema. Percuss and auscultate to expose tension pneumothorax and hemothorax. Apply supplemental oxygen. Prepare an advanced airway if the patient remains hypoxic with an oxygen saturation <90% despite administering 100% FiO_2.

Table 3. Normal Respiratory rate (Breaths per minute: bpm) [1].

Infant	30 – 60 bpm
Toddler	24 – 40 bpm
Preschool	22 – 34 bpm
School age	18 – 30 bpm
Adolescent	12 – 16 bpm

C: Circulation. Pallor and cyanosis provide the first clue about circulation. The lips, tongue, and mucus membranes reveal cyanosis that is otherwise difficult to observe in dark-skinned patients. Palpate peripheral and central pulses for at least 30 seconds to account for the expected variability in pediatric heart rate; note normal heart rate per age, as shown in Table **4**. Weak pulses, prolonged capillary refill > 2 seconds, and tachycardia are indicative of hypovolemia or hemorrhage. Measure blood pressure. Hypotensive values for age are shown in Table **5** .

Sinus tachycardia is a normal response to hemorrhage, hypovolemia, fever, and pain. Bradycardia is an ominous sign, and a heart rate < 60 beats per minute requires immediate attention in a distressed infant/child. First, assist oxygenation and ventilation in a bradycardic child. If the heart rate fails to improve with ventilation or if the child is unconscious, start chest compressions while treating the underlying etiology [13].

Table 4. Normal Heart Rate [7].

Age	Heart Rate – Awake	Heart Rate - Asleep
Newborn – 3 months	85 – 205	80 – 160
3 months – 2 years	100 – 190	75 – 160
2 – 10 years	60 – 140	60 – 90
> 10 years	60 – 100	50 - 90

Table 5. Hypotension [7].

Age	Systolic BP
0 – 4 weeks	< 60 mmHg
1 – 12 months	< 70 mmHg
1 – 10 years	< 70 + (age x 2)
> 10 years	< 90 mmHg

Obtain intravascular access. If unsuccessful after 2 attempts or 90 seconds, establish intraosseous access. Common Insertion Sites for Intraosseous Access (Fig. **1**)

- Proximal Tibia: 1-2 cm medial + inferior to the tibial tuberosity
- Distal Tibia: 1-2 cm superior to the medial malleolus
- Proximal Humerus: 1 cm superior to the surgical neck
- Distal Femur: 0-1 cm proximal to patella + 1-2 cm medial to the midline while displacing soft tissue

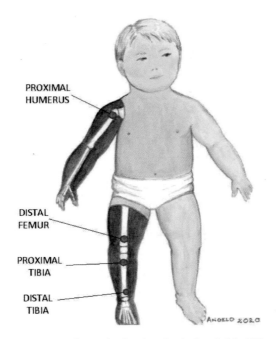

Fig. (1). Intraosseous insertion sites. Illustration by Angelo Andonakakis, DO.

Resuscitation with fluids and blood is initiated at this time and is discussed in detail in this chapter under the management of shock.

D: Disability + Neurologic Evaluation. The mnemonic AVPU is a rapid, simple tool to evaluate if the patient is **A**lert, responds to **V**oice, responds to **P**ain, or is **U**nconscious. The Glasgow Coma Scale (GCS) provides another quick, objective mechanism to evaluate consciousness with increased detail (Table **6**). The GCS assigns a numerical value to each of three parameters: eye-opening, verbal response, and motor response, and ranges from 3 (deeply unconscious) to 15 (fully conscious). A GCS score >12 is associated with mild injury [9 - 12] reflects a conscious patient with a moderate injury, and <9 correlates with severe head trauma and poor outcomes. It is best to establish a baseline that can be used for comparison prior to sedating or intubating medications, and motor function should be assessed on the least affected limb. Because young children are unable to perform certain tasks, a modified scale is used for children <2 years (Table 7). Common causes of diminished consciousness in children include hypoglycemia, intoxication, and inadequate oxygenation, ventilation, or perfusion. If these have been excluded, traumatic brain injury should be considered the etiology until proven otherwise [8].

Table 6. Glasgow Coma Scale [9].

	EYES	VERBAL	MOTOR
1	Closed	None	none
2	Opens to pain	Makes sounds	Decerebrate posturing: extension to painful stimuli
3	Opens to sound	Speaks words	Decorticate posturing: abnormal flexion to painful stimuli
4	Spontaneous	Confused	Flexion/withdrawal to painful stimuli
5	-	Oriented	Localizes to painful stimuli
6	-	-	Obeys commands

Table 7. Glasgow Coma Scale Modified for Infants and Young Children.

	EYES	VERBAL	MOTOR
1	Closed	None	None
2	Opens to pain	Moans in response to painful stimuli	Decerebrate posturing: abnormal extension to painful stimuli
3	Opens to sound	Cries with response to painful stimuli, inconsistently consolable	Decorticate posturing: abnormal flexion to painful stimuli
4	Spontaneous	Cries but consolable	Withdraws from painful stimuli
5	-	Coos + babbles	Withdraws from touch
6	-	-	Spontaneous, purposeful movement

E: Exposure + Environmental Control. The patient should be completely undressed and exposed. This removes potentially harmful substances retained in the patient's clothing and ensures that injuries are not missed. Hypothermia is prevented by covering the patient with warm blankets or using warming devices.

Table 8. Primary Survey.

A: Airway	Confirm airway patency Maintain c-spine immobilization Chin lift: place thumb under the chin and lift forward Jaw thrust: lace fingers behind angle of mandible, push anterior + superior
B: Breathing	Evaluate breathing, ventilation, and oxygenation Apply oxygen to hypoxic patients Treat tension pneumothorax, open pneumothorax, and hemothorax when present
C: Circulation	Check pulses (presence, quality, rate; first distal, then central if needed) Check capillary refill (reassuring when <2 seconds) Observe for pallor + cyanosis Identify obvious hemorrhage, control with direct pressure or tourniquet Obtain IV or IO access Administer crystalloid: 20 mL/kg bolus if evidence of hypovolemia Transfuse blood: 10 mL/kg bolus if not responsive to crystalloid
D: Disability and Neurologic Status	Determine Glasgow Coma Scale (GCS) Check pupil size and response Identify signs of increased intracranial pressure/impending cerebral herniation
E: Exposure + Environmental Control	Completely remove clothing to evaluate injuries Warm with blanket + warming devices Check temperature

SECONDARY SURVEY

Traumatic injuries are not always immediately apparent. ATLS guided assessment continues with the secondary survey for all trauma patients to decrease missed injuries and facilitate early treatment. Like the primary survey, resuscitation is initiated at any time it is needed during this assessment.

The secondary survey begins with a history, which can be obtained from the patient when age and condition permit but often requires input from family members (optimal) or EMS (if others are unavailable or unable).

The **SAMPLE** mnemonic guides a quick and focused history:

Obtaining detailed events of the injury reduces missed injuries. For example, a lower extremity fracture resulting from a motor vehicle accident raises suspicion of blunt force injuries to the abdomen and thorax, while the same injury obtained while evacuating a fire raises concern for inhalational injuries and hazardous chemical exposure.

A focused physical exam follows, first evaluating unstable and injured systems, followed by a thorough physical exam [11].

Head and neck: Visualize and palpate the scalp for hematoma, skull depression, or laceration. Assess pupil size and response, and identify periorbital ecchymosis (raccoon eyes). Blood or cerebrospinal fluid (CSF) drainage in the ear canal indicates a basilar skull fracture with CSF leak (avoid nasal airways and nasogastric tubes for risk of penetrating the anterior cranial fossa). Observe the ears for hemotympanum or retro-auricular ecchymosis. Presume cervical spine injury in blunt force trauma until proven otherwise. Inspect and palpate the neck for external injuries, being sure to look under the collar.

Chest: Palpate the chest wall for crepitus. Auscultate the heart and lungs. Sternal or clavicle fractures require substantial forces and raise concern for intrathoracic injuries.

Abdomen: Examine the abdomen for distention and tenderness. Bruising, especially the presence of a seatbelt sign, suggests evolving intraabdominal injuries.

Perineal Exam: Visually inspect the perineum. Gross blood at the rectal vault suggests a bowel injury, while blood at the urethral meatus suggests a urethral injury. When blood is present at the meatus, perform a retrograde urethrogram prior to insertion of a bladder catheter. Perform a rectal exam; diminished sphincter tone is concerning for spinal cord injury.

Pelvis: Palpate the pubis and anterior iliac spines for instability, and observe for ecchymosis.

Extremities: Palpate each extremity for tenderness. Immobilize injured joints and obtain radiographs. Assess uninjured joints for passive and active range of motion. Evaluate vascular function by examining pulses and capillary refill.

Neurologic: Assess sensory and motor function. Repeat the Glasgow Coma Scale.

Skin: Examine for lacerations, abrasions, ecchymosis, and hematomas. Give particular attention to the scalp, folds (axillary, abdominal, gluteal), perineum, and back.

Missed injuries are frequently present in the following scenarios:

• Blunt trauma: bowel injury, pancreatic injury, duodenal injury, diaphragmatic rupture

- Penetrating trauma: rectal injury
- Extremity trauma: compartment syndrome, distal extremity fractures.

AIRWAY MANAGEMENT

Noninvasive Airway Management: Airway obstruction is one of the most pressing concerns in a trauma patient, requiring swift assessment and intervention to prevent asphyxia. Pediatric airways are smaller and narrower, and therefore more susceptible to obstruction. Blood, emesis, edema, displaced pharyngeal tissue, bones, or cartilage, hematoma formation, and foreign bodies are frequent causes of airway obstruction. Initial maneuvers include oropharyngeal suctioning, chin lift, jaw thrust, and insertion of oral and nasal airways. Nasal airways (and nasogastric tubes) should be avoided if a basilar skull fracture is suspected (blood or CSF drainage in the ear canal), due to the risk of penetrating the anterior cranial fossa. Apply oxygen, and initiate bag-mask ventilation for patients needing assistance. Simultaneously, the cervical spine is immobilized by an assistant using two-hand manual axial stabilization.

Indications for Definitive Airway Management: When noninvasive airway management is insufficient, definitive airway control with a cuffed endotracheal tube or surgical airway is indicated (Table **9**). Intubation is appropriate for airway protection in the following scenarios: GCS <9, severe maxillofacial fractures, laryngeal or tracheal injury, evolving neck hematoma, or inhalation injury. Definitive airway control is also indicated for hypoxia or hypercarbia unresolved by the noninvasive oxygen therapy, shock, multiple severe injuries, and the need to induce anesthesia. Early endotracheal intubation is recommended before edema develops in victims with inhalation injuries. Early intubation and mechanical ventilation in children <16 years with severe head injuries and developing intracranial hypertension have improved mortality in retrospective studies. The surgical airway is performed when definitive airway control is necessary, and the patient cannot be intubated.

Tracheal placement of an airway must be **confirmed by capnography or exhaled carbon dioxide** in patients with a perfusing rhythm (level IIa evidence) [2].

Table 9. Indications for definitive airway management.

-	Indications for Definitive Airway Management
Unable to protect the airway	GCS< 9 Severe maxillofacial fractures Laryngeal/ tracheal injury Evolving neck hematoma Inhalation injury

(Table 9) cont.....

-	Indications for Definitive Airway Management
Inadequate oxygenation/ ventilation	Apnea Hypoxia: SpO_2 <90% despite FiO_2 100% Hypercarbia Respiratory distress
Surgical Airway	Need for definitive airway control when the patient cannot be intubated

Full Stomach: Trauma patients are considered to have full stomachs irrespective of the fasting interval because heightened sympathetic tone impedes gastric emptying, and swallowed blood and foreign bodies are common. The goal during airway management is to decrease the interval from loss of consciousness to secured airway. Rapid sequence induction (RSI) after adequate preoxygenation with 100% oxygen is appropriate unless there is a compelling contraindication, such as anticipated or known difficult airway. For the purpose of preventing aspiration, the application of **cricoid pressure** can distort the anatomy and make intubation difficult because pediatric tracheas are more compressible and easily obscured compared to adults. **Cricoid manipulation**, or external airway manipulation at the level of the cricoid cartilage guided by the intubating practitioner, can improve the laryngeal view and facilitate intubation. Cricoid pressure can be considered, but should not be performed at the expense of increasing the time interval to intubation. Awake intubation with topical anesthesia with or without sedation is appropriate when a difficult airway is anticipated. After intubation, the stomach should be decompressed with an orogastric or nasogastric (if no evidence of basilar skull fracture) tube.

LMAs: While the presence of a full stomach precludes elective laryngeal mask airway (LMA) use, they serve valuable roles in select clinical circumstances. LMAs are lifesaving rescue devices for cannot intubate, cannot ventilate scenarios. They are also useful guides for fiberoptic intubation. Temporary ventilation with an LMA can provide time to prepare advanced airway equipment or to prepare for a surgical airway in the setting of a difficult airway. The use of LMAs should be limited, as they do not protect against aspiration.

Cervical Spine Precautions: Cervical spine injury is assumed for any patient presenting blunt force trauma and any trauma resulting in the loss of consciousness. The cervical spine should be stabilized throughout airway management to prevent flexion, extension, and rotation. This can be achieved with manual in-line stabilization, collars, hardboard with sandbags, or traction pins. The gold standard for neck stabilization is the combined use of a hardboard, collar, sandbags, and tape or straps, which limits movement to 5% of the normal range [14, 16]. This is ideal for patient transport but impedes airway management. The majority of intubations with this technique resulted in a grade III-IV view on laryngoscopy. A practical approach for intubation is achieved using a two-person manual axial stabilization. The anterior hard collar is removed to improve mouth opening while an assistant stands at the head or side of the bed and uses both hands to stabilize the occipital and mastoid processes during intubation. While direct laryngoscopy is often successful with this technique, video laryngoscopy is helpful to improve the view of the larynx without neck extension. After endotracheal tube placement is confirmed, the collar should be replaced on the patient before performing further care.

As long as the child is alert, a clinical assessment is satisfactory to clear the cervical spine, there is no midline tenderness, there is no neurologic deficit, there are no distracting injuries, there is no intoxication, and there is no unexplained hypotension. Children < 3 years must have a GCS > 13. Additionally, the mechanism of an injury must not be a motor vehicle accident, a fall > 10 feet, or nonaccidental trauma. When the above criteria are not met, the cervical spine should be imaged. The type of imaging remains a topic of debate, and there is no good evidence to support x-ray *versus* CT scan. Researchers are exploring combined clinical clearance with plain film x-rays for most patients and limiting focused CT scans to high-risk patients. This aims to balance the immediate risk of missed spinal cord injury with the future risk of malignancy from radiation exposure. It is reasonable to defer to local institutional policies combined with the clinical judgment of the neurosurgical, orthopedic, and trauma specialists until additional evidence is available.

Pediatric Anatomy and Physiology: There are fundamental differences between a pediatric and an adult airway. These differences impact mask ventilation, laryngoscopy, and intubation, but can be overcome by modifying techniques and equipment. Pediatric patients have an increased basal metabolic rate and consume more oxygen per kilogram compared to adults. Their increased rate of oxygen consumption is further elevated in the setting of tachycardia, fever, or agitation. The result is a decreased apnea-to-hypoxia interval. Therefore, one must prepare equipment, medications, algorithms, backup plans, and personnel to safely secure a pediatric airway, especially in the setting of trauma, where airway management is complicated by the presenting injuries.

Difficult Airways: Pediatric trauma patients are at risk for having difficult airways due to baseline features, as described in Table **10** (obesity, short neck, recessed mandible, large tongue, and congenital facial deformities) and due to direct airway trauma. Maxillofacial injuries make visualization during laryngoscopy difficult due to being obscured by blood and debris and due to expanding edema and hematomas of the oropharynx. Bilateral mandibular condylar fractures make mouth opening difficult. Blunt or penetrating neck injuries distort pharyngeal and laryngeal anatomy, and edema and hematomas both make visualization of the cords and passage of an endotracheal tube difficult. Edema and hematomas can also cause abrupt airway obstruction due to the loss of tone with neuromuscular blockade, impeding both ventilation and intubation [17].

Management options for the difficult airway must be individualized to prioritize the patient's injuries, including airway and cervical spine injuries, current airway status, hemodynamic stability, and aspiration risk, weighing each risk against the other. Decisions must also consider institutional resources, the provider's skill set, and location. When time permits (if hemodynamically stable and without acute hypoxia), consider transportation to the operating room for airway management with emergency tracheostomy equipment and a surgeon available. Clinical judgment is used to decide whether direct laryngoscopy, video laryngoscopy (GlideScope ®), awake or sedated fiberoptic bronchoscopy, or surgical airway is most appropriate. If difficult ventilation and intubation are expected, muscle relaxants should be withheld until after endotracheal tube placement.

Table 10. Key characteristics of the pediatric airway, their clinical implication, and techniques to facilitate airway management [2].

Key Characteristics	Clinical Implications	Techniques to Facilitate Airway Management
Large occiput	- Increased risk for airway obstruction with neck flexion - Alignment of the oropharynx/larynx/trachea during laryngoscopy can be difficult, making it more difficult to visualize the vocal cords	- Position with neck extension using a folded towel/blanket under the shoulders
Large tongue + tonsils	- Airway obstruction - Difficult to visualize vocal cords during laryngoscopy	- Jaw thrust with in-line neck stabilization - Mask ventilation with oral or nasopharyngeal airways - Straight laryngoscope blade - Video laryngoscopy
Omega shaped epiglottis	- An obscured view of vocal cords during laryngoscopy	- Consider straight blade for laryngoscopy

Key Characteristics	Clinical Implications	Techniques to Facilitate Airway Management
Higher larynx, cricoid at the level of C4	- The acute angle of vocal cords increases the difficulty of laryngoscopy/intubation	- Infants: roll under shoulders - Child: sniffing position with a towel under the head - Video laryngoscopy - Stylet ETT with bend

(Table 10) cont.....

Key Characteristics	Clinical Implications	Techniques to Facilitate Airway Management
Smaller, conical-shaped larynx (vs. cylindrical); with the narrowest opening at the level of cricoid (below cords)	- Difficulty passing an endotracheal tube	- Prepare multiple ETT sizes, consider downsizing ½ size with a cuffed ETT
Compressible trachea	- At risk for tracheal compression with cricoid pressure	- Apply gentle cricoid, release if visualization is obscured. - Decrease time from induction to intubation to minimize aspiration risk without applying cricoid
Developing teeth	- Susceptible to injury, avulsion, aspiration	- Gentle mouth opening + intubation, suction available
Short apnea to hypoxia interval	- Increased basal metabolic rate leads to increased oxygen consumption and decreased time to hypoxia during the period of apnea	- Pre-oxygenate - Skilled airway provider - Multiple equipment sizes - Familiarity with the difficult airway algorithm

MANAGEMENT OF SHOCK: FLUIDS, BLOOD, AND TXA

Hemorrhage is the most common cause of shock in the setting of trauma and the leading cause of mortality in pediatric trauma patients with solid organ injuries. Frank bleeding is a telltale sign, but blood can accumulate undetected in an infant's expandable head and open fontanelles, in the pelvis, or the abdomen. The small absolute blood volume in very young children risks underestimation of the percentage of blood loss. Less frequent causes of shock include pericardial tamponade, blunt myocardial injury (myocardial contusion, coronary artery injury, rupture of the cardiac wall, septum, or valve), pneumo- or hemothorax, and neurogenic shock.

Children have heightened sympathetic tone and peripheral vasoconstriction, allowing them to maintain near-normal blood pressure until 25-35% of their circulating blood volume is lost. Tachycardia, delayed capillary refill >2 seconds, and thready pulses are better indicators of an impending shock than blood pressure alone. Patients with evidence of hypovolemia or hemorrhage should be administered a bolus of **20 mL/kg** of warmed **isotonic crystalloid.** If the patient does not improve with 1 bolus of crystalloid due to persistent hypovolemia or hemorrhage, new recommendations advise a bolus of **10 mL/kg of blood.** This recommendation deviates from the previously recommended 2 boluses of crystalloid because most children who require a second bolus of crystalloid also require a blood transfusion. By administering blood earlier in resuscitation, oxygen-carrying capacity is improved, coagulopathy is minimized, and the adverse effects of excess crystalloid, including pulmonary edema and intraabdominal hypertension, are mitigated [18, 19].

Whole Blood: The use of whole blood is gaining popularity in adult trauma care. Whole blood decreases the total number of blood products needed, exposing the patient to fewer donors, decreasing the allergen exposure and infection risk. It is associated with improved survival in adults when administered at the site of injury, compared with crystalloid or blood components. Its use in pediatrics is limited but demonstrates promise. Two trauma centers currently administer whole blood to pediatric patients. The University of Texas at San Antonio transfuses whole blood in children ages 5 and above in the field or upon arrival at the hospital, and the University of Pittsburgh administers it to children over age 2. Other facilities offer whole blood on a trial basis. The use of whole blood is evolving, and it is anticipated to play a larger role in pediatric resuscitation as more data becomes available [20].

Massive Transfusion: Balanced resuscitation of packed red blood cells (PRBCs), plasma, and platelets in a 1:1:1 or similarly defined ratio is the accepted standard for the management of adult hemorrhage. The trials in pediatric hemorrhaging patients are limited to small, nonrandomized studies or retrospective/database reviews. When comparing the administration of blood products with set ratios compared to the administration of blood products at the discretion of the physician, there was **no difference in mortality**. At this time, there is no evidence that a rigid 1:1:1 transfusion ratio of PRBCs:plasma:platelets will improve mortality. However, larger studies are needed. It is possible that mortality will be impacted, or additional outcome measures such as morbidity, duration of mechanical ventilation, or hospital length of stay, will justify a particular resuscitation strategy with additional evidence [21, 22].

TXA: Tranexamic acid (TXA), while not well studied in pediatric trauma, has proven beneficial for reducing blood loss and transfusion requirements for pediatric cardiac surgery, scoliosis surgery, and craniosynostosis repair. TXA has been studied in adult trauma patients and is associated with reduced mortality; it saves 1/67 adult lives in patients with hemodynamic instability and bleeding.

There is no physiologic reason to suggest that children would not have a similar benefit.

A primary concern with TXA is a thromboembolism; however, relative to adults, pediatric patients have healthier vascular systems and are at reduced risk. TXA doses used for scoliosis and cardiac surgery are larger than for trauma, and even at these high TXA doses, thrombosis is not reported. The most common side effects are self-limiting, including gastrointestinal complaints, hypotension resulting from a rapid injection, headache, muscle spasms and pain, and convulsions (associated with high doses) [24-28].

The massive hemorrhage protocol devised by the Hospital for Sick Children recommends TXA for pediatric trauma patients who require a blood transfusion and have one of the following indicators of severe shock: obvious significant bleeding, poor blood pressure response to crystalloid bolus, or systolic hypotension (<80 mmHg in children under 5, and <90 mmHg in children 5 and older). Children 12 years and older receive the adult dose of 1g, while children <12 are dosed 15 mg/kg up to 1g infused IV over 10 minutes [23].

Additional Etiologies: Definitive source control in the operating room or interventional radiology should be sought for patients requiring ongoing volume resuscitation. However, when patients fail to improve despite volume resuscitation and source control, or when clinical signs are present, other etiologies of shock must be considered, tension pneumo- or hemothorax, cardiac tamponade, myocardial injury, or neurogenic shock.

Tension Pneumothorax: Tension pneumothorax results from lung injury that creates a one-way valve, trapping increased amounts of air in the pleural space between the lung and chest wall each time the patient takes a breath. There should be high suspicion for tension pneumothorax in patients suffering from **blunt chest trauma** with ipsilateral loss of breath sounds, hypotension, and increased ventilation pressures. Neck vein distension supports the diagnosis but is often diminished in the setting of hypovolemia. Tracheal deviation occurs late, and its absence does not negate the diagnosis. Needle thoracostomy in the midclavicular second intercostal space must be performed urgently, followed by chest tube placement.

Pericardial Tamponade: Pericardial effusion leading to cardiac tamponade occurs from **penetrating chest trauma** more frequently than blunt trauma. The diagnosis is supported by muffled heart sounds, pulsus paradoxus, electrical alternans, and distended neck veins. The treatment is pericardiocentesis.

Neurogenic Shock: Spinal cord injuries result in a loss of sympathetic tone below the level of the injury, causing vasodilation. When this occurs above T6, the loss of sympathetic tone leads to hypotension and bradycardia, and vasogenic shock.

Initial therapy is volume resuscitation, and pharmacologic vasopressor support is recommended when the volume is insufficient. No single agent is standard. Phenylephrine, a pure alpha-1 agonist, is an effective vasoconstrictor but causes reflex bradycardia in patients already suffering from bradycardia and should be used cautiously. The selection of an agent with alpha and beta activity, such as norepinephrine or epinephrine, will both vasoconstrict and increase heart rate and contractility.

PHARMACOTHERAPY

Induction

There is no evidence-based practice that supports the use of a particular medication over another for the induction of a trauma patient. The goal is to produce rapid unconsciousness and paralysis to facilitate endotracheal intubation without exacerbating the injury. It is important to consider critical conditions, including hemorrhagic shock and increased intracranial/intraocular pressure that can be worsened by induction agents.

Patients suffering cardiac arrest do not warrant medications for intubation. Patients who are near cardiac arrest with agonal breathing or are unconscious without an intact gag reflex do not require medications to induce unconsciousness but may benefit from a neuromuscular blocking (NMB) agent. The use of an NMB remains controversial and requires a clinical decision based on the unique circumstances.

Etomidate: RSI Induction: 0.2-0.4 mg/kg IV

Etomidate is an imidazole that binds to the $GABA^A$ receptors and induces rapid unconsciousness, with an onset of action of 30-60 seconds. The duration of action is terminated through redistribution from the plasma after 3-5 minutes, and it is metabolized by hepatic and plasma esterases with a half-life of roughly 75 minutes. Etomidate has minimal impact on sympathetic tone, myocardial function, heart rate and mean arterial pressure. It causes a transient decrease in intracranial pressure (ICP) and intraocular pressure (IOP). For these reasons, it is frequently used in the setting of hemorrhagic shock, head injury, and eye injuries. Undesirable outcomes include pain on injection and myoclonic movements during induction. It lowers the seizure threshold in patients with a known seizure disorder. Post-op nausea and vomiting have been reported, and the reported incidence is slightly worse than Propofol and slightly better than barbiturates. Etomidate reversibly inhibits 11 β-hydroxylase, which blocks steroid synthesis and results in adrenal insufficiency [29, 30].

Ketamine: RSI Induction: 1.5-2 mg/kg IV

Ketamine is a phencyclidine derivative (PCP) that causes dissociative amnesia. The onset is rapid, inducing anesthesia roughly 30 seconds after IV administration, with a duration of 10-15 minutes. It preserves airway reflexes, causes bronchodilation, and causes minimal respiratory depression. It increases oropharyngeal secretions, which can be offset with an anticholinergic such as glycopyrrolate. Ketamine has intrinsic analgesic properties, which is beneficial for patients with painful injuries. Ketamine is a sympathomimetic, increasing heart rate, blood pressure, and cardiac output, and is advantageous in the setting of hypotension and shock. It has traditionally been avoided in patients with head and eye trauma due to the exacerbation of intracranial and intraocular hypertension. However, emerging research suggests that ventilated pediatric patients with intact CSF flow (*i.e.* no CSF outflow obstruction) and venous circulation adequately compensate, and increases in MAP and CPP do not increase ICP with ketamine [31, 37].

Additional research is necessary to determine if ketamine is safe in patients with acute head trauma. Hallucinations upon emergence are an adverse effect of ketamine, though children are at decreased risk compared to adults. Risk factors for hallucinations include patients > 15 years, female, personality disorders, and large doses >2 mg/kg IV; these can be offset with adjunct benzodiazepine use. Ketamine has both proconvulsive and anticonvulsant properties. It should be used cautiously in patients with a history of epilepsy, and anticonvulsants should be considered prior to ketamine use in epileptic patients.

Propofol: 1.5-3 mg/kg IV

Propofol is a lipophilic sedative-hypnotic that binds to $GABA^A$ receptors to rapidly induce general anesthesia. The onset is 40 seconds (one arm-brain circulation), and the duration is 10-15 minutes when the effects are terminated by redistribution. Induction doses cause transient apnea, respiratory depression, peripheral vasodilation, and cardiac depression. This results in decreased MAP, ICP, and IOP. Consider a different agent or reduced dose for patients with cardiovascular instability due to cardiac depression and peripheral vasodilation. Propofol causes pain with an injection, which can be minimized with lidocaine premedication. Propofol increases the seizure threshold [39].

NEUROMUSCULAR BLOCKING AGENTS

Neuromuscular blocking agents are used to facilitate the rapid securing of a definitive airway. They do not cause amnesia or anesthesia and are administered after an induction agent or natural loss of consciousness.

Succinylcholine: 1-2 mg/kg total body weight IV, 4 mg/kg IM

Succinylcholine is a depolarizing neuromuscular blocker (NMB). It binds to the same motor end-plate postsynaptic nicotinic cholinergic receptors as acetylcholine does. This causes calcium release from the sarcoplasmic reticulum and depolarization of the motor end-plate [38]. Unlike acetylcholine, it does not rapidly dissociate but instead remains bound to the receptors, interrupting repolarization and the normal depolarization in response to acetylcholine. The onset is 60 seconds with IV administration and 2-3 minutes after IM administration. The duration is 4-6 minutes, and it is terminated by rapid hydrolysis and metabolism by plasma pseudocholinesterase. It is specific to neuromuscular receptors and has no activity on the smooth and cardiac muscle.

Stimulation of the skeletal muscle causes hyperkalemia, increasing serum potassium by an average of 0.5 mEq/L. However, certain conditions upregulate acetylcholine receptors, which exacerbates potassium release with succinylcholine use, precipitating acute hyperkalemia, ventricular arrhythmias, and cardiac arrest. Succinylcholine should be avoided 48 hours or more after large denervating injuries such as spinal cord trauma, stroke, multisystem trauma, large body surface area burns, and rhabdomyolysis. The risk of hyperkalemia increases over time and typically peaks at 7-10 days. It is also contraindicated in patients with personal or family histories of skeletal muscle myopathies, such as muscular dystrophy, myotonia, and occult myopathies. Because personal and family history only identifies some patients with underlying myopathies, and previously healthy pediatric patients have suffered cardiac arrest from succinylcholine administration, controversy continues about elective use of succinylcholine in the pediatric population. Thus, succinylcholine use should be reserved in pediatrics for emergency intubations or instances where immediate airway control is necessary, such as laryngospasm, full stomach, or for intramuscular use when a suitable vein/intraosseous line is inaccessible [40-42].

Side effects include masseter muscle spasms, which can occur in isolation or conjunction with malignant hyperthermia. Bradycardia is common, with increased risk in younger patients and in patients receiving repeated doses [43]. Bradycardia can progress to asystole but can be mitigated by an anticholinergic such as atropine. Succinylcholine causes a transient increase in intracranial pressure and intraocular pressure. In patients with intracranial injuries and penetrating eye trauma, the need to rapidly secure an airway should be weighed against the risk of a transient increase in intracranial and intraocular pressure [43].

The dose of succinylcholine is based on **total body weight** rather than ideal or adjusted body weight. This can lead to under-dosing in the obese population if caution is not taken. The recommended doses are as follows:

2 mg/kg IV infants + young children

1-1.5 mg/kg IV older children

4 mg/kg IM, maximum dose 150 mg IM [43]

Rocuronium: 0.6-1.2 mg/kg IV

Rocuronium is an aminosteroid non-depolarizing neuromuscular blocking agent. It competes with acetylcholine at the nicotinic cholinergic receptor to induce neuromuscular paralysis. Like succinylcholine, the onset of action is rapid at 60-90 seconds, but the duration is much longer and can last 30-45 minutes after the rapid sequence induction (RSI) dose of 1.2 mg/kg IV. The most common side effect is an allergic reaction. It is excreted mostly unchanged in bile with approximately 30% in urine.

A summary of induction agents and neuromuscular relaxants is presented in Table **11**.

Table 11. Induction Medications and Muscle Relaxants used in Rapid Sequence Induction (RSI).

Medication	Mechanism	Clearance	Induction Dose*	Indications/ Advantages	Contraindications/ Adverse Effects
Etomidate [32]	Imidazole targets	Effects	0.2-0.4 mg/kg IV	- Minimal	- Reversibly inhibits
	GABA^A receptors	terminated by		cardiovascular	11 $^®$- hydroxylase
	to induce rapid	redistribution.		depression	$\rightarrow$ adrenal
	sedation	Highly protein		- Rapid onset, short	suppression
		bound in		duration	- Nausea/vomiting
		plasma,		- Decreases ICP	- Myoclonic activity
		metabolized by		while maintaining	- Decreased seizure
		hepatic +		MAP	threshold
		plasma			-
		esterases.			-

(Table 11) cont.....

Medication	Mechanism	Clearance	Induction Dose*	Indications/ Advantages	Contraindications/ Adverse Effects
Ketamine [33]	Phencyclidine derivative causes dissociative amnesia	Hepatic metabolism: *N*-demethylation	1.5-2 mg/kg IV	- Bronchodilation - Preserved respiratory reflexes - Minimal respiratory depression - Analgesia - Sympathomimetic: preserves BP, HR, CO	- Increases ICP - Increases IOP - Increased airway secretions - proconvulsive and anticonvulsant properties
Propofol [39]	GABA-A agonist, sedative-hypnotic	Effects terminated by redistribution. Ultimately hepatic metabolism	2.5 mg/kg (1-3.6 mg/kg) IV	- Rapid onset, short duration - Increases seizure threshold	- Vasodilation, cardiac depressant
Succinylcholine [43]	Depolarizing NMB	Rapid hydrolyzation and clearance by plasma esterases	1-2 mg/kg **total** body weight IV	- Rapid onset - Rapid termination of effects	- Hyperkalemia - Transient ↑ IOP, ICP - Malignant hyperthermia - Masseter spasm - bradycardia
Rocuronium [45]	Aminosteroid nondepolarizing NMB	Largely excreted unchanged in bile, 30% renal excretion	0.6-1.2 mg/kg IV	- at doses 1-1.2 mg/kg onset mimics succinylcholine - rapid reversal possible with Sugammadex	- large induction doses lead to prolonged duration of action - allergic reaction

* Dosing recommendations provide a guideline for what constitutes a reasonable dose in the average patient. This should not take the place of clinical judgment, and doses should be adjusted to avoid toxicity (especially in hemodynamically unstable patients) and to avoid subtherapeutic effects such as recall and pain (especially in patients with tolerance, anxiety, and hemodynamic stability).

REVERSAL

Sugammadex: 2-16 mg/kg total body weight IV

Succinylcholine is the neuromuscular blocking agent of choice for emergency airway management due to its rapid onset and short duration. Rocuronium also has a rapid onset, but a much longer duration. Due to the adverse effects of succinylcholine, it is plausible that rocuronium will gain preference when rapid rocuronium reversal becomes universally available. The introduction of sugammadex makes this a real possibility.

Sugammadex is a selective aminosteroidal neuromuscular blocker binding agent that was approved by the FDA for adult use in the United States in December 2015 [44]. It encapsulates rocuronium and vecuronium to form a complex and separate them from the nicotinic receptor, rapidly reversing neuromuscular blockade. It is the first noncompetitive antagonist for neuromuscular blockade reversal. Unlike acetylcholinesterase inhibitors, such as neostigmine, it is effective for the rapid reversal of neuromuscular blockade at any depth of muscle relaxation.

Sugammadex has not yet gained FDA approval in the pediatric population. While there are few pediatric prospective studies, multiple case reports of sugammadex use for cannot intubate, cannot ventilate scenarios have reported successful outcomes. Emerging data support the safety and efficacy of sugammadex in children of any age and with any depth of the neuromuscular block, and a 2019 study supports the dose of 4 mg/kg for the reversal of deep rocuronium-induced neuromuscular block (1-2 post-tetanic counts, no twitch response on train of four) for any age including infants and children.16 mg/kg sugammadex is recommended for the reversal of neuromuscular blockade with 1.2 mg/kg rocuronium within 3 minutes of administration. With growing evidence, and when sugammadex becomes readily available across institutions, it is possible that rocuronium plus sugammadex will replace succinylcholine as the preferred agent for rapid airway management [45 - 49].

Naloxone: 0.1 mg/kg up to 2 mg IV.

Naloxone is a pure opioid antagonist without agonist properties and should be administered when opioid intoxication is suspected. IV administration has an onset of action < 2 minutes and a duration of 20-60 minutes. The American Academy of Pediatrics recommends 0.1 mg/kg IV from birth through age 5 or 20 kg, up to 2 mg. AAP does not recommend subcutaneous or IM administration in pediatrics due to erratic absorption and delayed onset [50]. Patients should be observed for 24 hours after administration to ensure that re-sedation does not occur; doses can be repeated if the duration of intoxication exceeds the duration of naloxone [52].

Flumazenil: 0.01 – 0.02 mg/kg IV, maximum single dose 0.2 mg

Flumazenil is a competitive benzodiazepine antagonist that inhibits activity at the GABA/ benzodiazepine receptor. It reverses benzodiazepine intoxication, including sedation, amnesia, and respiratory depression. Rapid onset is observed in 1-2 minutes, reaching peak effect within 6-10 minutes. The recommended dose

is 0.01 – 0.02 mg/kg IV up to 0.2 mg and can be repeated at 1-minute intervals up to 0.05 mg/kg or 1 mg, whichever is lower. The duration is dose dependent and is affected by the plasma concentration of benzodiazepines. Patients should be monitored for at least 2 hours after administration to ensure that re-sedation does not occur [52, 53].

ADJUNCT MEDICATIONS

Lidocaine: 1.5 mg/kg IV

Lidocaine is administered as a premedication to blunt the sympathetic stimulation associated with intubation. It can be considered for patients in whom increases in blood pressure, heart rate, and intracranial pressure are deleterious, such as intracranial bleed, eye injury, or vascular injury [54]. However, its effectiveness has been inconsistent in studies. Because it has a potential benefit with minimal toxicity, its use is reasonable but lacks definitive supporting evidence. Its use should not delay intubation in the setting of hypoxia or hypercarbia, as the evidence clearly shows that these worsen intracranial and intraocular pressure.

Midazolam: Oral: 0.25 mg/kg, IV: 0.15 mg/kg

Midazolam is a benzodiazepine with anxiolytic and amnestic properties. It is a valuable adjunct in the stable patient but must be used cautiously in the patient with unstable and evolving injuries due to side effects, including myocardial depression, decreased systemic vascular resistance, and respiratory depression with apnea. Midazolam has variable bioavailability, so the administration of a low initial dose such as 0.25 mg/kg oral and 0.15 mg/kg IV with titration to effect is appropriate [55].

Opioids:

Opioids have potent analgesic and sedative properties, making them beneficial to trauma patients. They induce a dose-dependent respiratory depression, decrease sympathetic tone, decrease SVR, and cause hypotension. Dosing should be incremental with titration to effect, with cautious use in patients with hemodynamic instability.

Fentanyl is lipophilic and has a rapid onset (1-2 minutes) and short duration (30 minutes). It is associated with chest wall rigidity, especially with rapid injection, and compared to morphine, causes less histamine release. A reasonable analgesic dose is 0.5-1 mcg/kg/dose IV and can be repeated at 3-5 minute intervals until the desired effect is achieved. A dose of 3 mcg/kg is appropriate to blunt sympathetic tone during intubation in a stable patient.

Morphine is slower in onset with longer duration and increased histamine release compared to fentanyl. A reasonable dose is 0.05-0.2 mg/kg/dose IV administered at 5-15 minute intervals.

In consideration of the global care of the trauma patient, one should acknowledge the risk of developing a substance use disorder after opioid exposure. Adolescents who are treated for a traumatic injury are at 56% increased risk for developing a substance use disorder within 3 years of their injury in retrospective studies. This does not suggest that opioids should be withheld from injured patients, but one must be judicious when dosing opioids and consider analgesic adjuvants when appropriate [56].

RESUSCITATIVE MEDICATIONS

Epinephrine: 0.01 mg/kg IV or IO, 0.1 mg/kg tracheal

Epinephrine is an α- and β-adrenergic endogenous catecholamine. It causes intense vasoconstriction and cardiac contractility. It is indicated for cardiac arrest and severe symptomatic hypotension, bradycardia, or bronchospasm not responsive to other measures. IV, IO, or IM administration is preferred. Tracheal administration is acceptable but has unpredictable absorption. The recommended dose is 0.01 mg/kg IV or IO and 0.1 mg/kg tracheal and can be repeated at 3-5 minute intervals [15]. Higher doses failed to show improved benefit and had increased adverse effects such as increased myocardial oxygen consumption, myocardial dysfunction, tachycardia, hypertension, and ventricular ectopy [57]. An infusion of 0.1-0.2 µg/kg/ minute can be initiated after the return of spontaneous circulation during cardiac arrest.

Atropine: 0.02 mg/kg IV

Atropine is indicated to treat bradycardia. Previous recommendations suggested that all children <10 years must receive it as premedication before induction, but the data has not supported this requirement [58]. However, it should be immediately available and used to treat bradycardia, which is common with laryngoscopy due to the stimulation of parasympathetic laryngeal receptors. It can also occur with repeated doses of succinylcholine due to the stimulation of cardiac muscarinic receptors. The dose of 0.02 mg/kg IV is acceptable even in children <5 kg, disputing the previous recommendation of a minimum dose of 0.1 mg [59]. Additionally, a common cause of pediatric bradycardia is hypoxia, and it is important to ensure adequate oxygenation as part of the treatment. [21 - 31].

MAINTENANCE OF ANESTHESIA

Volatile Agents: For hemodynamically stable patients with hemorrhage source control, volatile agents are well tolerated [64]. The choice of agent should be determined by the duration of the procedure and institutional availability. In patients with unstable hemodynamics, volatile agents are poorly tolerated due to their negative inotropic effects. For patients suffering from head trauma, the goal is to prevent ischemic injury by maintaining adequate cerebral blood flow without exacerbating intracranial pressure. Volatile agents cause a decrease in the cerebral metabolic rate of oxygen consumption ($CMRO_2$), providing some protection from ischemic injury [60]. They also cause dose-dependent cerebral vasodilation that causes an increase in cerebral blood flow (CBF) and intracranial pressure (ICP). Sevoflurane maintains cerebral blood flow up to 1 MAC (at doses >1 MAC, CBF increases), and cerebral autoregulation is maintained up to 1.5 MAC. Thus, sevoflurane is the preferred volatile agent for patients with head injuries, limiting administration to <1 MAC.

Nitrous Oxide: Nitrous oxide is best avoided in trauma patients, especially in children whose injuries are not entirely identified. It is more soluble than nitrogen, allowing it to diffuse into closed air spaces and expand their volume. This is particularly dangerous for patients suffering from a pneumothorax, bowel injury, intracranial injury, or intraocular injury [61].

TIVA: A total intravenous anesthetic (TIVA) is an acceptable alternative to volatile agents. This is critical for patients at risk for malignant hyperthermia and serves as an acceptable alternative to volatile agents for patients with intracranial injuries. The selection of agents is determined by procedure length, hemodynamic stability of the patient, and institutional availability. IV agents decrease $CMRO_2$ and decrease CBF with the exception of ketamine. IV agents are selected based on the patient's condition, institutional availability, and procedure length and are frequently used in combination. Commonly selected agents include propofol, dexmedetomidine, ketamine (caution with a head injury), opioids (remifentanil is advantageous for its short context-sensitive half-life, while fentanyl and sufentanil are also frequent infusion choices).

INTRAOPERATIVE   MANAGEMENT   MONITORING   AND THERMOREGULATION

Monitors: Routine ASA monitors (blood pressure, pulse oximeter, capnography, electrocardiography, and temperature) are indicated for all trauma patients.

The addition of arterial, central, and bladder catheters benefit patients with extensive injuries, hemodynamic instability, head trauma, or anticipated prolonged operative procedures. Arterial catheters allow continuous blood pressure monitoring and frequent arterial blood gas sampling, providing acid-base, electrolyte, and hemoglobin data. Central catheters permit rapid infusion of fluid and blood products, provide CVP, and allow venous blood sampling. Bladder catheters provide indirect information about volume status. Additional monitors are appropriate in unique circumstances. Transesophageal echo (TEE) provides direct information about volume status and intrathoracic injuries. Somatosensory evoked potential monitors allow spinal cord monitoring of spinal cord injuries. Intracranial pressure (ICP) monitors provide additional information for patients with head trauma.

Temperature: Heat loss results from exposure at the scene of trauma, infusion of fluid and blood products, and exposure of wounds and surgical sites. Hypothermia leads to coagulopathies, acid-base disturbances, the leftward shift of the oxyhemoglobin saturation curve, myocardial dysfunction, and arrhythmias. Continuous temperature monitoring is critical. Steps to prevent hypothermia include covering the patient with warm blankets, warming the room, warming IV fluids and blood products, and using radiant warmers and forced-air warming devices. Hypothermia provides cerebral protection after cardiac arrest in patients who do not regain consciousness, and the benefits of warming should be balanced against the benefits of maintaining hypothermia in these patients [62].

INJURY MANAGEMENT

Head Injuries: Traumatic brain injury is the leading cause of morbidity and mortality in children [1]. Severity ranges from a mild concussion to severe injury, including intracranial hemorrhage with midline shift and brain herniation. A clinical neurological exam prior to sedation and muscle relaxation is critical to establish a baseline. Computed tomography (CT) scans are performed rapidly and provide information about depressed skull fractures, ventricle distortions, hematomas, and midline shifts. MRI is more sensitive for ischemic damage but impractical and expensive and rarely used in the acute traumatic setting [65].

Children suffering TBIs often require operative intervention, both neurosurgical intervention and surgical treatment of abdominal, chest, and orthopedic injuries unrelated to the TBI. In either instance, the perioperative goals are similar; maintain cerebral oxygen delivery to prevent ischemic injury, and prevent parenchymal injury and ischemia from tissue compression or herniation [69]. This is achieved by maintaining cerebral perfusion pressure (CPP) and avoiding intracranial hypertension. ICP is optimally monitored *via* ventriculostomy, which also allows for CSF drainage if the pressure becomes elevated, but can also be achieved with a subarachnoid bolt when an intraventricular catheter cannot be placed. CBF is evaluated *via* doppler. Hypoxia must be avoided to prevent increased cerebral vasodilation and increased ICP. Hyperventilation leads to hypocarbia, causing temporary cerebral vasoconstriction and decreased ICP. In ventilated patients, a target $PaCO_2$ 35-38 is appropriate. MAP should be maintained to prevent a decrease in CPP (CPP = MAP – ICP). The patient's head should remain elevated at 30 degrees unless surgical intervention precludes this. Hyperosmolar therapy with mannitol or hypertonic saline creates an osmotic gradient to shift water from the brain parenchyma into the vascular compartment, shrinking the brain and reducing ICP by reducing intracranial volume. It requires an intact blood-brain barrier. Caution is needed with mannitol use in hypovolemic patients as it can lead to hypotension *via* diuresis. Hypertonic saline alternatively increases intravascular volume, MAP, and CPP, but the risks include central pontine myelinolysis, electrolyte abnormalities, and hypervolemia [62].

The anesthetic selection must account for the impact of each agent on ICP. Succinylcholine causes a transient increase in ICP. The need to rapidly secure an airway and prevent hypoxia- or hypercarbia-induced intracranial hypertension should be weighed against this transient medication-induced elevation [44]. Nondepolarizing muscle blockers have no direct impact on ICP but they may decrease it in the setting of histamine release and hypotension. All volatile agents cause dose-dependent cerebral vasodilation, resulting in increased CBF and ICP while decreasing $CMRO_2$. Sevoflurane does not significantly increase CBF at <1 MAC; therefore, it is the preferred inhalational agent for patients with TBI. It should be limited to <1 MAC, as CBF and ICP are increased at greater doses [62]. Nitrous oxide is best avoided as it is a potent cerebrovasodilator and increases CBF and ICP, with debated increases in $CMRO_2$. IV agents are commonly selected and require judicious administration to prevent hypotension with subsequent decreases in CPP. Propofol, etomidate, benzodiazepines and barbiturates reduce $CMRO_2$, CBF, and ICP. Opioids decrease CBF and ICP when ventilation is constant. Ketamine increases CBF, ICP, and $CMRO_2$ and is typically avoided [65].

Thoracic Trauma: One must have a strong suspicion for internal thoracic injuries when children present with rib, sternal, and scapular fractures. Compared to adults, children have more cartilaginous rib cages, and higher forces are required to cause fractures [66, 67]. While they are less susceptible to flail chest (four or more ribs fractured in two places from blunt force trauma resulting in paradoxical chest wall movement, impeding spontaneous ventilation), severe pulmonary contusion, pneumothorax, and hemothorax can occur despite the absence of rib fracture. Children also have more compliant chest cavities and greater mobility of the mediastinum, which makes them less susceptible to aortic rupture. Pulmonary

contusions, including pneumothorax and hemothorax, are the most common pediatric thoracic injury and impair gas exchange and ventilation [68].

Pneumothorax occurs when air collects in the pleural space between the lung and chest wall. A tension pneumothorax results from an injury to the visceral pleura, parietal pleura, or the tracheobronchial tree that creates a one-way valve. With each successive breath, additional air is trapped in the pleural space, expanding the pneumothorax and impeding ventilation and venous return. Patients present with ipsilateral loss of breath sounds, hypotension, increased ventilation pressures, neck vein distension (may be absent in the setting of hypovolemia), and tracheal deviation (occurs late). Hemothorax results from injury to intercostal vessels or lung parenchyma. Each hemithorax can hold up to 40% of a pediatric patient's lung volume and can lead to hemodynamic collapse, if undetected.

Because pneumo/hemothorax is life-threatening, clinical diagnosis predicated on history and physical exam is sufficient in unstable patients. When the patient is stable and the diagnosis is uncertain, a chest radiograph or CT confirms the diagnosis. Treatment rarely requires thoracotomy, and patients can typically be managed outside of the operating room. Immediate needle thoracostomy is performed in the midclavicular second intercostal space, and definitive treatment involves chest tube placement.

Abdominal Trauma: Children are vulnerable to abdominal injuries. Solid-organ injuries, including the liver, spleen, pancreas, and kidneys, are most common. The anatomy of children is such that the liver and spleen are less protected by the rib cage, and the body of the pancreas is situated in a position that makes it vulnerable to compression by a seat belt or bicycle handlebars. Hollow visceral organ injuries occur with the next highest frequency, and points of fixation such as the 3rd and 4th duodenum, terminal ileum, and sigmoid colon are particularly vulnerable. Hemodynamic instability is the primary indication for the operative management of intraabdominal injuries. Patients frequently require resuscitation with blood and fluid while surgical teams achieve hemorrhagic source control. Temporary hemodynamic vasopressor support is sometimes required to prevent critical organ ischemia while preparing transfusion or controlling the hemorrhage but should be limited to prevent exacerbation of the hemorrhage and organ ischemia. Increasingly, the development of new techniques allows interventional radiology to treat intraabdominal vascular injuries, decreasing the need for operative intervention [69].

Burns: Over 52% of all pediatric burns occur in patients aged 4 and younger.

Burns are defined by the depth of injury: 1st-degree burns are limited to the epidermis, 2nd-degree burns extend partially into the dermis, 3rd-degree burns

extend completely through the dermis, and 4th-degree burns involve muscle, fascia, or bone [70]. Morbidity and mortality are proportional to the affected total body surface area (TBSA, Fig. (**2**)). Burns involving >10% of TBSA are defined as critical and should be managed in a burn unit, as should burns that involve the face, hands, feet, genitalia, or across joints. Patients with burns >15% TBSA often require IV fluids, especially in children with increased insensible losses proportional to adults. When >20% TBSA is affected, complex fluid shifts occur and can produce shock unless aggressive resuscitation ensues. Fluid resuscitation is guided by a modified Parkland formula to estimate fluid requirements during the initial 24 hours.

Estimated 24 hour Fluid Volume = 3 x body weight (kg) x TBSA burn + standard pediatric maintenance fluids

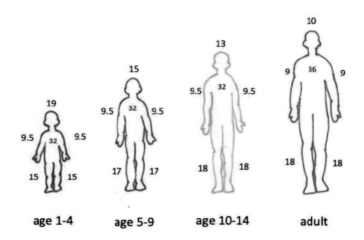

Fig. (2). Estimation of TBSA based on age [72]. Illustration by Kathleen Kwiatt.

The goal of fluid therapy is to achieve a urine output of 1 ml/kg/hour. More aggressive resuscitation leads to increased hydrostatic pressure in the setting of decreased osmotic pressure (protein losses), resulting in increased total body edema. Capillary leak and hydrostatic forces increase the incidence of pulmonary edema. Medications should be administered *via* IV or oral route, as the presence of edema results in unreliable subcutaneous and intramuscular uptake [72].

The mechanism of the burn is important to reduce missed injuries; burns occurring in closed spaces with smoke inhalation are associated with airway edema, while electrocution injuries often have minimal external injury despite extensive internal injuries. When carbon monoxide poisoning is suspected, the measurement of carboxyhemoglobin levels and co-oximetry assess carbon monoxide levels. Pulse oximetry is unreliable in the setting of carbon monoxide poisoning as it only detects oxygenated and deoxygenated hemoglobin and misinterprets carboxyhemoglobin as oxyhemoglobin, providing a false normal reading [71].

Many burn injury patients require repeated operative management for the debridement of their wounds. Ketamine is advantageous because of its sympathomimetic and analgesic properties. Etomidate is less ideal because of the risk of adrenal suppression with repeated dosing.

POST-OPERATIVE CARE

Immediate post-operative care mirrors initial care of trauma patients; monitoring and optimization of oxygenation and ventilation, circulation, temperature, neurologic function, coagulation, and fluid, electrolyte, and acid-base status. Pain control is important not just for patient comfort but also to optimize pulmonary function. Patients should be monitored for complications including abdominal and extremity compartment syndrome, hemorrhage, coagulopathy, renal failure, pulmonary failure, and thromboembolism.

While the overall incidence of thromboembolism is less in pediatric patients compared to adults, children recovering from traumatic injuries are at particular risk. Risk factors related to trauma include immobility > 5 days, GCS < 9, spinal cord injury, complex lower extremity fracture, open pelvic fracture, use of inotropes, and resuscitation requiring CPR. The incidence of thromboembolism occurs with the greatest frequency in children <1 and >13 years [72, 73]. The decision to anticoagulate must be weighed against the individualized risk for hemorrhage.

The goal of rehabilitation is to provide each child the opportunity to achieve his or her greatest potential. Multidisciplinary care is critical to this goal. Physical, occupational, cognitive, speech, play, and psychological therapy are essential to optimize a patient's potential. Behavioral health and psychiatric intervention can mitigate post-traumatic stress disorders. Child services must be contacted when non-accidental trauma is suspected.

CONCLUSION

Pediatric trauma has devastating consequences for children, their families, and society. The anesthesiologist can mitigate these by coordinating a team approach and systematically caring for each patient. Emphasis on ATLS protocols and adherence to evidence-based practice in the diagnostic approach, airway and intraoperative management, and resuscitative efforts improves outcomes with lasting benefits for the patient, family, and society.

ABBREVIATIONS

ATLS Advanced Trauma Life Support

CBF Cerebral blood flow

CPP Cerebral perfusion pressure

CSF Cerebrospinal fluid

CT Computed tomography

EMS Emergency medical services

FDA Food and Drug administration

GABA Gamma-aminobutyric acid

IOP Intraocular pressure

ICP Intracranial pressure

IV Intravenous

MAP Mean arterial pressure

MAC Mean alveolar concentration

g Milligram

MRI Magnetic resonance imaging

Kg Kilogram

TBSA Total body surface area

TIVA Total intravenous anesthesia

CONSENT FOR PUBLICATION

Not applicable.

CONFLICT OF INTEREST

The author declares no conflict of interest, financial or otherwise.

ACKNOWLEDGEMENTS

Declared none.

REFERENCES

[1]   Sathya C, Alali AS, Wales PW, *et al.* Mortality Among Injured Children Treated at Different Trauma Center Types. JAMA Surg 2015; 150(9): 874-81.
[http://dx.doi.org/10.1001/jamasurg.2015.1121] [PMID: 26106848]

[2]   Britnell S, Koziol-McLain J. Weight estimation in paediatric resuscitation: a hefty issue in New Zealand. Paediatric Emergency Medicine 2015. [http://dx.doi.org/10.1111/1742-6723.12389]

[3]   So TY, Farrington E, Absher RK. Evaluation of the accuracy of different methods used to estimate weights in the pediatric population. Pediatrics 2009; 123(6): e1045-51.
[http://dx.doi.org/10.1542/peds.2008-1968] [PMID: 19482737]

[4]   Planas JH, Waseem M. Trauma Primary Survey. StatPearls Treasure Island, FL: StatPearls Publishing 2020.https://www.ncbi.nlm.nih.gov/books/NBK430800/

[5]   American Heart Association PALS Pocket Reference Card. 2016.

[6]   Capan L, Miller S. Anesthesia for trauma and burn patients. Clinical Anesthesia. 6th ed. Philadelphia, PA: Lippincott Williams & Wilkins 2009; pp. 889-926.

[7]   Teasdale G, Murray G, Parker L, Jennett B. Adding up the Glasgow Coma Score. Acta Neurochir Suppl (Wien). 1979; 28: pp. (1)13-6.
[http://dx.doi.org/10.1007/978-3-7091-4088-8_2]

[8]   Wilberger J, Mao G. Traumatic Brain Injury 2019.https://www.merckmanuals.com/professional/injuries-poisoning/traumatic-brain-injury-tbi/traumatic-b rain-injury-tbi#CHDEHEFH

[9]   Trauma I – ABCs of Trauma. American College of Surgeons Division of Education. https://www.facs.org/-/media/files/education/core-curriculum/trauma_i_initial_eval.ashx

[10]   Zemaitis MR, Planas JH, Shah N, Waseem M. Trauma Secondary SurveyStatPearls. Treasure Island, FL: StatPearls Publishing 2020.https://pubmed.ncbi.nlm.nih.gov/28722931/

[11]   Mlcak R, Cortiella J, Desai MH, Herndon DN. Emergency management of pediatric burn victims. Pediatr Emerg Care 1998; 14(1): 51-4. [http://dx.doi.org/10.1097/00006565-199802000-00013].
[PMID: 9516633].
[http://dx.doi.org/10.1097/00006565-199802000-00013] [PMID: 9516633]

[12]   Suominen P, Baillie C, Kivioja A, Ohman J, Olkkola KT. Intubation and survival in severe paediatric blunt head injury. Eur J Emerg Med 2000; 7(1): 3-7.
[http://dx.doi.org/10.1097/00063110-200003000-00002] [PMID: 10839372]

[13]   American Heart Association ECC Guidelines Pediatric Advanced Life Support Circulation 102(suppl 1)2000;

[14]   Heath KJ. The effect of laryngoscopy of different cervical spine immobilisation techniques. Anaesthesia 1994; 49(10): 843-5.
[http://dx.doi.org/10.1111/j.1365-2044.1994.tb04254.x] [PMID: 7802175]

[15]   Kreyekes N, Longshore S, Petty J. Guidelines in Focus: Pediatric Cervical Spine Pediatric Trauma Society Guidelines https://pediatrictraumasociety.org/resources/pcs-guidelines.cgi

[16]   Hannon M, Mannix R, Dorney K, Mooney D, Hennelly K. Pediatric cervical spine injury evaluation after blunt trauma: a clinical decision analysis. Ann Emerg Med 2015; 65(3): 239-47.
[http://dx.doi.org/10.1016/j.annemergmed.2014.09.002] [PMID: 25441248]

[17]   Rosenblatt WH, Sukhupragarn W. Airway management. Clinical Anesthesia. 6th ed. Philadelphia, PA: Lippincott Williams & Wilkins 2009; pp. 751-92.

[18]   Whittaker B, Christiaans SC, Altice JL, *et al.* Early coagulopathy is an independent predictor of mortality in children after severe trauma. Shock 2013; 39(5): 421-6.
[http://dx.doi.org/10.1097/SHK.0b013e31828e08cb] [PMID: 23591559]

[19] Polites SF, Nygaard RM, Reddy PN, *et al.* Multicenter study of crystalloid boluses and transfusion in pediatric trauma-When to go to blood? J Trauma Acute Care Surg 2018; 85(1): 108-12.
[http://dx.doi.org/10.1097/TA.0000000000001897] [PMID: 29538238]

[20] Zhu CS, Pokorny DM, Eastridge BJ, *et al.* Give the trauma patient what they bleed, when and where they need it: establishing a comprehensive regional system of resuscitation based on patient need utilizing cold-stored, low-titer O+ whole blood. Transfusion 2019; 59(S2): 1429-38.
[http://dx.doi.org/10.1111/trf.15264] [PMID: 30980748]

[21] 2019.https://www.mayoclinic.org/medical-professionals/trauma/news/resuscitation-scheme-chang-ng-for-pediatric-patients/mac-20464846

[22] Maw G, Furyk C. Pediatric Massive Transfusion: A Systematic Review. Pediatr Emerg Care 2018; 34(8): 594-8.
[http://dx.doi.org/10.1097/PEC.0000000000001570] [PMID: 30080793]

[23] Grassin-Delyle S, Couturier R, Abe E, Alvarez JC, Devillier P, Urien S. A practical tranexamic acid dosing scheme based on population pharmacokinetics in children undergoing cardiac surgery. Anesthesiology 2013; 118(4): 853-62.
[http://dx.doi.org/10.1097/ALN.0b013e318283c83a] [PMID: 23343649]

[24] McLeod LM, French B, Flynn JM, Dormans JP, Keren R. Antifibrinolytic use and blood transfusions in pediatric scoliosis surgeries performed at US children's hospitals. J Spinal Disord Tech 2015; 28(8): E460-6.
[http://dx.doi.org/10.1097/BSD.0b013e3182a22a54] [PMID: 24091932]

[25] Basta MN, Stricker PA, Taylor JA. A systematic review of the use of antifibrinolytic agents in pediatric surgery and implications for craniofacial use. Pediatr Surg Int 2012; 28(11): 1059-69.
[http://dx.doi.org/10.1007/s00383-012-3167-6] [PMID: 22940882]

[26] Shakur H, Roberts I, Bautista R, *et al.* Effects of tranexamic acid on death, vascular occlusive events, and blood transfusion in trauma patients with significant haemorrhage (CRASH-2): a randomised, placebo-controlled trial. Lancet 2010; 376(9734): 23-32.
[http://dx.doi.org/10.1016/S0140-6736(10)60835-5] [PMID: 20554319]

[27] Beno S, Ackery AD, Callum J, Rizoli S. Tranexamic acid in pediatric trauma: why not? Crit Care 2014; 18(4): 313.
[http://dx.doi.org/10.1186/cc13965] [PMID: 25043066]

[28] Royal College of Paediatrics and Child Health: Evidence statement Major trauma and the use of tranexamic acid in children 2012.https://www.rcem.ac.uk/docs/External%20Guidance/

[29] Bergen JM, Smith DC. A review of etomidate for rapid sequence intubation in the emergency department. J Emerg Med 1997; 15(2): 221-30.
[http://dx.doi.org/10.1016/S0736-4679(96)00350-2] [PMID: 9144065]

[30] Forman SA. Clinical and molecular pharmacology of etomidate. Anesthesiology 2011; 114(3): 695-707.
[http://dx.doi.org/10.1097/ALN.0b013e3181ff72b5] [PMID: 21263301]

[31] Sinner B, Graf BM. KetamineModern Anesthetics. 2008. [http://dx.doi.org/10.1007/978-3-540-74-06-9_15]

[32] Bar-Joseph G, Guilburd Y, Tamir A, Guilburd JN. Effectiveness of ketamine in decreasing intracranial pressure in children with intracranial hypertension. J Neurosurg Pediatr 2009; 4(1): 40-6.https://thejns.org/pediatrics/view/journals/j-neurosurg-pediatr/4/1/article-p40.xml
[http://dx.doi.org/10.3171/2009.1.PEDS08319] [PMID: 19569909]

[33] White PF, Way WL, Trevor AJ. Ketamine--its pharmacology and therapeutic uses. Anesthesiology 1982; 56(2): 119-36.
[http://dx.doi.org/10.1097/00000542-198202000-00007] [PMID: 6892475]

[34]   Greifenstein FE, Devault M, Yoshitake J, Gajewski JE. A study of a 1-aryl cyclo hexyl amine for anesthesia. Anesth Analg 1958; 37(5): 283-94.
[http://dx.doi.org/10.1213/00000539-195809000-00007] [PMID: 13583607]

[35]   Ferrer-Allado T, Brechner VL, Dymond A, Cozen H, Crandall P. Ketamine-induced electroconvulsive phenomena in the human limbic and thalamic regions. Anesthesiology 1973; 38(4): 333-44.
[http://dx.doi.org/10.1097/00000542-197304000-00006] [PMID: 4707578]

[36]   Celesia GG, Chen RC, Bamforth BJ. Effects of ketamine in epilepsy. Neurology 1975; 25(2): 169-72.
[http://dx.doi.org/10.1212/WNL.25.2.169] [PMID: 1167644]

[37]   2017.https://www.accessdata.fda.gov/drugsatfda_docs/label/2017/019627s066lbl.pdf

[38]   Hager   HH,   Burns   B.   Succinylcholine   Chloride   2019.https://www.ncbi.nlm. nih.gov/books/NBK499984/

[39]   Iwasaki H, Renew JR, Kunisawa T, Brull SJ. Preparing for the unexpected: special considerations and complications after sugammadex administration. BMC Anesthesiol 2017; 17(1): 140.
[http://dx.doi.org/10.1186/s12871- 017-0429-9] [PMID: 29041919]

[40]   Kent RS. Revised label regarding use of succinylcholine in children and adolescents: I and II. Anesthesiology 1994; 80: 244-5.
[http://dx.doi.org/10.1097/00000542-199401000-00049]

[41]   Anectine   drug   insert   Sandoz   Inc   2018.https://www.accessdata.fda.gov/drugsatfda_ docs/label/2018/008453s036lbl.pdf

[42]   Tran DT, Newton EK, Mount VA, Lee JS, Wells GA, Perry JJ. Rocuronium versus succinylcholine for rapid sequence induction intubation. Cochrane Database Syst Rev 2015; 10(10): CD002788.
[http://dx.doi.org/10.1002/14651858.CD002788.pub3] [PMID: 26512948]

[43]   Jain   A,   Maani   CV.   RocuroniumStatPearls   Treasure   Island,   FL: StatPearls   Publishing 2020.https://www.ncbi.nlm.nih.gov/books/NBK539888/

[44]   Adam JM, Bennett DJ, Bom A, *et al.* Cyclodextrin-derived host molecules as reversal agent for the neuromuscular blocker rocuronium bromide: synthesis and structure-activity relationships. J Med Chem 2002; 25:45(9): 1806-6.

[45]   Bridion   drug   insert   Updated   2018   Merck   and   Co,   Inc   https://www.merck.com/ product/usa/pi_circulars/b/bridion/bridion_pi.pdf

[46]   Wołoszczuk-Gębicka B, Zawadzka-Głos L, Lenarczyk J, Sitkowska BD, Rzewnicka I. Two cases of the "cannot ventilate, cannot intubate" scenario in children in view of recent recommendations. Anaesthesiol Intensive Ther 2014; 46(2): 88-91.
[PMID: 24858967]

[47]   Liu G, Wang R, Yan Y, Fan L, Xue J, Wang T. The efficacy and safety of sugammadex for reversing postoperative residual neuromuscular blockade in pediatric patients: A systematic review. Sci Rep 2017; 7(1): 5724.
[http://dx.doi.org/10.1038/s41598-017-06159-2] [PMID: 28720838]

[48]   Matsui M, Konishi J, Suzuki T, Sekijima C, Miyazawa N, Yamamoto S. Reversibility of Rocuronium-Induced Deep Neuromuscular Block with Sugammadex in Infants and Children-A Randomized Study. Biol Pharm Bull 2019; 42(10): 1637-40.https://www.jstage.jst.go.jp/ article/bpb/42/10/42_b19-00044/_article/-char/en
[http://dx.doi.org/10.1248/bpb.b19-00044] [PMID: 31406051]

[49]   Bridion Prescribing Information Merck Sharp & Dohme Corp, a subsidiary of Merck & Co, Inc 2018.https://www.merckconnect.com/static/pdf/ bridion-sugammadex-dosi- g-considerations.pdf

[50]   Naloxone   Hydrochloride   Injection   drug   insert   Hikma   Pharmaceuticals   USA   Inc 2020.https://www.accessdata.fda.gov/drugsatfda_docs/label/2007/020073s016lbl.pdf

[51]   American Academy of Pediatrics. Emergency drug doses for infants and children and naloxone use in newborns: clarification. Pediatrics 1989; 83(5): 803. https://pediatrics.aappublications.org/content/83/5/803
       [http://dx.doi.org/10.1542/peds.83.5.803] [PMID: 2717301]

[52]   Flumazenil drug insert Roche Pharmaceuticals 2007. https://www.accessdata.fda.gov/drugsatfda_docs/label/2007/020073s016lbl.pdf

[53]   Hegenbarth MA. Preparing for pediatric emergencies: drugs to consider. Pediatrics 2008; 121(2): 433-43.
       [http://dx.doi.org/10.1542/peds.2007-3284] [PMID: 18245435]

[54]   Lev R, Rosen P. Prophylactic lidocaine use preintubation: a review. J Emerg Med 1994; 12(4): 499-506.
       [http://dx.doi.org/10.1016/0736-4679(94)90347-6] [PMID: 7963397]

[55]   Reed MD, Rodarte A, Blumer JL, *et al.* The single-dose pharmacokinetics of midazolam and its primary metabolite in pediatric patients after oral and intravenous administration. J Clin Pharmacol 2001; 41(12): 1359-69.
       [http://dx.doi.org/10.1177/00912700122012832] [PMID: 11762564]

[56]   Bell TM, Raymond J, Vetor A, *et al.* Long-term prescription opioid utilization, substance use disorders, and opioid overdoses after adolescent trauma. J Trauma Acute Care Surg 2019; 87(4): 836-40.
       [http://dx.doi.org/10.1097/TA.0000000000002261] [PMID: 30889139]

[57]   Carpenter TC, Stenmark KR. High-dose epinephrine is not superior to standard-dose epinephrine in pediatric in-hospital cardiopulmonary arrest. Pediatrics 1997; 99(3): 403-8.
       [http://dx.doi.org/10.1542/peds.99.3.403] [PMID: 9041296]

[58]   McAuliffe G, Bissonnette B, Boutin C. Should the routine use of atropine before succinylcholine in children be reconsidered? Can J Anaesth 1995; 42(8): 724-9.
       [http://dx.doi.org/10.1007/BF03012672] [PMID: 7586113]

[59]   Barrington KJ. The myth of a minimum dose for atropine. Pediatrics 2011; 127(4): 783-4.
       [http://dx.doi.org/10.1542/peds.2010-1475] [PMID: 21382950]

[60]   Reynolds P, Scattoloni JA, Gadepalli SK, Ehrlich P, Cladis FP, Davis PJ. Anesthesia for the Pediatric Trauma Patient. 2017.

[61]   O'Sullivan I, Benger J. Nitrous oxide in emergency medicine. Emerg Med J 2003; 20(3): 214-7.
       [http://dx.doi.org/10.1136/emj.20.3.214] [PMID: 12748131]

[62]   Topjian AA, de Caen A, Wainwright MS, *et al.* Pediatric Post-Cardiac Arrest Care: A Scientific Statement From the American Heart Association. Circulation 2019; 140(6): e194-233.
       [http://dx.doi.org/10.1161/CIR.0000000000000697] [PMID: 31242751]

[63]   Rangel-Castilla L, Gopinath S, Robertson CS. Management of intracranial hypertension [published correction appears in Neurol Clin. 2008 Aug;26(3):xvii. Rangel-Castillo, Leonardo [corrected to Rangel-Castilla, Leonardo]]. Neurol Clin 2008; 26(2): 521-x.
       [PMID: 18514825]

[64]   Stoelting RK. Basics of Anesthesia. 5th ed. China: Elsevier 2007; p. 456.

[65]   Miller MT, Pasquale MD, Bromberg WJ, Wasser TE, Cox J. Not so FAST. J Trauma 2003; 54(1): 52-9.
       [http://dx.doi.org/10.1097/00005373-200301000-00007] [PMID: 12544899]

[66]   Harrison BP, Roberts JA. Evaluating and managing pneumothorax. Emerg Med 2005; 37: 18-25.

[67]   Grisoni ER, Volsko TA. Thoracic injuries in children. Respir Care Clin N Am 2001; 7(1): 25-38.
       [http://dx.doi.org/10.1016/S1078-5337(05)70021-6] [PMID: 11584803]

[68]   Sharma A, Jindal P. Principles of diagnosis and management of traumatic pneumothorax. J Emerg Trauma Shock 2008; 1(1): 34-41.
[http://dx.doi.org/10.4103/0974-2700.41789] [PMID: 19561940]

[69]   Reynolds P, Scattoloni JA, Gadepalli SK, Ehrlich P, Cladis FP, Davis PJ. Anesthesia for the Pediatric Trauma Patient. Smith's Anesthesia for Infants and Children. 9th edition. Elsevier 2017; 37: pp. 969-.

[70]   Hansbrough JF, Hansbrough W. Pediatric burns. Pediatr Rev 1999; 20(4): 117-23.
[http://dx.doi.org/10.1542/pir.20.4.117] [PMID: 10208084]

[71]   Hampson NB. Pulse oximetry in severe carbon monoxide poisoning. Chest 1998; 114(4): 1036-41.
[http://dx.doi.org/10.1378/chest.114.4.1036] [PMID: 9792574]

[72]   Landisch RM, Hanson SJ, Cassidy LD, Braun K, Punzalan RC, Gourlay DM. Evaluation of guidelines for injured children at high risk for venous thromboembolism: A prospective observational study. J Trauma Acute Care Surg 2017; 82(5): 836-44.
[http://dx.doi.org/10.1097/TA.0000000000001404] [PMID: 28430759]

[73]   Stein PD, Kayali F, Olson RE. Incidence of venous thromboembolism in infants and children: data from the National Hospital Discharge Survey. J Pediatr 2004; 145(4): 563-5.
[http://dx.doi.org/10.1016/j.jpeds.2004.06.021] [PMID: 15480387]

CHAPTER 9

Pediatric and Neonatal Resuscitation

Melissa Lester[1] and **Grace Dippo**[1]

[1] *Department of Anesthesiology, Cooper Medical School of Rowan University, Cooper University Health Care, Camden, NJ, USA*

Abstract: Because of the expansive differences between the anatomy and physiology of the pediatric *versus* the adult patient, the management of cardiorespiratory arrest and shock states in pediatric patients has many unique complexities. A detailed understanding of the etiology of the most common pathologies leading to these clinical scenarios both outside and inside the operating room enables providers to treat these patients in a systematic and goal-directed fashion and can lead to improved outcomes. The basics of cardiopulmonary resuscitation theory and technique, medication management, vascular access, monitoring, and post-resuscitation care are discussed. A special emphasis is placed on cardiac resuscitation during anesthesia care. Advanced techniques, including temporary extracorporeal life support, are also described so that providers will be able to recognize the clinical scenarios where these treatments may be indicated and enlist the appropriate resources.

Keywords: 2020 AHA PALS, Anaphalyxsis, Cardiac arrest, Cardiac bypass, Cardiogenic shock, Cardiopulmonary resuscitation, Cardioversion, Defibrillation, Distributive shock, Endotracheal medication administration, Extracorporeal life support, H's and T's, Hypovolemic shock, Obstructive shock, Pacing, Pediatric Perioperative Cardiac Arrest Registry, Phases of cardiac arrest, Return of spontaneous circulation, Succinylcholine induced bradycardia, Targeted temperature management, Ventricular assist device.

CARDIOPULMONARY ARREST IN THE PEDIATRIC PATIENT

Epidemiology

Cardiopulmonary arrest in the pediatric patient is distinct in many ways from adult cardiac arrest. Though the incidence of arrests is lower compared with adults, there are still many children affected. Pediatric patients account for 16,000 out-of-hospital cardiac arrests yearly in the United States [1, 2]. According to the

---

* **Corresponding author Bharathi Gourkanti**: Department of Anesthesiology, Cooper Medical School of Rowan University, Cooper University Health Care, Camden, NJ, USA; E-mail: gourkantibharathi@cooperhealth.edu

Bharathi Gourkanti, Irwin Gratz, Grace Dippo, Nathalie Peiris and Dinesh K. Choudhry (Eds.)
All rights reserved-© 2022 Bentham Science Publishers

Resuscitation Outcomes Consortium Registry, an incidence of 1-20/100,000 in a cohort study of eleven Canadian and US hospitals has been reported [3]. Sudden cardiac arrest has been attributed to multiple cardiac, respiratory, and vascular pathologies, including inherited heart rhythm disorders, coronary disease, hypertrophic cardiomyopathy, and left ventricular myopathy [4, 5]. Left ventricular hypertrophy has been associated with sudden cardiac death in children with otherwise unremarkable hearts on autopsy [6]. The etiology of cardiac arrest in pediatric patients often remains unclear in 50% of cases [7]. With the increasing prevalence of childhood diabetes, hypertension, and obesity, it is concerning that at least one of these factors has been found in 58% of sudden cardiac arrests in youth [6].

The pediatric arrest can occur in the hospital and out of the hospital. The clinical characteristics of in-hospital and out-of-hospital patients are different. In-hospital arrest patients are more likely to have preexisting conditions [1]. Interestingly, sports-related sudden cardiac arrests account for only a small portion (14%) of overall cases [6].

The low incidence would render mass screening a low-yield effort; however, certain individual characteristics could warrant further workup, including "exercise-associated syncope, non-vasopressor syncope, family history of sudden unexpected death or family history of hypertrophic cardiomyopathy" [8, p120B]. The outcomes of pediatric arrest vary. Post-arrest brain injury can result from cortical hypoperfusion after nine minutes [1]. Out-of-hospital arrests are more likely to cause death from neurological injury as well [1].

ANESTHESIA-RELATED CARDIAC ARREST

According to the Pediatric Perioperative Cardiac Arrest (POCA) Registry (1998-2004), cardiac etiology of cardiac arrest under anesthesia was the most prevalent, second to respiratory causes [9]. The most common cardiac cause was hypovolemia due to blood loss, with secondary contributors including the underestimation of blood loss and inadequate vascular access [9]. These patients were more likely to be ASA Class 3 to 5 [9]. Respiratory, medication-related and equipment-related events were also contributors to the registry. 58% of cardiac arrests took place during maintenance of anesthesia, 24% were during induction/preinduction, and 19% occurred after emergence including up until recovery [9]. Airway surgery was more likely to precipitate respiratory events. Cardiac surgery, neurosurgery, and spine procedures preceded most cardiac events [9].

According to the POCA (1998-2004), 61% of patients with cardiac arrest under anesthesia had no injury. In pediatric patients undergoing surgery with congenital or acquired heart disease, including aortic stenosis and cardiomyopathy, Ramamoorthy *et al.* found that the mortality rate was higher than for patients without heart disease [10].

DIAGNOSIS OF CARDIAC ARREST

Early recognition of impending acute circulatory failure is crucial to improving patient outcomes. Four phases of cardiac arrest are described in Table **1** including pre-arrest, no-flow, low-flow, and post-resuscitation [1, 11].

Table 1. Four Phases of Cardiac Arrest [1, 11]

Phase	Definition	Crucial Management Steps
Pre-arrest	Events prior to cardiac arrest	Determine and treat precipitating factors
No-flow	Untreated cardiac arrest	Identification of cardiac arrest and initiation of CPR
Low-flow	Initiation of CPR	High-quality chest compressions Determine shockable rhythms
Post-resuscitation	Achievement of ROSC	Initiation of targeted temperature management

The pre-arrest phase consists of pathologic states, including shock (Table **2**), bradyarrhythmia, tachyarrhythmia, and arrhythmia (Table **3**).

Sinus bradycardia, junctional bradycardia and atrioventricular block are noted to affect pediatric patients and can lead to cardiac arrest [13]. Hypervagotonia, apnea, bradycardia of the premature newborn, and infectious causes such as Lyme disease or Chagas disease are also possible etiologies [13]. Management of bradycardia depends on symptoms and whether or not there is hemodynamic compromise. If there is a cardiopulmonary compromise, CPR is initiated, and atropine and epinephrine are administered for persistent bradycardia.

Table 2. Shock States [12]

Shock State	Cause	Treatment
Hypovolemic	Burns GI or renal loss Hemorrhage	Isotonic crystalloid 20 ml/kg
Obstructive	Tension Pneumothorax Pericardial Tamponade	Relief of Obstruction
Cardiogenic	Cardiomyopathy Congenital Heart Disease Myocarditis	Cold/wet: Inotropes Warm/wet: diuretics or inodilators

(Table 2) cont.....

Shock State	Cause	Treatment
Distributive	Sepsis Anaphylaxis	Antibiotics Removal of the offending agent, supportive care, epinephrine

Table 3. Dysrhythmias leading to cardiac arrest [11].

Arrhythmia	Etiology	Treatment
Bradycardia Sinus bradycardia Junctional bradycardia Atrioventricular block Congenital complete heart block Tachycardia Supraventricular tachycardia atrial flutter, intraatrial reentrant tachycardia, ectopic atrial tachycardia and atrial fibrillation VT, VF	Increased Vagal tone AV block Apnea Prematurity Abnormal Conduction predisposition including reentrant circuits	Atropine Epinephrine CPR Temporary pacing Permanent pacing Vagal Maneuvers Adenosine Defibrillation or> cardioversion if a shockable rhythm

Supraventricular tachycardia is the most common tachyarrhythmia in children and adolescents [2]. Ventricular tachycardia and ventricular fibrillation are shockable cardiac arrest rhythms. Arrhythmia in the newborn is another special consideration. As with older children, SVT is also the most common tachyarrhythmia for neonates [2, 14]. It is usually associated with reentry, such as Wolff-Parkinson-White syndrome [14]. The first-line treatment for atrioventricular reentrant tachycardia is adenosine triphosphate [15].

CARDIOPULMONARY RESUSCITATION: MECHANISM OF ACTION

Cardiopulmonary resuscitation decreases the no-flow phase of CPR and starts the low flow phase [1]. The main objective is the delivery of oxygen to the brain through the management of the airway, breathing and circulation. Assessment of the airway includes determining patency and checking for breathing. Medical providers should start with a jaw-thrust and chin-lift/head tilt, assuming there is no obvious trauma [1, 16]. Ventilations should be immediately started if the patient is apneic, or gasping, or obstructing. This can take the form of mask ventilation or an invasive airway. CO_2 monitoring is used to confirm the correct placement of an endotracheal tube or laryngeal mask airway. Depending on whether the performer of CPR is alone or in a pair, compression-ventilation should start at a ratio of 30:2 or 15:2; compression-ventilation for neonates should be performed in a ratio of 3:1 [17] (Table **4**).

For infants, compressions should encircle the chest if there are two providers and only two fingers for one provider; for older children, either can be used [17]. High-quality chest compressions should have a depth of 1/3 anterior-posterior diameter of the chest and should minimize interruptions. Please see the AHA PALS resuscitation algorithms for further details.

Table 4. Pediatric compression to ventilation ratio.

Patient	Compression/ventilation ratio (solo provider)	Compression/ventilation ratio (with a partner)
Neonate	3:1	3:1
Child	30:2	15:2

DEFIBRILLATION AND CARDIOVERSION

The differentiation of shockable and nonshockable rhythms is essential for effective CPR. In otherwise healthy children, sudden cardiac arrest is associated with ventricular fibrillation, pulseless ventricular tachycardia, or arrhythmia [14]. Defibrillation is based on countershock, which involves using a high-intensity current to allow the myocardium to simultaneously depolarize [19, 20]. Pediatric dosing for defibrillation is 2 J/kg, which can be increased to 4 J/kg. Pediatric dosing for cardioversion is less than for defibrillation with 0.5 to 1 J/kg for the initial dose increasing to up to 4 J/kg (Table **5**) [22]. According to AHA, pad placement is acceptable anterolateral, anteroposterior, or apex posterior in order to maximize current flow to the heart [22], as illustrated in Fig. (**1**) below.

Table 5. Pediatric Dosing for Defibrillation and Cardioversion [22].

-	Initial Energy Dose (J/kg)	Subsequent Energy Dose (J/kg)
Cardioversion	0.5 to 1	Up to 2
Defibrillation	2 to 4	4*

*do not exceed 10 J/kg or the highest adult dose

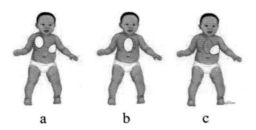

Fig. (1). a) Anterolateral, **b)** anteroposterior and **c)** apex posterior positioning of cardioversion or defibrillator pads. It is important to ensure that pads do not overlap or touch when placed on the patient. Illustration by Grace Dippo MD.

MONITORING DURING CPR

In the field, monitoring of the pediatric patient post-cardiac arrest includes ECG, pulse oximetry, capnography, noninvasive blood pressure, and point of care glucose [22]. ICU level monitoring includes cardiac telemetry, pulse oximetry, continuous capnography, continuous temperature, urine output, arterial/venous blood gasses, serum electrolytes, glucose, calcium lactate, and chest X-ray. If the patient requires intubation, CO_2 monitoring is needed to confirm the placement of the advanced airway.

EMERGENCY VASCULAR ACCESS AND FLUID ADMINISTRATION

IV access in the pediatric population can be difficult. Common peripheral intravascular sites include dorsum of hand and leg, antecubital, great saphenous vein, external jugular, and scalp veins [23]. Intraosseous access is indicated when the provider is unable to secure an intravascular cannula. The onset of action and dosing are similar between IV and IO administered medications [21]. Contraindications to IO insertion include long bone fractures, local vascular injury, local infection, or local burn [21]. Sites in pediatric patients include distal humerus, ulna, femur, and tibia; an illustration is shown in Part I Chapter 8 (Fig. **1**): Intraosseous insertion sites [20]. Complications, though <1% [24, 25], include extravasation, compartment syndrome, cellulitis, skin abscesses. Neonatal IV access includes an umbilical vein catheter, which can be inserted up to two weeks of age. Central venous access is indicated for difficult peripheral access; however, there is a risk of pneumothorax, arterial puncture hematoma, arrhythmias, and infection [26].

MEDICATIONS USED DURING CPR

Most medications used in adult CPR are also administered to pediatric and neonatal patients with dosing changes, as listed below in Tables **6** and **7**.

Table 6. PALS AHA Antiarrhythmics.

Medication	Mechanism of Action	Dosage/Route
Atropine [28]	Block acetylcholine at parasympathetic sites	Neonatal Bradycardia IV, Intraosseous: 0.02 mg/kg/dose Endotracheal .04-.06mg/kg/dose Pediatric Bradycardia IV, Intraosseous: .02 mg/kg/dose Endotracheal: .04-.06/mg/kg
Amiodarone [31]	Class III antiarrhythmic	Neonatal supraventricular tachycardia Oral: loading 10-20 mg/kg/day in 2 divided doses 7-10 days Tachyarrhythmia Loading dose IV: 5 mg/kg over 60 minutes Continuous: Initial 5 mcg/kg/minute 5 to 15 mcg/kg/minute
Lidocaine [32]	Class Ib antiarrhythmic	Neonatal Ventricular fibrillation or pulseless ventricular tachycardia, shock-refractory IV, intraosseous: Loading dose: 1 mg/kg/dose Continuous infusion: 20-50 mcg/kg/minute ETT: Loading dose: 2-3 mg/kg/dose Pediatric Ventricular fibrillation or pulseless ventricular tachycardia, shock-refractory IV, intraosseous Loading dose: 1 mg/kg/dose Continuous IV infusion: 20 to 50 mcg/kg/min Endotracheal: 2 to 3 mg/kg/dose

Table 7. PALS AHA Medications.

Medication	Mechanism of Action	Dosage/Route
Epinephrine [27]	Activates alpha, beta 1, and beta 2 adrenergic receptors	Neonatal IV, Intraosseous: .01-.03 mg/kg 3-5 minutes each dose Endotracheal: .05 to 1 mg/kg 3-5min each dose

(Table 7) cont.....

Medication	Mechanism of Action	Dosage/Route
		Pediatric IV, Intraosseous: .01 mg/kg 3-5 each dose Endotracheal: .1 mg/kg 3-5 min Anaphylaxis: *IM preferredIM, SubQ .01 mg/kg/dose of 1mg/mL solutionPrepubertal: .3 mg/dose Adolescent .5 mg/doseAdministered every 5-15 minutes
Sodium Bicarbonate [29]	Bicarbonate ion neutralizes H+; raises blood/urine pH	Neonatal Metabolic acidosis 1-2 mEq/kg/dose Pediatric Cardiac arrest IV, Intraosseous: 1 mEq/kg/dose
Dextrose [30]	Source of calories Stimulates transient uptake of potassium by cells	Neonatal Hypoglycemia IV: 0.2 g/kg/dose; 5 to 8 mg/kg/minute Hyperkalemia IV 0.4g/kg/dose, 0.2-0.4g/kg/hr Pediatric Hypoglycemia IV, Intraosseous Infants/children: D25 0.5 to 1 g/kg/dosets: D50 0.5-1g/kg/dose max: 25 g/dose

ENDOTRACHEAL MEDICATION ADMINISTRATION

Medications can be administered through the endotracheal tube utilizing the absorptive surface of the pulmonary capillaries [33]. Absorption is best at the alveolar level. Particularly, for neonates in the delivery room, endotracheal tube placement and administration is faster than securing an umbilical venous catheter [34]. The preferred agent is epinephrine. Dosing is 0.1 to 0.3 mL/kg of 1:10,000 solution every 3-5 minutes [35, 36]. Endotracheal naloxone can be given at a dose of 0.1 mg/kg [35]; however, this route has not been well studied in neonates. It is not recommended to give sodium bicarbonate through the endotracheal tube because of the high pH. Endotracheal calcium and norepinephrine can result in tissue necrosis [36].

SPECIAL SITUATIONS

Perioperative cardiac arrest includes several unique etiologies compared to out of the hospital or in hospital arrests, as shown in Table **8** [9]:

Table 8. Anesthesia-related causes of cardiac arrest [9].

Etiology	Mechanism	Treatment
Cardiac	Hypovolemia related to blood loss Hyperkalemia due to transfusion	Volume repletion including blood products* Judicious use of blood products, Monitoring intraoperative blood loss, autologous transfusions, intraoperative blood salvage, antifibrinolytics, using fresh red blood cells, saline washing of irradiated blood Cardiac protection: calcium gluconate Glucose/Insulin Sodium Bicarbonate Dialysis
Respiratory	Laryngospasm	IM succinylcholine, deepening of anesthetic
Medication Induced	Volatile gas-induced cardiovascular depression Succinylcholine induced bradycardia Anaphylaxis	Sevoflurane used over halothane Atropine Epinephrine, supportive care
Equipment Related	Injury to lung parenchyma or vascular injury during central line placement	Ultrasound guidance recommended

*See trauma chapter for transfusion guidelines.

Anaphylaxis

Anaphylaxis is a systemic allergic reaction that can rapidly develop into cardiac arrest [37]. Symptoms include rash involving skin or mucosa, angioedema, respiratory compromise, hypotension, hypotension, tachycardia, gastrointestinal symptoms, or decreased blood pressure after known exposure to an allergen [37]. Management includes supporting the airway, breathing, and circulation. The preferred treatment is intramuscular or IV epinephrine, 0.01 mg/kg redosed every 5 to 15 minutes [27, 37]. Place the patient in a recumbent position with lower extremities elevated. Patients may require continuous epinephrine infusion. Antihistamines are a second-line treatment. Diphenhydramine may be administered, 1 mg/kg^{-2} mg/kg, up to 50 mg. Corticosteroids may be administered but have a slower onset of action. Pediatric dosing is 1.0 to 2.0 mg/kg per dose of methylprednisolone every six hours. Medication treatment for anaphylaxis is summarized in Table **9**.

Table 9. Treatment of Anaphylaxis.

First line: IM or IV epinephrine .01 mg/kg every 5 to 15 minutes, continuous infusion may be required
Antihistamines *i.e.*, diphenhydramine 1-2 mg/kg up to 50 mg
Corticosteroids *i.e.*, methylprednisolone 1.0-2.0 mg/kg every 6 hours

Hs/Ts

Hs and Ts are a mnemonic to determine the reversible causes of cardiac arrest. The mechanisms and treatments for each pathology are listed in Table **10a** and **10b** [38]:

Table 10a. Hs of Reversible cardiac arrest.

Etiology	Mechanism	Signs, symptoms, and diagnosis	Treatment
Hypoxia	Asthma Pneumonia Drowning Anemia Airway Obstruction	Decreased oxygen saturation or partial pressure of oxygen	Treat underlying etiology Ventilate Supplemental oxygen
Hypovolemia	Trauma Burns Diarrhea/vomiting	Decreased urine output Tachycardia hypotension	Start with 20 mg/kg bolus and assess volume status [39]
Hypo/Hyperkalemia	Hyperkalemia: impaired kidney excretion, drugs, metabolic acidosis Hypokalemia: GI loss Medications Metabolic alkalosis Mg loss	Hyperkalemia: peaked T waves, widened QRS, first- degree heart block Hypokalemia: u waves, flat T waves	Hyperkalemia: Cardiac protection: calcium gluconate Glucose/Insulin Sodium Bicarbonate Dialysis Hypokalemia Replete potassium
Hyper/Hypothermia	Hypothermia: Core temperature less than 35 degrees Celsius. Leads to bradycardia and asystole Hyperthermia (Heat exhaustion/heat stroke)	Varies depending on the clinical scenario	Hypothermia: Remove from the cold environment Passive rewarming Hyperthermia: Ice packs, Cold IV fluids

Table 10b. Ts of reversible cardiac arrest.

Etiology	Mechanism	Signs, symptoms, and diagnosis	Treatment
Thrombosis	Pulmonary Embolism	Hypoxia Dyspnea	Extracorporeal CPR Surgical embolectomy and mechanical thrombectomy
Cardiac Tamponade	Pericardial sac fills with fluid	Hemodynamic instability Blunt or penetrating trauma Visualize with ultrasound	Thoracotomy Pericardiocentesis
Toxins	Benzodiazepines Tricyclic antidepressants Local anesthetics Cocaine	Altered mental status Suspicion varies based on clinical scenario	Flumazenil is not routinely used – may increase the risk of seizure Sodium bicarbonate 20% Lipid emulsion

(Table 10b) cont.....

Etiology	Mechanism	Signs, symptoms, and diagnosis	Treatment
Tension Pneumothorax	Intrapleural air mass causing hemodynamic instability	Hypotension Respiratory distress Unilateral breath sounds Subcutaneous emphysema Clinical diagnosis	Needle decompression Thoracostomy

Extracorporeal Membrane Oxygenation (ECMO) should be considered when a multistoried treatment approach including fluids, inotropes, and vasopressors does not stabilize the patient [18]. In the PICU setting, ECMO after ROSC can decrease mortality by 87% [40].

Neonatal respiratory failure is associated with postpartum (low Apgar scores, NICU admission), antepartum (hypertension, oligohydramnios, infection), and intrapartum (preterm delivery, breech presentation, emergency C-section) events [41]. In one study, preterm delivery had an unadjusted positive likelihood ratio of

>10 for PPV-ETT utilization [41]. After a neonate is asystolic for 10 minutes, the chance of survival decreases even with therapeutic hypothermia.Table **11** lists several other advanced life support methods for the pediatric population.

Table 11. Supplementary Techniques.

Therapy	Mechanism of Action	Indications	Contraindications
Extracorporeal Membrane Oxygenation [42]	After cannulation, blood is oxygenated outside the body and returned *via* venous or arterial access veno-arterial (VA) ECMO veno-venous (VV) ECMO if cardiac pump function preserved	Cardiac arrest or any cause refractory to CPR Cardiac arrest after cardiac surgery	lethal chromosomal or syndromic abnormalities irreversible brain injury multiorgan injury
Cardiac Bypass [43, 44]	After venous and arterial cannulation, blood drained to a reservoir outside the body, oxygenated, and pumped back into the arterial system	Perioperative cardiothoracic arrest Cardiac arrest refractory to CPR	-
Ventricular Assist Device [45, 46]	Mechanical pump for the heart	Advanced heart failure	Systemic infection, extreme prematurity, <2.0 kg weight, significant neurologic damage, congenital anomalies with poor prognosis, and chromosomal aberrations

(Table 11) cont.....

Therapy	Mechanism of Action	Indications	Contraindications
Intra-aortic Balloon [47, 48]	The balloon is placed in	Acute heart Failure,	Aortic regurgitation
Pump [55-56]	descending aorta, inflation and	Refractory Left	Aortic dissection
-	deflation is timed with cardiac	Ventricular Failure	Sepsis
-	cycle to decrease afterload	-	Bleeding diathesis

Adequate chest compressions ensure perfusion to the heart and brain [49]. Active compression-decompression works by "active lifting of the anterior chest wall" during decompression with a hand-held suction cup device [49]. This creates a vacuum in the thorax, which increases cardiac preload [50]. Benefits of active compression-decompression include decreased rescuer fatigue and complete chest recoil [49].

POST-CARDIAC ARREST CARE AND STABILIZATION

Post cardiac arrest syndrome in children is a pathologic state characterized by "brain injury, myocardial dysfunction, systemic ischemic/reperfusion response, and persistent precipitating pathophysiology" [18]. Brain injury is believed to result in part from hypoxemia along with reactive oxygen species. It can cause "coma, cerebral edema, seizures, myoclonus, sympathetic hyperarousal, long term neurobehavioral and functional deficits" [18]. The exact pathophysiology of post-arrest myocardial dysfunction remains unclear and can happen even without a cardiac cause of arrest. It is estimated that 95% of children with in-hospital cardiac arrest in the ICU have resulting myocardial dysfunction (Berg RA, Sutton). When out-of-hospital cardiac arrest patients have elevated troponins and decreased ventricular shortening fraction, there is increased mortality [59]. Myocardial dysfunction can present with hypotension, ventricular dysfunction, decreased cardiac output, and pulmonary edema [18]. Systemic ischemia and reperfusion response results in the increase of cytokines, endotoxins, and alterations to coagulation pathways [1, 52]. No studies in children have endorsed the use of prophylactic antiarrhythmics after achieving ROSC [18]. Critical illness hyperglycemia results from a post-arrest insulin-resistant state, which can decrease survival [53 - 54]. The multisystem ischemia and reperfusion can lead to capillary leak, intravascular hypovolemia, vasoplegia, adrenal insufficiency, and impaired oxygen usage [18].

Once ROSC is achieved, targeted temperature management is initiated [18]. It requires hypothermia 24-32 degrees Celsius and normothermia 36-37.5 degrees Celsius. There are 4 phases of targeted temperature management [18]:

1. Immediate: 0 to 20 minutes after ROSC
2. Early: 20 minutes to 6-12 hours
3. Intermediate: 12-72 hours
4. Recovery: 72 hours to day 7

The immediate phase can be complicated by hypokalemia, hypomagnesemia, hypocalcaemia, hyperglycemia, bradycardia, and hypotension [18]. Shivering can be controlled with opioids. Neuroprognostication occurs during the intermediate or recovery phase and can include EEG and neuroimaging.

Post ROSC, seizures can occur in 10-50% of patients who are encephalopathic [55, 56]. Seizures require prompt control as they can increase metabolic demand along with increasing intracranial pressure [18]. Treatments include benzodiazepines, levetiracetam, and phenytoin.

2020 AHA PALS GUIDELINES UPDATE

The 2020 American Heart Association Pediatric Life Support Updates include several updates to the standard of practice which are summarized below [22]:

Pre-arrest Care [22]:

- Crystalloid both balanced and unbalanced and colloid fluids can be administered for sepsis resuscitation.
- Reassess the patient after each fluid bolus Intra-Arrest Care [22]
- Family members are recommended to have the option to be present during resuscitation
- A respiratory rate of 20-30 breaths per minute is recommended in patients with an advanced airway or who have both a pulse and are receiving rescue breaths.
- Earlier administration of epinephrine for patients with non-shockable rhythms can improve patient survival.
- If there is suspected cervical spinal injury, jaw thrust without head tilt is recommended to manage the airway.
- Cuffed endotracheal tubes are recommended to decrease the need for tube exchange
- Routine use of cricoid pressure does not decrease the risk of regurgitation
- There is no evidence that naloxone has a role for patients in cardiac arrest.
- Use of "CPR mode" on hospital beds is recommended if available.
- Consider ECPR for patients with cardiac pathology in centers with available resources

Post Arrest Care [22].

- After ROSC is achieved, unconscious patients require further care that may include TTM and EEG for the detection of seizures.
- Maintain systolic blood pressures to the fifth percentile for age using fluids, inotropes, vasoactive drugs.
- Continuous arterial pressure monitoring is recommended for hypotension management
- All patients should be evaluated for rehabilitation

CONCLUSION

Due to the differences between the pediatric and adult patient, there are nuances to managing cardiorespiratory arrest and shock states. This chapter reviewed the common pathologies along with the systematic treatments both inside and outside the operating room. Both the basics of cardiopulmonary resuscitation and advanced techniques were described.

CONSENT FOR PUBLICATION

Not applicable.

CONFLICT OF INTEREST

The author declares no conflict of interest, financial or otherwise.

ACKNOWLEDGEMENTS

Declared none.

REFERENCES

[1]   Tress EE, Kochanek PM, Saladino RA, Manole MD. Cardiac arrest in children. J Emerg Trauma Shock 2010; 3(3): 267-72.
[http://dx.doi.org/10.4103/0974-2700.66528] [PMID: 20930971]

[2]   Marino B, Tabbutt S, MacLaren G, Hazinski M, Adatia I, Atkins D, *et al.* Cardiopulmonary Resuscitation in Infants and Children With Cardiac Disease: A Scientific Statement From the American Heart Association. Circulation : Journal of the American Heart Association 2018; 137(22): e691-782.
[http://dx.doi.org/10.1161/CIR.0000000000000524]

[3]   Atkins DL, Everson-Stewart S, Sears GK, *et al.* Epidemiology and outcomes from out-of-hospital cardiac arrest in children: the Resuscitation Outcomes Consortium Epistry-Cardiac Arrest. Circulation 2009; 119(11): 1484-91.
[http://dx.doi.org/10.1161/CIRCULATIONAHA.108.802678] [PMID: 19273724]

[4]   Fishman GI, Chugh SS, Dimarco JP, *et al.* Sudden cardiac death prediction and prevention: Report from a national heart, lung, and blood institute and heart rhythm society workshop. Circulation 2010; 122(22): 2335-48.
[http://dx.doi.org/10.1161/CIRCULATIONAHA.110.976092] [PMID: 21147730]

[5]   Chugh SS, Jui J, Gunson K, *et al.* Current burden of sudden cardiac death: multiple source surveillance

versus retrospective death certificate-based review in a large U.S. community. J Am Coll Cardiol 2004; 44(6): 1268-75.2004;
[http://dx.doi.org/10.1016/j.jacc.2004.06.029]

[6]   Jayaraman R, Reinier K, Nair S, *et al.* Risk Factors of Sudden Cardiac Death in the Young: Multiple-Year Community-Wide Assessment. Circulation 2018; 137(15): 1561-70.
[http://dx.doi.org/10.1161/CIRCULATIONAHA.117.031262] [PMID: 29269388]

[7]   Cunningham Taylor, *et al.* Initially Unexplained Cardiac Arrest in Children and Adolescents: A National Experience from the Canadian Pediatric Heart Rhythm Network. Heart Rhythm.
[http://dx.doi.org/10.1016/j.hrthm.2020.01.030]

[8]   Driscoll DJ, Edwards WD. Sudden unexpected death in children and adolescents. J Am Coll Cardiol 1985; 5(6) (Suppl.): 118B-21B.
[http://dx.doi.org/10.1016/S0735-1097(85)80540-4] [PMID: 3998328]

[9]   Bhananker SM, Ramamoorthy C, Geiduschek JM, *et al.* Anesthesia-related cardiac arrest in children: update from the Pediatric Perioperative Cardiac Arrest Registry. Anesth Analg 2007; 105(2): 344-50.
[http://dx.doi.org/10.1213/01.ane.0000268712.00756.dd] [PMID: 17646488]

[10]   Ramamoorthy Chandra. "Anesthesia-Related Cardiac Arrest in Children with Heart Disease". Anesthesia & Analgesia 110(5): 1376-82.2010;
[http://dx.doi.org/10.1213/ANE.0b013e3181c9f927]

[11]   Berg MD, Nadkarni VM, Zuercher M, Berg RA. In-hospital pediatric cardiac arrest. Pediatr Clin North Am 2008; 55(3): 589-604, x.
[http://dx.doi.org/10.1016/j.pcl.2008.02.005] [PMID: 18501756]

[12]   Mendelson J. Emergency Department Management of Pediatric Shock. Emergency Medicine Clinics of North America. WB Saunders Co 2018; 36: pp. (2)427-0.
[http://dx.doi.org/10.1016/j.emc.2017.12.010]

[13]   Baruteau AE, Perry JC, Sanatani S, Horie M, Dubin AM. Evaluation and management of bradycardia in neonates and children. Eur J Pediatr 2016; 175(2): 151-61.
[http://dx.doi.org/10.1007/s00431-015-2689-z] [PMID: 26780751]

[14]   Ban JE. Neonatal arrhythmias: diagnosis, treatment, and clinical outcome. Korean J Pediatr 2017; 60(11): 344-52.
[http://dx.doi.org/10.3345/kjp.2017.60.11.344] [PMID: 29234357]

[15]   Camm AJ, Garratt CJ. Adenosine and supraventricular tachycardia. N Engl J Med 1991; 325(23): 1621-9.
[http://dx.doi.org/10.1056/NEJM199112053252306] [PMID: 1944450]

[16]   Harless J, Ramaiah R, Bhananker SM. Pediatric airway management. Int J Crit Illn Inj Sci 2014; 4(1): 65-70.
[http://dx.doi.org/10.4103/2229-5151.128015] [PMID: 24741500]

[17]   International Liaison Committee on Resuscitation. 2005 International consensus on cardiopulmonary resuscitation and emergency cardiovascular care science with treatment recommendations. Part 6: pediatric basic and advanced life support. Resuscitation 2005; 67(2-3): 271-91.
[PMID: 16324992]

[18]   Topjian AA, de Caen A, Wainwright MS, *et al.* Pediatric Post-Cardiac Arrest Care: A Scientific Statement From the American Heart Association. Circulation 2019; 140(6): e194-233.
[http://dx.doi.org/10.1161/CIR.0000000000000697] [PMID: 31242751]

[19]   Mower MM, Mirowski M, Spear JF, Moore EN. Patterns of ventricular activity during catheter defibrillation. Circulation 1974; 49(5): 858-61.
[http://dx.doi.org/10.1161/01.CIR.49.5.858] [PMID: 4828606]

[20]   Zipes DP, Fischer J, King RM, Jolly WW, Jolly WW. Termination of ventricular fibrillation in dogs by depolarizing a critical amount of myocardium. Am J Cardiol 1975; 36(1): 37-44.

[http://dx.doi.org/10.1016/0002-9149(75)90865-6] [PMID: 1146696]

[21]   Rosetti VA, Thompson BM, Miller J, Mateer JR, Aprahamian C. Intraosseous infusion: an alternative route of pediatric intravascular access. Ann Emerg Med 1985; 14(9): 885-8.
[http://dx.doi.org/10.1016/S0196-0644(85)80639-9] [PMID: 4025988]

[22]   Topjian , Alexis A, *et al.* Part 4: Pediatric Basic and Advanced Life Support: 2020 American Heart Association Guidelines for Cardiopulmonary Resuscitation and Emergency Cardiovascular Care. Circulation 142: S469-523.2020;
[http://dx.doi.org/10.1161/CIR.0000000000000901]

[23]   Naik Vibhavari M, *et al.* Vascular access in children. Indian journal of anaesthesia 63(9): 737-45.2019;
[http://dx.doi.org/10.4103/ija.IJA_489_19]

[24]   Luck RP, Haines C, Mull CC. Intraosseous access. J Emerg Med 2010; 39(4): 468-75.
[http://dx.doi.org/10.1016/j.jemermed.2009.04.054] [PMID: 19545966]

[25]   Fiser DH. Intraosseous infusion. N Engl J Med 1990; 322(22): 1579-81.
[http://dx.doi.org/10.1056/NEJM199005313222206] [PMID: 2186277]

[26]   Ares G, Hunter CJ. Central venous access in children: indications, devices, and risks. Curr Opin Pediatr 2017; 29(3): 340-6.
[http://dx.doi.org/10.1097/MOP.0000000000000485] [PMID: 28323667]

[27]   Epinephrine. In: Pediatric and Neonatal Lexi-drugs online [database on the Internet]. Hudson (OH): Lexicomp Inc.; 2016 [updated 4 June 2020; cited 8 June 2020]. Available from:. http://online.lexi.com

[28]   Atropine. In: Pediatric and Neonatal Lexi-drugs online [database on the Internet]. Hudson (OH): Lexicomp Inc.; 2016 [updated 18 May 2020; cited 8 June 2020]. Available from:. http://online.lexi.com

[29]   Bicarbonate S. . In: Pediatric and Neonatal Lexi-drugs online [database on the Internet]. Hudson (OH): Lexicomp Inc.; 2016 [updated 4 June 2020; cited 8 June 2020]. Available from:. http://online.lexi.com

[30]   In: Pediatric and Neonatal Lexi-drugs online [database on the Internet]. Hudson (OH): Lexicomp Inc.; 2016 [updated 5 June 2020; cited 8 June 2020]. Available from:. http://online.lexi.com

[31]   Amiodarone. In: Pediatric and Neonatal Lexi-drugs online [database on the Internet]. Hudson (OH): Lexicomp Inc.; 2016 [updated 4 June 2020; cited 8 June 2020]. Available from:. http://online.lexi.com

[32]   Lidocaine. In: Pediatric and Neonatal Lexi-drugs online [database on the Internet]. Hudson (OH): Lexicomp Inc.; 2016 [updated 5 May 2020; cited 8 June 2020]. Available from:. http://online.lexi.com

[33]   Greenberg MI. The use of endotracheal medication in cardiac emergencies. Resuscitation 1984; 12(3): 155-65.
[http://dx.doi.org/10.1016/0300-9572(84)90001-7] [PMID: 6096940]

[34]   Wyckoff MH, Wyllie J. Endotracheal delivery of medications during neonatal resuscitation. Clin Perinatol 2006; 33(1): 153-160, ix.
[http://dx.doi.org/10.1016/j.clp.2005.11.013] [PMID: 16533641]

[35]   Kattwinkel J, Niermeyer S, Nadkarni V, *et al.* Resuscitation of the newly born infant: an advisory statement from the Pediatric Working Group of the International Liaison Committee on Resuscitation. Resuscitation 1999; 40(2): 71-88.
[http://dx.doi.org/10.1016/S0300-9572(99)00012-X] [PMID: 10225280]

[36]   Powers RD, Donowitz LG. Endotracheal administration of emergency medications. South Med J 1984; 77(3): 340-341, 346.
[http://dx.doi.org/10.1097/00007611-198403000-00018] [PMID: 6322354]

[37]   Sampson HA, Muñoz-Furlong A, Campbell RL, *et al.* Second symposium on the definition and management of anaphylaxis: summary report--Second National Institute of Allergy and Infectious Disease/Food Allergy and Anaphylaxis Network symposium. J Allergy Clin Immunol 2006; 117(2):

391-7.
[http://dx.doi.org/10.1016/j.jaci.2005.12.1303] [PMID: 16461139]

[38]   Truhlář A, Deakin CD, Soar J, *et al*. European Resuscitation Council Guidelines for Resuscitation 2015: Section 4. Cardiac arrest in special circumstances. Resuscitation 2015; 95: 148-201.
[http://dx.doi.org/10.1016/j.resuscitation.2015.07.017] [PMID: 26477412]

[39]   de Caen AR, Berg MD, Chameides L, *et al*. Part 12: Pediatric Advanced Life Support: 2015 American Heart Association Guidelines Update for Cardiopulmonary Resuscitation and Emergency Cardiovascular Care. Circulation 2015; 132(18) (Suppl. 2): S526-42.
[http://dx.doi.org/10.1161/CIR.0000000000000266] [PMID: 26473000]

[40]   de Mos N, van Litsenburg RR, McCrindle B, Bohn DJ, Parshuram CS. Pediatric in-intensive-care-unit cardiac arrest: incidence, survival, and predictive factors. Crit Care Med 2006; 34(4): 1209-15.
[http://dx.doi.org/10.1097/01.CCM.0000208440.66756.C2] [PMID: 16484906]

[41]   Aziz K, Chadwick M, Baker M, Andrews W. Ante- and intra-partum factors that predict increased need for neonatal resuscitation. Resuscitation 2008; 79(3): 444-52.
[http://dx.doi.org/10.1016/j.resuscitation.2008.08.004] [PMID: 18952348]

[42]   Erdil T, Lemme F, Konetzka A, *et al*. Extracorporeal membrane oxygenation support in pediatrics. Ann Cardiothorac Surg 2019; 8(1): 109-15.
[http://dx.doi.org/10.21037/acs.2018.09.08] [PMID: 30854319]

[43]   Cochran JB, Tecklenburg FW, Lau YR, Habib DM. Emergency cardiopulmonary bypass for cardiac arrest refractory to pediatric advanced life support. Pediatr Emerg Care 1999; 15(1): 30-2.
[http://dx.doi.org/10.1097/00006565-199902000-00009] [PMID: 10069309]

[44]   Whiting D, Yuki K, DiNardo JA. Cardiopulmonary bypass in the pediatric population. Best Pract Res Clin Anaesthesiol 2015; 29(2): 241-56.
[http://dx.doi.org/10.1016/j.bpa.2015.03.006] [PMID: 26060033]

[45]   Burki S, Adachi I. Pediatric ventricular assist devices: current challenges and future prospects. Vasc Health Risk Manag 2017; 13: 177-85.
[http://dx.doi.org/10.2147/VHRM.S82379] [PMID: 28546755]

[46]   Shin YR, Park YH, Park HK. Pediatric Ventricular Assist Device. Korean Circ J 2019; 49(8): 678-90.
[http://dx.doi.org/10.4070/kcj.2019.0163] [PMID: 31347320]

[47]   Paul Collison S, Singh Dagar K. The role of the Intra-aortic balloon pump in supporting children with acute cardiac failure. Postgrad Med J 2007; 83(979): 308-11.
[http://dx.doi.org/10.1136/pgmj.2006.053611] [PMID: 17488858]

[48]   Murli K. MBBS FRCA FFPMRCA, Kai Zacharowski, MD PhD FRCA, Principles of intra-aortic balloon pump counterpulsation. Contin Educ Anaesth Crit Care Pain 2009; 9(1): 24-8.
[http://dx.doi.org/10.1093/bjaceaccp/mkn051]

[49]   Udassi JP, Udassi S, Lamb MA, *et al*. Improved chest recoil using an adhesive glove device for active compression-decompression CPR in a pediatric manikin model. Resuscitation 2009; 80(10): 1158-63.
[http://dx.doi.org/10.1016/j.resuscitation.2009.06.016] [PMID: 19683849]

[50]   Wolcke BB, Mauer DK, Schoefmann MF, *et al*. Comparison of standard cardiopulmonary resuscitation *versus* the combination of active compression-decompression cardiopulmonary resuscitation and an inspiratory impedance threshold device for out-of-hospital cardiac arrest. Circulation 2003; 108(18): 2201-5.
[http://dx.doi.org/10.1161/01.CIR.0000095787.99180.B5] [PMID: 14568898]

[51]   Checchia PA, Sehra R, Moynihan J, Daher N, Tang W, Weil MH. Myocardial injury in children following resuscitation after cardiac arrest. Resuscitation 2003; 57(2): 131-7.
[http://dx.doi.org/10.1016/S0300-9572(03)00003-0] [PMID: 12745180]

[52]   Parenica J, Jarkovsky J, Malaska J, *et al*. GREAT Network. Infectious complications and immune/inflammatory response in cardiogenic shock patients: a prospective observational study.

Shock 2017; 47(2): 165-74.
[http://dx.doi.org/10.1097/SHK.0000000000000756] [PMID: 27749762]

[53]   Nayak PP, Davies P, Narendran P, *et al.* Early change in blood glucose concentration is an indicator of mortality in critically ill children. Intensive Care Med 2013; 39(1): 123-8.
[http://dx.doi.org/10.1007/s00134-012-2738-2] [PMID: 23103955]

[54]   Bhutia TD, Lodha R, Kabra SK. Abnormalities in glucose homeostasis in critically ill children. Pediatr Crit Care Med 2013; 14(1): e16-25.
[http://dx.doi.org/10.1097/PCC.0b013e3182604998] [PMID: 23249786]

[55]   Topjian AA, Sánchez SM, Shults J, Berg RA, Dlugos DJ, Abend NS. Early electroencephalographic background features predict outcomes in children resuscitated from cardiac arrest. Pediatr Crit Care Med 2016; 17(6): 547-57.
[http://dx.doi.org/10.1097/PCC.0000000000000740] [PMID: 27097270]

[56]   Abend NS, Topjian A, Ichord R, *et al.* Electroencephalographic monitoring during hypothermia after pediatric cardiac arrest. Neurology 2009; 72(22): 1931-40.
[http://dx.doi.org/10.1212/WNL.0b013e3181a82687] [PMID: 19487651]

CHAPTER 10

Pediatric Emergency Surgeries

Michael R. Schwartz[1] and **Yue Monica Li**[1]

[1] *Department of Anesthesiology, Cooper Medical School of Rowan University, Cooper University Health Care, Camden, NJ, USA*

Abstract: This chapter will explore common pediatric emergency surgeries and situations that many anesthesiologists may face in their careers. Although there are specialized pediatric hospitals and pediatric anesthesiologists in practice, pediatric emergencies arise at secondary and tertiary centers, where staff may not be familiar with these situations. Sometimes there is time to triage patients to a higher level of care, but in some emergencies, a pediatric anesthesiologist may not be available right away, or there is not enough time to transfer the patient. This chapter will go over special considerations that any anesthesiologist should be aware of when providing care to patients in these situations.

Keywords: Anesthesia, Appendicitis, Epiglottitis, Esophageal Foreign Body, Hydrocephalus, Intra-abdominal emergencies, Intussusception, Open Globe Injury, Pediatric Emergencies, Pediatric Trauma, Tonsillar Hemorrhage, Tracheal Foreign Body, Volvulus.

INTRA-ABDOMINAL EMERGENCIES

There are numerous intra-abdominal processes that may present in adolescence that may require surgical correction. Often, they present with abdominal pain, nausea, and vomiting, loss of appetite, change in bowel habits but can progress to bowel obstruction, mesenteric infarction, bowel perforation, and sepsis. Some processes are more common than others, but anesthesiologists should be familiar with their presentation and concerns associated with them when performing anesthesia.

VOLVULUS

Volvulus is caused by malrotation of the intestines, which, if left untreated, can lead to bowel ischemia. Fig. **(1)** shows examples of midgut volvulus with malrota-

* **Corresponding author Bharathi Gourkanti:** Department of Anesthesiology, Cooper Medical School of Rowan University, Cooper University Health Care, Camden, NJ, USA; E-mail: gourkantibharathi@cooperhealth.edu

Bharathi Gourkanti, Irwin Gratz, Grace Dippo, Nathalie Peiris and Dinesh K. Choudhry (Eds.)
All rights reserved-© 2022 Bentham Science Publishers

tion. Volvulus usually occurs in infancy but can occur at any age. It usually presents bilious vomiting, abdominal distention, and pain, but older children tend to present more vague complaints, and onset is more insidious [1]. If it progresses, it can lead to hypovolemia, metabolic acidosis, electrolyte abnormalities, bowel infarction and perforation, sepsis and hemodynamic instability. Non-surgical endoscopic decompression may be attempted in mild cases to resolve volvulus, but if any signs of peritonitis or ischemia are present, then surgical management with anesthesia is needed. The open Ladd's procedure was the gold standard for volvulus management, but the laparoscopic approach has gained popularity in recent years [2]. If patients are distended, septic or there are concerns for dead and friable bowel, then laparoscopic may not be ideal, and an open approach may be easier to perform.

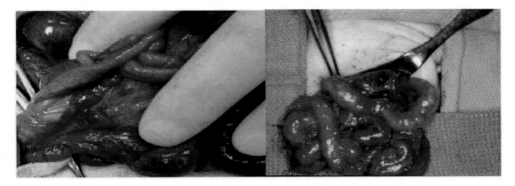

Fig. (1). Midgut Volvulus with Malrotation. Permission: Katz, D. Camden, NJ: Cooper University Hospital.

INTUSSUSCEPTION

Intussusception is caused when a bowel segment envelops, invaginates or "telescopes" into another segment. Fig. (**2**) shows examples of intussusception pathology. It usually occurs at the junction between the small and large intestine but may occur anywhere along the tract. This pathology eventually leads to bowel obstruction, abdominal pain and cramps, nausea and vomiting, rectal bleeding, and if left untreated, can eventually lead to bowel necrosis and sepsis. It can occur at any age but usually occurs in children from 3 months to 3 years [3]. Intussusception can usually be diagnosed by physical exam in combination with a bedside abdominal ultrasound. Initial management of intussusception revolves around fluid resuscitation and electrolyte repletion. Sometimes, the obstruction can be relieved by attempting a radiological reduction using a contrast enema. If this procedure fails, then surgery is necessary to either reduce the intussusception or excise the affected bowel. Surgery can be performed either open or *via* laparoscopy. Benefits of laparoscopy may include shorter operative time, shorter time to full feeds, lower requirement for intravenous (IV) narcotics, and earlier discharges [4]. However, as with volvulus repair, the open approach may be more beneficial to those patients exhibiting severe symptoms.

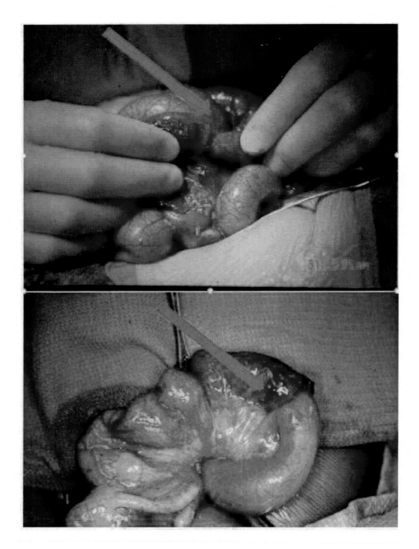

Fig. (2). Intussusception with invagination of bowel. Permission: Katz, D. Camden, NJ: Cooper University Hospital.

APPENDICITIS

Appendicitis is caused by inflammation of the appendix. Fig. (**3**) shows an inflamed appendix during an open repair. It usually presents sharp abdominal pain, which starts near the navel and then moves to the right side. This pain is often associated with fever, bloating, anorexia, change in bowels, nausea and vomiting. If left untreated, an inflamed appendix can rupture, leading to infection, abscesses and sepsis. Appendicitis is usually diagnosed via history, physical findings, and radiographic imaging. If an infected appendix is found *via* ultrasound or CT scan, then repair should be undertaken as soon as possible. However, if the appendix is found to already be ruptured, then surgery is usually delayed for a later time (interval appendectomy), and the patient is placed on antibiotics, fluids and pain medications to treat symptoms [5].

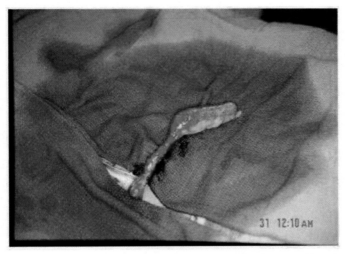

Fig. (3). Open repair of appendicitis. Permission: Katz, D. Camden, NJ: Cooper University Hospital.

As with the other two pathologies, there has been an increase in using a laparoscopic approach to treat appendicitis. Aziz *et al.* performed a meta-analysis on open *versus* laparoscopic appendectomy that showed that laparoscopy reduced overall complications [6]. Main benefits included reduced wound infection, ileus, and hospital length of stay. However, operating times and postoperative fevers were similar, whereas intra-abdominal abscess formation was actually higher in the laparoscopic group. Finally, based on a recent Cochrane Review, the evidence that there is a significant clinical difference in pain between open and laparoscopic approaches is still uncertain [7].

PREOPERATIVE EVALUATION

Preoperatively, patients should be evaluated for the severity of the disease. Many children, who are otherwise healthy, do not require preoperative labs. However, if there are concerns for hypovolemia, electrolyte abnormalities, or sepsis, then a complete blood count and basic metabolic panel may help guide treatment. In cases of bowel obstruction, persistent nausea and vomiting can lead to electrolyte loss leading to hypovolemic, hypokalemic, and hypochloremic acidosis. Inflamed bowels can also lead to an increase in protein loss and hypoalbuminemia. If this volume contraction persists, it can lead to hypoperfusion and an increase in lactic acid, which can lead to acidosis. Patients should be volume resuscitated and their electrolytes repleted as needed. Broad-spectrum antibiotics should be started as soon as possible to mitigate infection. Depending on the extent of vomiting, a nasogastric tube (NGT) may be placed preoperatively, however, most patients at our institute do not maintain them postoperatively unless deemed necessary by the surgeon.

INTRAOPERATIVE MANAGEMENT

Inside the operating room (OR), patients should be placed on standard ASA monitors. The need for advanced monitors such as arterial lines and central venous catheters is dependent on patients' underlying comorbidities or concerns for severe sepsis. However, if patients are otherwise healthy, no additional monitoring is usually necessary. If there are concerns for severe sepsis, then additional IV access, as well as an arterial line, may be useful for hemodynamic monitoring with a need for the administration of vasopressors, as well as a frequent blood draw to monitor electrolytes, hemoglobin, and lactic acid.

Acute abdominal processes may alter gastrointestinal motility, especially if an obstruction is present. These patients are often considered at a full stomach regardless of NPO status and at an increased risk for pulmonary aspiration. Although in some cases with minor symptoms, laryngeal mask airways have been used, intubation with rapid sequence induction has been found to be safe and effective [8]. If there are concerns for aspiration or unknown NPO status, the airway should be secured with a rapid sequence induction (RSI). If not already present, an NGT should be placed to decompress the stomach, especially if laparoscopy is to be performed. A foley catheter should be placed to monitor urine output, as ongoing fluid resuscitation is likely. However, urine production may not be accurate due to concomitant use of anesthesia, positioning, and pneumoperitoneum [9]. Anesthesiologists should be aware of high intra-abdominal pressures and maintain adequate hydration in order to prevent renal vascular hypoperfusion and subsequent renal impairment.

Use of either succinylcholine or non-depolarizing muscle relaxants is safe for paralysis unless the patients have any absolute contraindications to their use. Depending on the surgeon, some of these procedures may be quick, so the use of long-acting muscle relaxants may not be needed. If the patient's hemodynamics can tolerate a deeper anesthetic, the muscle relaxation from volatile anesthetics may be enough for adequate surgical exposure. However, with the increase in use and availability of sugammadex, the ability to reverse paralysis for a short procedure is possible. Regardless, some form of peripheral nerve monitoring, whether train of four (TOF) or accelerometry, should be utilized to prevent postoperative muscle weakness.

Without the use of antiemetics, the incidence of postoperative nausea and vomiting (PONV) when undergoing anesthesia is about 20-30%. However, laparoscopic procedures may have an increased risk of PONV, with some studies showing that it may be as high as 25-75 [10 - 12]. PONV can lead to retching, which can lead to pain and tension on the incisional sites, which may lead to suture rupture and the need for further surgical repair. Therefore, anesthesiologists should make every attempt to reduce PONV. There are many antiemetics available that work on different receptors, which can help reduce PONV. Another method may be to utilize TIVA, which has been shown to decrease PONV [13]. PONV is also related to the overall amount of narcotics given during an anesthetic, so any analgesic modalities that can be used to limit narcotics may be beneficial. It is usually easier to prevent PONV than it is to treat it, so anesthesiologists should attempt to use every tool available to help reduce PONV.

A big concern for patients undergoing these procedures is postoperative pain control. Although it is considered a minor procedure, up to a third of children undergoing laparoscopic appendectomy report substantial postoperative pain [14]. As mentioned earlier, the difference in pain between open and laparoscopic approaches in children is minimal, if not clinically insignificant, but other considerations have led to an increase in the laparoscopic approach. Regardless, efforts to provide adequate pain control are essential to improving surgical outcomes and patient and family satisfaction. Liu *et al.* showed that patients undergoing laparoscopic appendectomy benefited from a multimodal approach to pain management, which included local anesthesia infiltration, patient-controlled administration (PCA) of opioids, NSAIDs, and oral acetaminophen/hydrocodone to help reduce postoperative pain [15]. Several studies have looked at the use of local anesthesia to help reduce IV opioid requirements. Bergmans *et al.* showed that transversus abdominis plane (TAP) blocks may help reduce pain and opioid use in patients undergoing certain abdominal procedures [16]. Other studies have shown that pain scores and opioid consumption are likely to decrease whether TAP blocks or trocar site infiltration are used compared to nothing, however, the difference between the two methods may not be significant [17, 18]. Regardless, some type of local anesthetic added to a multimodal analgesic approach is likely beneficial for pain outcomes.

FOREIGN BODY ASPIRATION

Foreign body aspiration is a not uncommon airway emergency seen in the pediatric population, especially in children under three years old [19]. Despite more parental awareness, education, and advanced technology in children's safety, the incidence of aspiration still remains high as developing children discover their environment. Aspirated objects are usually organic (such as nuts and seeds), occur in the bronchial tree (right more than left), and occur in boys more than girls [20]. There are many types of aspirated foreign bodies, including small toys, plastic, and food. Fig. (**4**) shows some aspirated objects removed at our institution. Despite advances in the medical field, the risks of severe morbidity and mortality are still present. The goal of management in these patients is quick recognition of airway compromise and removal of foreign bodies before complications arise. Complications associated with tracheal foreign bodies include laryngeal edema, bronchospasm, pneumothorax, pneumomediastinum, aspiration, lung abscess, tracheal and bronchial laceration, cardiac arrest, hypoxia, hypercarbia, hypoxic brain injury and death [20, 21]. Anesthesiologists must be aware that complications may also present while performing anesthesia during removal. Due to the shared airway, it is imperative that the anesthesiologist is in constant communication with the ENT surgeon during the procedure.

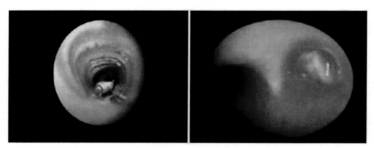

Fig. (4). Aspirated foreign bodies. 1. Metal screw above the carina. 2. Peanut in the right mainstem bronchus. Permission: Solomon, D. Camden, NJ: Cooper University Hospital.

PREOPERATIVE EVALUATION

Early recognition of aspiration is essential in reducing complications. This includes diagnosis through a combination of history, physical exam, and imaging. Aspiration may be witnessed but may only be noticed when symptoms occur. Symptoms commonly include coughing, choking, gagging, throat clearing and respiratory distress. They may be less specific and more insidious, including fever, pneumonia, stridor, hemoptysis, throat and sternal discomfort and restlessness, which may not present right away, especially if aspiration is unwitnessed [20]. The physical examination will often show coughing, choking, or respiratory distress. Lung auscultation will usually reveal one-sided breath sounds and may present wheezing and/or rhonchi. Imaging studies are often used for diagnosis, but a strong history and physical exam may preclude the need for them. Posteroanterior and lateral chest x-rays are the most common imaging used but may miss foreign bodies. Imaging studies may show localized emphysema and air trapping, atelectasis, infiltrate, and mediastinal shift [22]. Food aspiration may cause increased secretions and may lead to inflammation and increased airway reactivity. Some children may require anxiolytics prior to proceeding, however, the anesthesiologist must consider the amount of airway obstruction present and the need to maintain vigilance that a secured airway may be needed imminently. Anticholinergics may be given preoperatively or on induction to help reduce secretions which may help reduce laryngospasm and improve visualization during airway management.

INTRAOPERATIVE MANAGEMENT

All patients should have standard ASA monitors applied. Depending on the cooperation of the child, an IV may or may not be present for induction. NPO guidelines should be considered for all patients unless concerns for airway obstruction are serious. Also, the benefits of rapid sequence induction to prevent aspiration must be weighed against the risk of maintaining a patent airway with spontaneous ventilation. The best type of ventilation during the procedure has been debated extensively. There have been numerous studies evaluating whether spontaneous ventilation or controlled ventilation is superior in providing adequate procedure conditions [23 - 25]. Proponents of spontaneous ventilation advocate that maintaining airway patency decreases the risk of airway obstruction. However, there is a risk of patient movement, coughing, and laryngospasm development during the procedure. Ensuring adequate depth of anesthesia and topicalization of the larynx, trachea, and vocal cords by the surgeon can help reduce coughing, laryngospasm and reduce anesthetic requirements. Proponents of controlled ventilation advocate that in conjunction with muscle relaxants, controlled ventilation allows the procedure to occur without movement and reduces the need for a deeper anesthetic. With controlled ventilation, the anesthesiologist should ensure the ability to ventilate the patient prior to paralyzing the patient. Other risks that may occur with controlled ventilation include forcing the foreign object further down into the airway due to positive pressure, as well as air trapping due to decreased ability for air to escape.

The other debate regarding anesthetic management is the type of anesthesia to provide for the procedure. Foreign body removal can be safely performed using volatile anesthetics or with total intravenous anesthesia (TIVA) [26 - 28]. The use of volatiles provides some level of analgesia as well as smooth muscle relaxation. Volatiles may also allow for faster induction and recovery [29]. However, with the use of a rigid bronchoscope, there is a risk of environmental pollution and inadequate ventilation. Due to air leak, ventilation/perfusion mismatches, and possible frequent disconnections, the use of TIVA may allow for a more steady state of anesthesia. If TIVA is used, the anesthesiologist might consider placing a second IV. Bispectral index monitoring may be beneficial to maintain anesthetic depth since end-tidal volatile concentration is not monitored. However, the ability to prevent recall is not guaranteed, and it does not fully reflect the synergistic effect of opioids with hypnotic agents [30].

Regardless of the anesthetic technique, the anesthesiologist and proceduralist should be in constant communication due to the shared airway. Rigid bronchoscopy is the preferred method for foreign body retrieval with patients going under general anesthesia. Fig. (**5**) shows the airway obstructed by forceps being used with a rigid bronchoscope. Anesthesiologists must be aware of what is going on at all times, as the loss of airway may be possible at any point. Often during object retrieval, the object may get stuck in a different location. If ventilation becomes difficult or if end-tidal carbon dioxide ($ETCO_2$) is lost, it may be because the object has become lodged in the main stem. If the foreign body is unable to be moved upwards, the best option is to push it into the right mainstem bronchus to allow for ventilation of at least one lung. Anesthesiologists should be aware of any injuries to the airway tract, as trauma from either the aspirated object or from the rigid bronchoscope may lead to bleeding or to the need for a more invasive surgery. Injury may lead to the need for thoracotomy or tracheostomy [31]. If the obstruction is severe or serious injury does occur, patients may need to remain intubated or be placed on extracorporeal membrane oxygenation (ECMO) to allow for adequate oxygenation and further treatment [32 - 34].

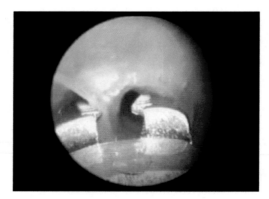

Fig. (5). Shared airway for foreign body removal.Permission: Solomon, D. Camden, NJ: Cooper University Hospital.

POSTOPERATIVE MANAGEMENT

If extubation is possible, patients can usually be transported to the postanesthesia care unit (PACU) for standard recovery. The biggest concern for anesthesiologists postoperatively is airway management. Due to possible trauma and swelling, patients should be closely monitored on pulse oximetry, and supplemental oxygen should be available. Usually, the procedure to remove the foreign body is not painful, so postoperative pain can typically be managed with non-opioids, such as NSAIDs and acetaminophen. If opioids are required for breakthrough pain, short-acting analgesics should be administered to limit respiratory depression. Other concerns in the PACU can include wheezing and bronchospasm, as well as croup from swelling. Bronchodilators, as well as racemic epinephrine, should be available to treat any symptoms that may arise. In some cases of foreign body extraction, due to the size of the object or unexpected trauma to the airway, the patient may not be able to be extubated. In this case, patients may require an ICU admission for postoperative ventilation and sedation for further airway management. In some instances of life- threatening aspiration, patients may even need ECMO, which will require ICU management and possibly a transfer to a center with ECMO utilization.

ESOPHAGEAL FOREIGN BODY

As with tracheal foreign bodies, curious children will find ways to put objects that they find in their mouth. More often than not, they pass through the esophagus and gastrointestinal (GI) tract unnoticed and without any issue. However, approximately 20% may get stuck in the GI tract, especially at transition points. Common sites of obstruction include the upper, middle and lower esophagus, as well as the pylorus, ileocecal valve and rectosigmoid colon [35]. Common objects that are ingested and may become stuck include coins, magnets, jewelry, toys, batteries and food [36]. Fig. (**6**) shows several objects removed endoscopically at our institute.

Foreign body ingestion is not always observed. Symptoms from retained foreign bodies in the GI tract include dysphagia, cough, hypersalivation, sensation of something being stuck, vomiting and hematemesis [37]. More serious complications may include difficulty breathing, hypoxemia, esophageal puncture or tear, bowel obstruction, bowel perforation, bronchoesophageal fistula, mediastinitis, esophageal diverticulum and one case report reported a death as a result of an aortoesophageal fistula with uncontrollable bleeding [38]. Ingested batteries, in particular, can cause caustic injury due to hydroxide created by hydrolyzed water, which can lead to rupture and sepsis. These serious complications can be due to chronically retained objects, acute perforations from sharp objects, or from the actual endoscopic removal.

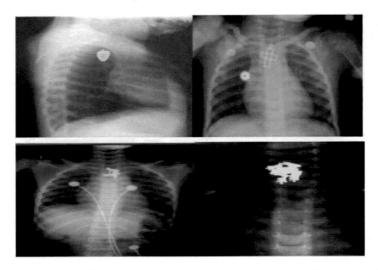

Fig. (6). Heart pendant, cross necklace and small toys stuck in the esophagus. Permission: Solomon, D. Camden, NJ: Cooper University Hospital.

Due to the risk of rupture, corrosion, obstruction, and possible airway compromise, foreign bodies should be evaluated promptly, and the need for surgical intervention be determined as soon as possible. Most of the pediatric cases of a foreign body or food impaction in our institution are done under general anesthesia with an endotracheal tube (ETT). However, some institutes will perform these cases under sedation in the appropriate pediatric population.

PREOPERATIVE EVALUATION

All patients who present with a known or suspected esophageal foreign body should get a thorough history and physical exam. Sometimes, when the incident is witnessed, the child or caretaker may be able to tell what object was swallowed which can facilitate and expedite treatment. The majority of patients receive plain films to show the location and type of object; but, if the object is radiolucent, it may not be visualized. Physical examination should focus mostly on the cardiorespiratory system, and signs of respiratory distress should be noted. All patients should have pulse oximetry attached to them throughout the evaluation and supplemental oxygen should be available, if necessary. In rare cases where an object is causing compression of the trachea, securing the airway may be necessary. NPO status should be obtained, but if the object is in the esophagus, it may be assumed that the patient is at risk of aspiration, which is why in our practice, we prefer a secured airway for the operation. Anxiolytics, such as midazolam, may be given if the patient is uncomfortable but should be weighed against any risk of respiratory compromise. IV access should be obtained prior to induction.

INTRAOPERATIVE MANAGEMENT

Patients should be attached to standard ASA monitors. Endoscopic removal is a low-risk procedure, but if there are any concerns due to patient comorbidities or the surgeon is concerned for rupture and bleeding, then additional IV access and even an arterial line may be considered. As stated earlier, due to aspiration risks as well as a shared airway, we prefer general anesthesia with a rapid sequence induction. Securing the airway can prevent aspiration and laryngospasm. Adequate suction should be available, especially in cases where NPO status is unknown, or there is active hematemesis.

Induction is usually performed with propofol and succinylcholine, assuming no contraindications. An anticholinergic such as glycopyrrolate may be given to reduce secretions from hypersalivation, which may facilitate visualization during intubation as well as the actual endoscopy. During induction and intubation, the object may move into the oropharynx due to esophageal sphincter relaxation. Anesthesiologists should have Magill forceps on hand so that they can safely remove the object if possible. Even if the object is safely removed, an ETT should be placed as most proceduralists will still want to take a look at the GI tract to determine the location and extent of any injuries. Often with food impactions, the food is semi-digested and the proceduralist will often have to go in and out several times, and a short 10-minute procedure may take over an hour. In cases like this, a longer-acting non-depolarizing muscle relaxant may be given after intubation to facilitate removal. Also, due to muscle relaxation, under general anesthesia, objects may migrate down the GI tract, so they may not be visible during the endoscopy. Depending on the type of object and where it ends up, further evaluation or surgery may be indicated. The anesthesiologist should be aware of what is happening during the procedure at all times and conscious of any injuries that the object or the proceduralist may have caused to the GI tract. Any tears, perforations, or uncontrolled bleeding may require more invasive repair as well as hemodynamic support. In some cases, endoscopy may have to be converted to an open procedure or thoracotomy [39].

At the end of the procedure, the patient's stomach should be suctioned out and be wide awake for extubation to prevent aspiration. The patient should be fully reversed if long-acting muscle relaxants were used. These procedures are generally not too painful and can be controlled with acetaminophen and NSAIDs, but small doses of short-acting opioids may be necessary. Antiemetics should also be given to prevent PONV. Dexamethasone may also be given if there are concerns for airway edema.

POSTOPERATIVE MANAGEMENT

After the procedure, patients can be transported to the PACU with supplemental oxygen. Patients should be monitored for respiratory distress and any new or uncontrolled hematemesis. Patients will get follow-up radiographs to ensure removal of all ingested objects. If the objects can not be removed, additional imaging may be required to determine their location and what further treatment may be indicated.

EPIGLOTTITIS

Epiglottitis, also known as supraglottitis, is caused by inflammation of the epiglottis, which can lead to airway obstruction. Fig. (7) shows a secured patient's airway with an inflamed epiglottis. It is a pediatric airway emergency and is managed by securing the airway and providing antibiotics until symptoms resolve. Epiglottitis was historically more common in children from 3 to 5 years of age, and typically resulted from infection with *Haemophilus influenzae* type b (Hib). Due to the advent of the *Haemophilus* vaccine in 1985, the incidence in the pediatric population has dropped to less than 1 case per 100,000 and is now more likely due to group A *Beta-hemolytic Streptococci* [40]. Epiglottitis can also be multifactorial, with concurrent viral and bacterial etiologies [41]. Although the incidence of epiglottitis in the pediatric population has decreased due to the advent of the Hib vaccine, anesthesiologists should be aware of the symptoms and management of the condition.

Epiglottitis can also be caused by non-infectious causes such as trauma, chemical and inhalation burns, chemotherapy and radiation, as well as systemic diseases [42]. Thermal epiglottitis is usually caused by ingestion of hot foods or beverages or by inhalation of hot gasses. Symptoms of non-infectious epiglottis present similarly to those seen in infectious causes, and management is the same [43]. Thermal injuries may cause trauma to mouths and tongues, which may lead to more swelling of supraglottic structures and may add to the difficulty in airway assessment and management.

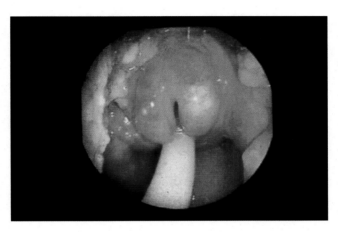

Fig. (7). Secured airway with epiglottitis. Permission: Solomon, D. Camden, NJ: Cooper University Hospital.

PREOPERATIVE EVALUATION

Epiglottitis in children usually presents acutely with high fevers, inspiratory stridor, shortness of breath, drooling and an overall toxic appearance. Children may maintain a "tripod position," with them sitting and leaning forward with their hands on their knees in order to maintain their airway. Other signs and symptoms may include drooling, hoarseness, dysphagia and coughing. Epiglottis should be differentiated from croup, which is more associated with a slow 2 to 3-day onset, coughing and stridor. Other differentials include but are not limited to angioedema, laryngitis, tonsillitis, and peritonsillar or retropharyngeal abscess.

Diagnosis is usually clinical, but neck radiographs may show swollen epiglottic folds known as the "thumbprint sign". Radiographs may differentiate between other airway issues such as croup which could show subglottic narrowing, also known as the "steeple sign." If radiographs are obtained, patients should be accompanied by an airway management expert and remain upright, as supine positioning can increase obstruction. Due to the risk of impending airway obstruction, radiographs should only be obtained if the diagnosis is still unclear. Bedside ultrasonography has also been used to diagnose epiglottitis, which may limit the need to transport patients unnecessarily [44, 45].

Patients with epiglottitis have a good prognosis if accurately diagnosed and managed by securing their airways. However, difficulty with airway management can lead to hypoxemia, anoxic brain damage, and death. Other complications with epiglottitis include pneumonia, cellulitis, otitis media, pneumothorax, tonsillar and epiglottic abscesses, meningitis, bacteremia and sepsis [46].

Any attempts at airway management should be performed in the OR. This often requires coordination between the anesthesiologist and ENT surgeon. The goal is to avoid complete airway obstruction, which could be triggered with any stimulation of the patient. IV access may be placed preoperatively, however, agitation in children may precipitate respiratory distress. The patient should not be sent for until the OR is fully equipped with anesthetic and ENT equipment and personnel. The anesthesiologist and ENT surgeon should be present during transportation, and at minimum, the patient should be placed on a portable pulse oximeter and emergency oxygen and airway equipment available.

INTRAOPERATIVE MANAGEMENT

Once in the OR, the patient should be attached to standard ASA monitors. An inhalation induction should be performed in order to maintain spontaneous ventilation. Sevoflurane is usually preferred as desflurane is more irritating to the airway and may cause bronchospasm and worsen airway reactivity [47]. Continuous pressure may be added by adjusting the pop-off valve in order to maintain airway patency. Once the patient is through the excitatory phase of stage 2 and at a proper depth of anesthesia, an IV line should be started, if not already in place. IV access is imperative if any complications such as laryngospasm, bronchospasm or complete airway obstruction are encountered prior to securing the airway. Once IV access is established, the airway should be secured with whatever equipment is deemed most appropriate. Consider placing a smaller than expected ETT as there will likely be swelling of the epiglottis and adjacent airway. A nasal ETT may also be beneficial to prevent dislodgement. All necessary emergency airway equipment should be in the room, and the ENT surgeon should be in the room in case emergent tracheostomy is necessary. After securing the airway, the patient may be paralyzed if needed. The next goals of management are to reduce swelling and control the source. Antibiotics and dexamethasone should be initiated at this time, if not already started. Usually, patients require several days of treatment, and they typically remain intubated and are sent to an intensive care unit postoperatively.

POSTOPERATIVE MANAGEMENT

Patients being managed for epiglottitis require frequent follow-up to determine the resolution of symptoms. Patients usually require 24 to 48 hours for acute toxemia to resolve and to be suitable for extubation. When deemed ready for extubation, an anesthesiologist and ENT surgeon should be present at the bedside. Direct visualization of the airway may be performed to determine if the swelling has adequately resolved. Some institutions may perform a leak test to determine the extent of the swelling but this may not be predictive of successful extubation

[48]. Emergency airway equipment and a tracheostomy kit should be available at the bedside. After extubation, patients may benefit from CPAP for a period of time to maintain airway patency.

ACUTE HYDROCEPHALUS

Hydrocephalus is caused by fluid accumulation in the brain due to cerebrospinal fluid (CSF) in the ventricular system. Normally CSF is produced in the walls of the ventricles and then flows to the brain surface, down the spinal cord, and is eventually absorbed into the bloodstream. CSF buildup can be caused by either overproduction, poor absorption from the bloodstream, or blockage in its flow from the ventricles. The Monro-Kellie doctrine theorizes that an increase in the volume of CSF will cause a decrease in blood or brain volume. However, in infants, skull size may increase if cranial suture fusion has not occurred. After suture fusion, an increase in CSF volume with an inability to compensate may lead to an increase in intracranial pressure (ICP).

Hydrocephalus can either be congenital or acquired. Congenital causes include Dandy-Walker syndrome, Maroteaux-Lamy syndrome, mucopolysaccharidoses, X-linked hydrocephalus, aqueduct of Sylvia stenosis, myelomeningocele, and in utero intraventricular hemorrhage. Acquired hydrocephalus may be due to space-occupying lesions, infections, intraventricular hemorrhage, trauma or failure of prior shunt placement [49]. Hydrocephalus in infancy is usually managed with a shunt procedure that diverts CSF from the ventricles, usually to the peritoneal cavity but may also lead to the pleura and right atrium. Ventriculoperitoneal (VP) shunts are the most common as they are associated with lower morbidity. Internal CSF drainage *via* endoscopic third ventriculostomy is another option in infants to relieve hydrocephalus. Anesthetic considerations for acute hydrocephalus will be discussed in this section.

PREOPERATIVE EVALUATION

Acute hydrocephalus may occur after VP shunt placement due to shunt failure, misplacement or children outgrowing them. Acute hydrocephalus after VP shunt failure may have variable presentations depending on the age of the patient. Infants may present cranial enlargement, fontanelle fullness, and irritability. Older children may present headaches, decreased consciousness, cranial nerve palsies, seizures, nausea and vomiting. They may also present Cushing's triad, which is a combination of hypertension, bradycardia, and apnea. Failure to recognize acute hydrocephalus and increased ICP can lead to devastating neurological outcomes and, in the worst cases, cerebral herniation can lead to death. When evaluating these patients, symptoms of increased ICP should be monitored, as patients who progress to severe symptoms may require urgent airway management. If hydrocephalus is associated with an underlying congenital syndrome, anesthesiologists should be aware of specific concerns associated with that syndrome, such as difficult airways or altered cardiopulmonary physiology. Due to the urgency of maintaining and controlling ICP, IV access should be obtained as quickly as possible. Premedication with sedatives should likely be avoided as altered consciousness may already be present, and any further respiratory depression and hypercapnia could make airway intervention more emergent. However, some patients may present to the operating room intubated, sedated, with IV access and ICP monitors already in place.

INTRAOPERATIVE MANAGEMENT

The main concern for anesthesiologists during these procedures is awareness and management of increased ICP. Depending on the degree of symptoms, patients may require an RSI due to progressive vomiting or loss of consciousness. In this case, attempts to avoid further increases in ICP should be undertaken. Regardless, intravenous induction is the preferred method due to faster onset and avoidance of increased cerebral blood flow seen with inhalation inductions. Induction can usually be performed with propofol which can ideally help decrease cerebral blood flow (CBF) and metabolism. Ketamine, which increases CBF and metabolism and, in turn, ICP, should most likely be avoided. Increases in ICP can be attenuated with lidocaine and short-acting narcotics, such as fentanyl or remifentanil. Muscle relaxants should be used to avoid coughing and bucking with laryngoscopy, which may lead to increased ICP. Succinylcholine may produce an increase in ICP, but it is usually small and transient so as not to preclude its use [50].

Maintenance of anesthesia should also be dictated by the degree of ICP elevation. Although volatile anesthetics can usually be used for most shunt revisions, they do increase cerebral volume and CBF. However, nitrous oxide should probably be avoided due to increased CBF, cerebral metabolic activity ($CMRO_2$) and risk of expanding gas-filled spaces. If there are considerable concerns for increased ICP, a total intravenous anesthetic should be performed to help reduce CBF, CBV and $CMRO_2$. Ventilation should be adjusted to avoid hypercapnia. $ETCO_2$ should be maintained between 30-40 mmHg. Hyperventilation to decrease $ETCO_2$ in cases of acute ICP increases may be necessary prior to ventricular decompression. However, continuous hyperventilation to keep $ETCO_2$ below 30 mmHg has not been shown to be beneficial to patient outcomes [51].

Due to the high risk of infections seen with ventriculostomies and VP shunts, anesthesiologists should ensure the appropriate administration of antibiotics. Infections can lead to recurrent hydrocephalus, sepsis, worse neurological outcomes, and the need for shunt revision and further operations. Although most infections occur within a few months of the surgery, up to 10% of infections may occur even after one year [52].

Pain management usually consists of short-acting opioids to prevent over-sedation, as the goal for these patients is to have them extubated in order to obtain a thorough neurological examination as quickly as possible. Non-opioid adjuncts such as acetaminophen, ketorolac, and local anesthesia infiltration by the surgeon can help reduce overall narcotic administration. Oftentimes patients may require additional narcotics or increasing anesthetic depth during the tunneling aspect of the shunt procedure.

Extubation should be performed after adequate suctioning of the stomach and oropharynx. The patient should be fully awake from anesthesia and appropriately reversed from any muscle relaxants that were used. Attempts should be made to prevent coughing and bucking during extubation, which may increase ICP. However, if hydrocephalus is resolved, the impact of increased ICP should be minimal.

POSTOPERATIVE MANAGEMENT

After extubation, most patients are suitable for recovery in the PACU. Transport to the PACU should be accompanied by at minimum supplemental O_2. A thorough neurologic assessment is usually performed by the neurosurgeons in the PACU to ensure resolution of any increased ICP. Anesthesiologists should also be able to perform a basic assessment to ensure adequate mentation and respiratory drive. In some cases, patients may require ICU management due to the need for assisted ventilation or for ongoing neurologic deficits. If ICU care is necessary, patients should be transported with oxygen and fully monitored.

Pain management should revolve around non-opioid analgesics or short-acting narcotics to prevent over-sedation so frequent neurological assessment can be performed. Patients may also be at increased risk for respiratory depression and aspiration due to altered mental status postoperatively. Antiemetics may be helpful to prevent nausea and vomiting, which can increase ICP. However, anesthesiologists and PACU nurses should be aware that nausea and vomiting may be a side effect of recurrent hydrocephalus and not due to the anesthesia. Although unlikely to occur immediately postoperatively, shunt infection is still a high cause of morbidity in this population, so surgeons should be aware of monitoring patient's temperatures.

TONSILLAR HEMORRHAGE

Tonsillar hemorrhage can be a surgical emergency that usually occurs in patients that have recently undergone tonsillectomy. There are incidences of spontaneous tonsillar hemorrhage not associated with surgery, which usually evolves from chronic tonsillitis that has not been properly treated [50]. However, both types of hemorrhage are treated the same, so the anesthetic management of both is similar. Post-tonsillar hemorrhage can occur in up to 5% of the pediatric population. Minor bleeding may be a predecessor to more severe bleeding, so these patients are usually observed in the emergency department and admitted for monitoring. If severe bleeding occurs, the need for resuscitation and surgical evaluation should not be delayed [53].

There are two types of post-tonsillar bleeding. Primary post-tonsillar bleeding occurs within 24 hours (and usually within 6 hours) and tends to be more profuse and fatal. Secondary post-tonsillar bleeding occurs after 24 hours, sometimes up to 10-12 days after surgery, and is due to sloughing of the eschar clot. Complications from tonsillar bleeding include hematemesis, pulmonary aspiration of blood, anemia, hypovolemia and hypotension, respiratory distress, dysrhythmias and death [54]. It is essential that patients are promptly recognized and treated to prevent serious morbidity.

PREOPERATIVE EVALUATION

When evaluating bleeding tonsils, anesthesiologists should do a thorough history and physical exam. Patients are often hypovolemic due to ongoing blood loss, however, their vitals signs may show tachycardia and hypertension due to adrenaline and catecholamine surges. Oftentimes, patients and their families are worried and high levels of anxiety may be present. However, due to the increased risk of airway obstruction and respiratory depression, anxiolytics should probably not be administered. Patients should be reassured while continuing to assess their hemodynamics. It is imperative that intravenous access is established. Due to hypovolemia, this may require ultrasound or intraosseous access. Baseline labs including a complete blood count and type and crossmatch should be obtained as soon as possible. Patients should be resuscitated with crystalloid and blood products based on vital signs and ongoing blood loss. If the patient had their tonsillectomy at your institution, you should attempt to review their anesthesia record for any prior intubation difficulties. However, with ongoing hemorrhage, the airway may be more difficult this time.

INTRAOPERATIVE MANAGEMENT

In the OR, it is imperative that two sources of suction are available as copious blood may obstruct the airway or even clot off the tubing. As stated earlier, a review of an old record may give insight into airway management. However, multiple laryngoscope blades should be available, including video laryngoscopes. ENT should also be at the bedside for induction, as a surgical airway may be needed if trouble arises with intubation attempts.

Patient's should be placed on standard ASA monitors and preoxygenated with 100% oxygen in preparation for an RSI without ventilation if possible. Preferably, the most experienced provider should manage the airway to limit delays in securing the trachea. All patients should be assumed to have a full stomach as blood is often ingested during active hemorrhage. RSI can be performed with propofol, etomidate, or ketamine, but providers should be aware of post-induction hypotension due to hypovolemia. Succinylcholine or non-depolarizing muscle relaxants may be used safely for muscle relaxation. Aggressive resuscitation should continue throughout the procedure until bleeding is controlled and the patient is felt to be euvolemic.

Once the airway is secure, besides ongoing hemodynamic support, these procedures tend to be straightforward as most tonsillectomies. Since many patients presenting with hemorrhage had their tonsils removed due to obstructive sleep apnea, the same precautions used for those cases apply here. Anesthesiologists should focus on a multimodal approach to pain management as patients with OSA may have 10 times the respiratory complications postoperatively [55]. Adjuncts such as ketamine, acetaminophen, clonidine, dexmedetomidine, and dexamethasone may also help reduce pain and opioid consumption after tonsillectomy [56 - 62]. PONV is also a concern after tonsillectomy due to ingested blood, so antiemetics should also be given, and an orogastric tube should be passed by either ENT or anesthesia to fully suction out gastric contents. Patients should be fully reversed and wide awake for extubation to reduce the risk of aspiration.

POSTOPERATIVE MANAGEMENT

Most patients should be able to recover in the PACU. If concerns for severe OSA or underlying comorbidities, an ICU admission may be necessary. Due to concerns for respiratory depression, transportation should be done with supplemental oxygen and a portable pulse oximeter. Patients should continue to be monitored and may require extended recovery if OSA is present. Continuous respiratory monitoring is important, as well as frequent assessment for new-onset bleeding. Ongoing resuscitation may be required in recovery depending on the duration of the procedure and amount of blood loss. If there are any concerns, a postoperative CBC may be sent to guide therapy, although it may not be accurate in the setting of acute bleeding.

Pain management should be continued, and any non-opioid adjuncts not given in the OR should be administered if indicated. If opioids are needed, short-acting narcotics at lower doses should be given, and respiratory status should be frequently assessed afterwards. PONV should be assessed and treated as needed. Medications for croup, laryngospasm, and bronchospasm should also be available.

OPEN GLOBE INJURY

Open globe injuries refer to ocular trauma where the integrity of the ocular wall is breached. These injuries are usually caused by rupture, laceration, or penetration of the globe due to a variety of causes. The World Health Organization (WHO) estimated that about 200,000 open globe injuries occur annually. These injuries are more common in males than females. Pediatric anesthesiologists should be familiar with these injuries and their management; the peak incidence in males is between the ages of 15 and 24 years and in females, the peak is between the ages of 5 and 14 years. Compared to closed injuries, open globe injuries usually require surgery and can lead to serious morbidity, including a decrease and loss of vision. Although open globe injuries can often be delayed up to 6 to 8 hours to adjust for NPO fasting guidelines, the need for rapid primary closure within 24 hours of the injury is usually required to preserve eye function [63].

PREOPERATIVE EVALUATION

Despite the ability to delay repair up to 24 hours and waiting the necessary time to fulfill NPO fasting guidelines, most ocular trauma, which may be associated with polytrauma, should be considered a full stomach and a rapid-sequence induction should likely be performed. The obvious concern for anesthesiologists is the risks of elevated intraocular pressure (IOP) and its impact on extrusion of orbital contents and choroidal hemorrhage. Since eye trauma is often associated with polytrauma, patients should be assessed for other injuries which may impact anesthetic management. All attempts to avoid increases in IOP should be undertaken.

INTRAOPERATIVE MANAGEMENT

Open eye injuries in the pediatric population are usually due to trauma. Unless specific comorbidities are present, standard ASA monitors should be utilized for the procedures. If antibiotics have not been started, they should be administered prior to incision to prevent infection. If untreated, endophthalmitis can develop, which can lead to poor outcomes, including loss of vision in addition to the initial injury [64].

Due to the risk of aspiration, a rapid sequence induction should be performed unless other facial trauma increases the risk for difficult airway. In this case, awake fiberoptic intubation may be needed, but again the risks of airway management *versus* risk for elevation in IOP must be considered. IOP is decreased with the use of induction agents such as propofol, thiopental, and etomidate [65]. There were theoretical concerns with the use of etomidate and myoclonus-induced extrusion of ocular contents; however, they have not been clinically proven [66]. The use of ketamine in children at doses less than 4mg/kg has not been shown to significantly increase IOP clinically [67, 68]. However, in our practice, propofol is the preferred agent for induction. The use of narcotics, such as fentanyl, alfentanil, sufentanil and remifentanil, significantly decrease IOP on induction. Other adjuncts used during induction, such as lidocaine, dexmedetomidine, clonidine and gabapentin, have been shown to attenuate the response of IOP to laryngoscopy and intubation [69 - 73].

The type of muscle relaxant used on induction has been a controversial topic for years when it comes to open globe injuries. Succinylcholine has been shown to increase IOP by up to 10 mmHg, and theoretically, it could induce eye content extrusion [74]. However, its reliability and quick onset may be beneficial in the case of an RSI for a full stomach. One study of 73 patients with an open globe injury showed that despite succinylcholine administration, there was no loss of globe contents [75]. The use of rocuronium has been shown to be as reliable as succinylcholine within 60 seconds when used at higher doses greater than 0.9 mg/kg for RSI [76]. Regardless of the type of muscle relaxant used, IOP will likely increase with laryngoscopy and intubation. The use of rocuronium may attenuate this response [77]. Most of the concerns associated with succinylcholine are theoretical, and no clinically significant outcomes have been reported. The most critical concern is ensuring adequate relaxation to prevent coughing and bucking, which can severely increase IOP.

Several studies have looked at airway management and the impact of intubation on IOP. All types of laryngoscopy increase IOP, but several studies showed that videolaryngoscopy caused less increase than direct laryngoscopy with Macintosh or Miller blades. Also, IOP increases even more with subsequent intubation attempts [78 - 80]. The goal for anesthesiologists is to secure the airway as quickly as possible with as little hemodynamic fluctuation, coughing, and bucking as possible. Repeated attempts with possible coughing and bucking will likely increase IOP significantly more than any theoretical or clinical risk from any individual agent or technique. Our recommendation is to perform intubation with the induction agents and equipment you are most comfortable with to achieve these goals.

Anesthesia maintenance can be achieved with either volatile anesthetics or intravenous agents. As mentioned before, most intravenous agents decrease IOP, and all the volatile agents decrease it as well. Although nitrous oxide has no effect on IOP when used in conjunction with other volatiles and narcotics, its use in eye surgeries has fallen out of favor due to the risk of gas expansion and central retinal artery occlusion [81, 82]. Although volatiles decrease IOP, the use of TIVA may be beneficial due to its lower incidence of PONV [13]. Nausea and vomiting can lead to large increases in IOP, so anti-emetics such as aprepitant, ondansetron, and dexamethasone should be considered for the procedure.

At the end of the procedure, the goal for extubation is to minimize coughing, bucking on the ETT as well as PONV, which can lead to an elevation in IOP up to 30-40 mmHg [83]. Some places recommend deep extubation, but if concerns for aspiration are present, it is best to be avoided. Also, depending on the comfort of PACU staff, doing awake extubation in the OR may be more beneficial. The stomach and oropharynx should be suctioned out prior to emergence while the patient is still deep as to prevent movement. The patient should be fully reversed if long-acting muscle relaxants were used. Reversal of rocuronium with neostigmine and glycopyrrolate was shown to increase IOP, whereas sugammadex had no change in IOP [84]. Sugammadex has also been shown to decrease the risk of PONV compared to neostigmine [85]. Table **1** summarizes common anesthetic drugs that are used for open eye surgeries and their effects on IOP.

Table 1. Effects of common anesthetic drugs on IOP.

Anesthetic Drugs	Effect on IOP
Volatile Gasses	Decrease
Nitrous Oxide	May increase
Propofol	Decrease
Ketamine	May increase at doses >4 mg/kg
Etomidate	Decrease
Opioids	Decrease
Thiopental	Decrease
Succinylcholine	Increase
Rocuronium	Decrease (prior to intubation)

(Table 1) cont.....

Anesthetic Drugs	Effect on IOP
Glycopyrrolate	Decrease
Atropine	Decrease
Neostigmine	Increase
Sugammadex	No effect
Lidocaine	Attenuates increase

PEDIATRIC TRAUMA

Every year approximately 20% of all Emergency Department (ED) visits are from the pediatric population [86]. Unintentional injury, suicide and homicide were three of the four leading causes of death in the pediatric population in 2017 as per the Centers for Disease Control and Prevention (CDC) [87]. The majority of these injuries involved motor vehicle-related accidents. Other injuries, which may require surgery, include penetrating trauma, blunt force trauma, falls, and burns. A majority of children in the United States live within fifty miles of a level I or II trauma center. However, many in less populated areas do not have access to a trauma center within an hour [88]. Those with access to a children's hospital or a trauma center that manages pediatrics and adults have improved outcomes [89]. Lower pediatric mortality rates are seen in states where there is a pediatric trauma center [90]. The ability to triage and get pediatric patients appropriate care and resources can help improve outcomes. However, because of acuity and location, anesthesiologists should be aware of concerns with pediatric trauma patients.

Any pediatric trauma patient may require emergent surgery because of hemodynamic instability, open orthopedic fractures, vertebral fractures, spinal cord injuries, burns or crush injuries. Initial management of these patients should follow pediatric acute life support (PALS) guidelines for assessment, resuscitation, and treatment. For more information on PALS, pediatric resuscitation, and management of pediatric trauma patients, please refer to Chapter 8 and Chapter 9, respectively.

CONCLUSION

Pediatric surgical emergencies are not uncommon and may occur in hospitals that do not encounter these patients on a regular basis. This chapter described in depth the common pediatric surgical emergencies and the preoperative, intraoperative and postoperative anesthetic considerations. With these considerations in mind, one can provide safe and effective anesthetic care for pediatric patients.

CONSENT FOR PUBLICATION

Not applicable.

CONFLICT OF INTEREST

The author declares no conflict of interest, financial or otherwise.

ACKNOWLEDGEMENTS

Declared none.

REFERENCES

[1]   Reddy AS, Shah RS, Kulkarni DR. Laparoscopic ladd's procedure in children: challenges, results, and problems. J Indian Assoc Pediatr Surg 2018; 23(2): 61-5.
[http://dx.doi.org/10.4103/jiaps.JIAPS_126_17] [PMID: 29681694]

[2]   Arnaud AP, Suply E, Eaton S, *et al.* Laparoscopic Ladd's procedure for malrotation in infants and children is still a controversial approach. J Pediatr Surg 2019; 54(9): 1843-7.
[http://dx.doi.org/10.1016/j.jpedsurg.2018.09.023] [PMID: 30442460]

[3]   Lloyd DA, Kenny SE. The surgical abdomen Pediatric Gastrointestinal Disease: Pathophysiology, Diagnosis, Management. 4th ed. Ontario, Canada: BC Decker 2004; p. 604.

[4]   Hill S, Koontz CS, Langness SM, Wulkan ML. Laparoscopic *versus* open repair of congenital duodenal obstruction in infants. J Laparoendosc Adv Surg Tech A 2011; 21(10): 961-3.
[http://dx.doi.org/10.1089/lap.2011.0069] [PMID: 22129146]

[5]   Graffeo CS, Counselman FL. Appendicitis. Emerg Med Clin North Am 1996; 14(4): 653-71.
[http://dx.doi.org/10.1016/S0733-8627(05)70273-X] [PMID: 8921763]

[6]   Aziz O, Athanasiou T, Tekkis PP, *et al.* Laparoscopic *versus* open appendectomy in children: a meta-analysis. Ann Surg 2006; 243(1): 17-27.
[http://dx.doi.org/10.1097/01.sla.0000193602.74417.14] [PMID: 16371732]

[7]   Jaschinski T, Mosch CG, Eikermann M, Neugebauer EA, Sauerland S. Laparoscopic versus open surgery for suspected appendicitis. Cochrane Database of Systematic Reviews 2018; 11.
[http://dx.doi.org/10.1002/14651858.CD001546.pub4]

[8]   Fabregat-López J, Cook T. Airway management considerations for appendectomy. Canadian Journal of Anesthesia/Journal canadien d'anesthésie 2010; 1;57(5): 515-6.
[http://dx.doi.org/10.1007/s12630-010-9286-4]

[9]   Henny CP, Hofland J. Laparoscopic surgery: pitfalls due to anesthesia, positioning, and pneumoperitoneum. Surg Endosc 2005; 19(9): 1163-71.
[http://dx.doi.org/10.1007/s00464-004-2250-z] [PMID: 16132330]

[10] Bhakta P, Ghosh BR, Singh U, *et al.* Incidence of postoperative nausea and vomiting following gynecological laparoscopy: A comparison of standard anesthetic technique and propofol infusion. Acta Anaesthesiol Taiwan 2016; 54(4): 108-13.
[http://dx.doi.org/10.1016/j.aat.2016.10.002] [PMID: 28024715]

[11] Hargitai B, Stangl R, Szebeni Z, Nagy E, Darvas K, Kupcsulik P. The risk of PONV in patients undergoing laparoscopic cholecystectomy: A-41. Eur J Anaesthesiol 2006; 23: 11.
[http://dx.doi.org/10.1097/00003643-200606001-00039]

[12] Arslan M, Ciçek R, Kalender HÜ, Yilmaz H. Preventing postoperative nausea and vomiting after laparoscopic cholecystectomy: a prospective, randomized, double-blind study. Curr Ther Res Clin Exp

2011; 72(1): 1-12.
[http://dx.doi.org/10.1016/j.curtheres.2011.02.002] [PMID: 24648571]

[13]   Bayter MJ, Peña P, Marquez M, *et al.* Incidence of postoperative nausea and vomiting when total intravenous anaesthesia is the primary anaesthetic in the ambulatory patient population. Ambul Surg 2018; 24(1): 8-11.

[14]   Tomecka MJ, Bortsov AV, Miller NR, *et al.* Substantial postoperative pain is common among children undergoing laparoscopic appendectomy. Paediatr Anaesth 2012; 22(2): 130-5.
[http://dx.doi.org/10.1111/j.1460-9592.2011.03711.x] [PMID: 21958060]

[15]   Liu Y, Seipel C, Lopez ME, *et al.* A retrospective study of multimodal analgesic treatment after laparoscopic appendectomy in children. Paediatr Anaesth 2013; 23(12): 1187-92.
[http://dx.doi.org/10.1111/pan.12271] [PMID: 24112856]

[16]   Bergmans E, Jacobs A, Desai R, Masters OW, Thies KC. Pain relief after transversus abdominis plane block for abdominal surgery in children: a service evaluation. Local Reg Anesth 2015; 8: 1-6.
[PMID: 25897261]

[17]   Molfino S, Botteri E, Baggi P, *et al.* Pain control in laparoscopic surgery: a case-control study between transversus abdominis plane-block and trocar-site anesthesia. Updates Surg 2019; 71(4): 717-22.
[http://dx.doi.org/10.1007/s13304-018-00615-y] [PMID: 30569346]

[18]   Seyedhejazi M, Motarabbesoun S, Eslampoor Y, Taghizadieh N, Hazhir N. Appendectomy Pain Control by Transversus Abdominis Plane (TAP) Block in Children. Anesth Pain Med 2019; 9(1)e83975
[http://dx.doi.org/10.5812/aapm.83975] [PMID: 30881907]

[19]   Mahajan JK, Rathod KK, Bawa M, Rao KL. Tracheobronchial foreign body aspirations: lessons learned from a 10-year audit. J Bronchology Interv Pulmonol 2011; 18(3): 223-8.
[http://dx.doi.org/10.1097/LBR.0b013e31822386a4] [PMID: 23208564]

[20]   Fidkowski CW, Zheng H, Firth PG. The anesthetic considerations of tracheobronchial foreign bodies in children: a literature review of 12,979 cases. Anesth Analg 2010; 111(4): 1016-25.
[http://dx.doi.org/10.1213/ANE.0b013e3181ef3e9c] [PMID: 20802055]

[21]   Kendigelen P. The anaesthetic consideration of tracheobronchial foreign body aspiration in children. J Thorac Dis 2016; 8(12): 3803-7.
[http://dx.doi.org/10.21037/jtd.2016.12.69] [PMID: 28149580]

[22]   Zerella JT, Dimler M, McGill LC, Pippus KJ. Foreign body aspiration in children: value of radiography and complications of bronchoscopy. J Pediatr Surg 1998; 33(11): 1651-4.
[http://dx.doi.org/10.1016/S0022-3468(98)90601-7] [PMID: 9856887]

[23]   Mashhadi L, Sabzevari A, Gharavi Fard M, *et al.* Controlled *vs* spontaneous ventilation for bronchoscopy in children with tracheobronchial foreign body. Iran J Otorhinolaryngol 2017; 29(95): 333-40.
[PMID: 29383314]

[24]   Liu Y, Chen L, Li S. Controlled ventilation or spontaneous respiration in anesthesia for tracheobronchial foreign body removal: a meta-analysis. Paediatr Anaesth 2014; 24(10): 1023-30.
[http://dx.doi.org/10.1111/pan.12469] [PMID: 24975102]

[25]   Litman RS, Ponnuri J, Trogan I. Anesthesia for tracheal or bronchial foreign body removal in children: an analysis of ninety-four cases. Anesth Analg 2000; 91(6): 1389-91.
[http://dx.doi.org/10.1097/00000539-200012000-00015] [PMID: 11093985]

[26]   Farrell PT. Rigid bronchoscopy for foreign body removal: anaesthesia and ventilation. Paediatr Anaesth 2004; 14(1): 84-9.
[http://dx.doi.org/10.1046/j.1460-9592.2003.01194.x] [PMID: 14717878]

[27]   Dutta A, Shouche S. Study of efficacy of anaesthesia with propofol and fentanyl for rigid bronchoscopy in foreign body bronchus removal in children. Indian J Otolaryngol Head Neck Surg

2013; 65(3): 225-8.
[http://dx.doi.org/10.1007/s12070-011-0476-3] [PMID: 24427571]

[28] Shen X, Hu CB, Ye M, Chen YZ. Propofol-remifentanil intravenous anesthesia and spontaneous ventilation for airway foreign body removal in children with preoperative respiratory impairment. Paediatr Anaesth 2012; 22(12): 1166-70.
[http://dx.doi.org/10.1111/j.1460-9592.2012.03899.x] [PMID: 22694274]

[29] Liao R, Li JY, Liu GY. Comparison of sevoflurane volatile induction/maintenance anaesthesia and propofol-remifentanil total intravenous anaesthesia for rigid bronchoscopy under spontaneous breathing for tracheal/bronchial foreign body removal in children. Eur J Anaesthesiol 2010; 27(11): 930-4.--> [EJA]. [http://dx.doi.org/10.1097/EJA.0b013e32833d69ad]. [PMID: 20683333].
[http://dx.doi.org/10.1097/EJA.0b013e32833d69ad] [PMID: 20683333]

[30] Whyte SD, Booker PD. Monitoring depth of anaesthesia by EEG. BJA CEPD Reviews 2003; 3(4): 106-10.
[http://dx.doi.org/10.1093/bjacepd/mkg106]

[31] Hasdiraz L, Oguzkaya F, Bilgin M, Bicer C. Complications of bronchoscopy for foreign body removal: experience in 1,035 cases. Ann Saudi Med 2006; 26(4): 283-7.
[http://dx.doi.org/10.5144/0256-4947.2006.283] [PMID: 16883083]

[32] Park AH, Tunkel DE, Park E, et al. Management of complicated airway foreign body aspiration using extracorporeal membrane oxygenation (ECMO). Int J Pediatr Otorhinolaryngol 2014; 78(12): 2319-21.
[http://dx.doi.org/10.1016/j.ijporl.2014.10.021] [PMID: 25465455]

[33] Deng L, Wang B, Wang Y, Xiao L, Liu H. Treatment of bronchial foreign body aspiration with extracorporeal life support in a child: A case report and literature review. Int J Pediatr Otorhinolaryngol 2017; 94: 82-6.
[http://dx.doi.org/10.1016/j.ijporl.2017.01.011] [PMID: 28167019]

[34] Anton-Martin P, Bhattarai P, Rycus P, Raman L, Potera R. The Use of Extracorporeal Membrane Oxygenation in Life-Threatening Foreign Body Aspiration: Case Series, Review of Extracorporeal Life Support Organization Registry Data, and Systematic Literature Review. J Emerg Med 2019; 56(5): 523-9.
[http://dx.doi.org/10.1016/j.jemermed.2019.01.036] [PMID: 30879854]

[35] Schwartz GF, Polsky HS. Ingested foreign bodies of the gastrointestinal tract. Am Surg 1976; 42(4): 236-8.
[PMID: 1267274]

[36] Chinski A, Foltran F, Gregori D, Ballali S, Passali D, Bellussi L. Foreign bodies in the oesophagus: the experience of the Buenos Aires Paediatric ORL Clinic. Int J Pediatr 2010.
[http://dx.doi.org/10.1155/2010/490691]

[37] Athanassiadi K, Gerazounis M, Metaxas E, Kalantzi N. Management of esophageal foreign bodies: a retrospective review of 400 cases. Eur J Cardiothorac Surg 2002; 21(4): 653-6.
[http://dx.doi.org/10.1016/S1010-7940(02)00032-5] [PMID: 11932163]

[38] Gilchrist BF, Valerie EP, Nguyen M, Coren C, Klotz D, Ramenofsky ML. Pearls and perils in the management of prolonged, peculiar, penetrating esophageal foreign bodies in children. J Pediatr Surg 1997; 32(10): 1429-31.
[http://dx.doi.org/10.1016/S0022-3468(97)90554-6] [PMID: 9349761]

[39] Crysdale WS, Sendi KS, Yoo J. Esophageal foreign bodies in children. 15-year review of 484 cases. Ann Otol Rhinol Laryngol 1991; 100(4 Pt 1): 320-4.
[http://dx.doi.org/10.1177/000348949110000410] [PMID: 2018291]

[40] Briere EC, Rubin L, Moro PL, Cohn A, Clark T, Messonnier N. Prevention and control of haemophilus influenzae type b disease: recommendations of the advisory committee on immunization practices (ACIP). MMWR Recomm Rep 2014; 63(RR-01): 1-14.

[PMID: 24572654]

[41] Shah KM, Carswell KN, Paradise Black NM. Prolonged Stridor and Epiglottitis With Concurrent Bacterial and Viral Etiologies. Clin Pediatr (Phila) 2016; 55(1): 91-2.
[http://dx.doi.org/10.1177/0009922815584221] [PMID: 25926662]

[42] Lichtor JL, Roche Rodriguez M, Aaronson NL, Spock T, Goodman TR, Baum ED. Epiglottitis: It Hasn't Gone Away. Anesthesiology 2016; 124(6): 1404-7.
[http://dx.doi.org/10.1097/ALN.0000000000001125] [PMID: 27031010]

[43] Inaguma Y, Matsui S, Kusumoto M, Kurosawa H, Tanaka R. Thermal epiglottitis: Acute airway obstruction caused by ingestion of hot food. Pediatr Int 2019; 61(9): 927-9.
[http://dx.doi.org/10.1111/ped.13948] [PMID: 31569296]

[44] Ko DR, Chung YE, Park I, *et al.* Use of bedside sonography for diagnosing acute epiglottitis in the emergency department: a preliminary study. J Ultrasound Med 2012; 31(1): 19-22.
[http://dx.doi.org/10.7863/jum.2012.31.1.19] [PMID: 22215764]

[45] Hung TY, Li S, Chen PS, *et al.* Bedside ultrasonography as a safe and effective tool to diagnose acute epiglottitis. Am J Emerg Med 2011; 29(3): 359.e1-3.
[http://dx.doi.org/10.1016/j.ajem.2010.05.001] [PMID: 20674236]

[46] Shah RK, Roberson DW, Jones DT. Epiglottitis in the Hemophilus influenzae type B vaccine era: changing trends. Laryngoscope 2004; 114(3): 557-60.
[http://dx.doi.org/10.1097/00005537-200403000-00031] [PMID: 15091234]

[47] Klock PA Jr, Czeslick EG, Klafta JM, Ovassapian A, Moss J. The effect of sevoflurane and desflurane on upper airway reactivity. Anesthesiology 2001; 94(6): 963-7.
[http://dx.doi.org/10.1097/00000542-200106000-00008] [PMID: 11465621]

[48] De Backer D. The cuff-leak test: what are we measuring? Crit Care 2005; 9(1): 31-3.
[http://dx.doi.org/10.1186/cc3031] [PMID: 15693980]

[49] Hamid RK, Newfield P. Pediatric neuroanesthesia. Hydrocephalus. Anesthesiol Clin North America 2001; 19(2): 207-18.
[http://dx.doi.org/10.1016/S0889-8537(05)70224-8] [PMID: 11469060]

[50] Ganjoo P, Kapoor I. Neuropharmacology. In: Prabhakar H, Ed. Essentials of Neuroanesthesia. Academic Press: Elsevier Inc. 2017; pp. 103-22.
[http://dx.doi.org/10.1016/B978-0-12-805299-0.00006-3]

[51] Zhang Z, Guo Q, Wang E. Hyperventilation in neurological patients: from physiology to outcome evidence. Curr Opin Anaesthesiol 2019; 32(5): 568-73.
[http://dx.doi.org/10.1097/ACO.0000000000000764] [PMID: 31211719]

[52] Kim YS, Hong SJ, Choi J, Lee SH, Kwon SY, Choi JH. Spontaneous tonsillar hemorrhage and post-tonsillectomy hemorrhage. Clin Exp Otorhinolaryngol 2010; 3(1): 56-8.
[http://dx.doi.org/10.3342/ceo.2010.3.1.56] [PMID: 20379405]

[53] Wall JJ, Tay KY. Postoperative Tonsillectomy Hemorrhage. Emerg Med Clin North Am 2018; 36(2): 415-26.
[http://dx.doi.org/10.1016/j.emc.2017.12.009] [PMID: 29622331]

[54] Fields RG, Gencorelli FJ, Litman RS. Anesthetic management of the pediatric bleeding tonsil. Paediatr Anaesth 2010; 20(11): 982-6.
[http://dx.doi.org/10.1111/j.1460-9592.2010.03426.x] [PMID: 20964765]

[55] McColley SA, April MM, Carroll JL, Naclerio RM, Loughlin GM. Respiratory compromise after adenotonsillectomy in children with obstructive sleep apnea. Arch Otolaryngol Head Neck Surg 1992; 118(9): 940-3.
[http://dx.doi.org/10.1001/archotol.1992.01880090056017] [PMID: 1503720]

[56] De Oliveira GS Jr, Almeida MD, Benzon HT, McCarthy RJ. Perioperative single dose systemic

dexamethasone for postoperative pain: a meta-analysis of randomized controlled trials. Anesthesiology 2011; 115(3): 575-88.
[http://dx.doi.org/10.1097/ALN.0b013e31822a24c2] [PMID: 21799397]

[57] Waldron NH, Jones CA, Gan TJ, Allen TK, Habib AS. Impact of perioperative dexamethasone on postoperative analgesia and side-effects: systematic review and meta-analysis. Br J Anaesth 2013; 110(2): 191-200.
[http://dx.doi.org/10.1093/bja/aes431] [PMID: 23220857]

[58] Schnabel A, Meyer-Frießem CH, Reichl SU, Zahn PK, Pogatzki-Zahn EM. Is intraoperative dexmedetomidine a new option for postoperative pain treatment? A meta-analysis of randomized controlled trials. Pain 2013; 154(7): 1140-9.
[http://dx.doi.org/10.1016/j.pain.2013.03.029] [PMID: 23706726]

[59] Tang C, Xia Z. Dexmedetomidine in perioperative acute pain management: a non-opioid adjuvant analgesic. J Pain Res 2017; 10(10): 1899-904.
[http://dx.doi.org/10.2147/JPR.S139387] [PMID: 28860845]

[60] Subramanyam R, Varughese A, Kurth CD, Eckman MH. Cost-effectiveness of intravenous acetaminophen for pediatric tonsillectomy. Paediatr Anaesth 2014; 24(5): 467-75.
[http://dx.doi.org/10.1111/pan.12359] [PMID: 24597962]

[61] Brui B, Lavandhomme P, Veyckemans F, Pendeville P. Clonidine effect on pain after pediatric tonsillectomy: systemic versus local administration: A-712. Eur J Anaesthesiol 2005; 22: 183-4.
[http://dx.doi.org/10.1097/00003643-200505001-00663]

[62] Bameshki SA, Salari MR, Bakhshaee M, Razavi M. Effect of Ketamine on Post-Tonsillectomy Sedation and Pain Relief. Iran J Otorhinolaryngol 2015; 27(83): 429-34.
[PMID: 26788487]

[63] Sinha A, Baumann BC. Anesthesia for ocular trauma. Curr Anaesth Crit Care 2010; 21: 184.
[http://dx.doi.org/10.1016/j.cacc.2010.05.001]

[64] Andreoli CM, Andreoli MT, Kloek CE, Ahuero AE, Vavvas D, Durand ML. Low rate of endophthalmitis in a large series of open globe injuries. Am J Ophthalmol 2009; 147(4): 601-608.e2.
[http://dx.doi.org/10.1016/j.ajo.2008.10.023] [PMID: 19181306]

[65] Kim SH, Lee SH, Shim SH, *et al.* Effects of Etomidate, Propofol and Thiopental Sodium on Intraocular Pressure during the Induction of Anesthesia. Korean J Anesthesiol 2000; 39(3): 309-13.
[http://dx.doi.org/10.4097/kjae.2000.39.3.309]

[66] Berry JM, Merin RG. Etomidate myoclonus and the open globe. Anesth Analg 1989; 69(2): 256-9.
[http://dx.doi.org/10.1213/00000539-198908000-00022] [PMID: 2764296]

[67] Nagdeve NG, Yaddanapudi S, Pandav SS. The effect of different doses of ketamine on intraocular pressure in anesthetized children. J Pediatr Ophthalmol Strabismus 2006; 43(4): 219-23.
[http://dx.doi.org/10.3928/01913913-20060701-03] [PMID: 16915900]

[68] Drayna PC, Estrada C, Wang W, Saville BR, Arnold DH. Ketamine sedation is not associated with clinically meaningful elevation of intraocular pressure. Am J Emerg Med 2012; 30(7): 1215-8.
[http://dx.doi.org/10.1016/j.ajem.2011.06.001] [PMID: 22169582]

[69] Drenger B, Pe'er J, BenEzra D, Katzenelson R, Davidson JT. The effect of intravenous lidocaine on the increase in intraocular pressure induced by tracheal intubation. Anesth Analg 1985; 64(12): 1211-3.
[http://dx.doi.org/10.1213/00000539-198512000-00016] [PMID: 4061906]

[70] Mowafi HA, Aldossary N, Ismail SA, Alqahtani J. Effect of dexmedetomidine premedication on the intraocular pressure changes after succinylcholine and intubation. Br J Anaesth 2008; 100(4): 485-9.
[http://dx.doi.org/10.1093/bja/aen020] [PMID: 18285392]

[71] Jaakola ML, Ali-Melkkilä T, Kanto J, Kallio A, Scheinin H, Scheinin M. Dexmedetomidine reduces intraocular pressure, intubation responses and anaesthetic requirements in patients undergoing

ophthalmic surgery. Br J Anaesth 1992; 68(6): 570-5.
[http://dx.doi.org/10.1093/bja/68.6.570] [PMID: 1351736]

[72]   Innemee HC, van Zwieten PA. The influence of clonidine on intraocular pressure. Doc Ophthalmol 1979; 46(2): 309-15.
[http://dx.doi.org/10.1007/BF00142620] [PMID: 477484]

[73]   Kaya FN, Yavascaoglu B, Baykara M, Altun GT, Gülhan N, Ata F. Effect of oral gabapentin on the intraocular pressure and haemodynamic responses induced by tracheal intubation. Acta Anaesthesiol Scand 2008; 52(8): 1076-80.
[http://dx.doi.org/10.1111/j.1399-6576.2008.01627.x] [PMID: 18840107]

[74]   Cook JH. The effect of suxamethonium on intraocular pressure. Anaesthesia 1981; 36(4): 359-65.
[http://dx.doi.org/10.1111/j.1365-2044.1981.tb10238.x] [PMID: 7246985]

[75]   Libonati MM, Leahy JJ, Ellison N. The use of succinylcholine in open eye surgery. Anesthesiology 1985; 62(5): 637-40.
[http://dx.doi.org/10.1097/00000542-198505000-00017] [PMID: 3994030]

[76]   Chiu CL, Jaais F, Wang CY. Effect of rocuronium compared with succinylcholine on intraocular pressure during rapid sequence induction of anaesthesia. Br J Anaesth 1999; 82(5): 757-60.
[http://dx.doi.org/10.1093/bja/82.5.757] [PMID: 10536557]

[77]   Vinik HR. Intraocular pressure changes during rapid sequence induction and intubation: a comparison of rocuronium, atracurium, and succinylcholine. J Clin Anesth 1999; 11(2): 95-100.
[http://dx.doi.org/10.1016/S0952-8180(99)00013-6] [PMID: 10386278]

[78]   Ahmad N, Zahoor A, Riad W, Al Motowa S. Influence of GlideScope assisted endotracheal intubation on intraocular pressure in ophthalmic patients. Saudi J Anaesth 2015; 9(2): 195-8.
[http://dx.doi.org/10.4103/1658-354X.152885] [PMID: 25829910]

[79]   Agrawal G, Agarwal M, Taneja S. A randomized comparative study of intraocular pressure and hemodynamic changes on insertion of proseal laryngeal mask airway and conventional tracheal intubation in pediatric patients. J Anaesthesiol Clin Pharmacol 2012; 28(3): 326-9.
[http://dx.doi.org/10.4103/0970-9185.98325] [PMID: 22869938]

[80]   Watcha MF, Chu FC, Stevens JL, White PF. Intraocular pressure and hemodynamic changes following tracheal intubation in children. J Clin Anesth 1991; 3(4): 310-3.
[http://dx.doi.org/10.1016/0952-8180(91)90226-D] [PMID: 1910800]

[81]   Goyagi T, Sato T, Horiguchi T, Nishikawa T. The Effect of Nitrous Oxide on the Intraocular Pressure in Patients Undergoing Abdominal Surgery under Sevoflurane and Remifentanil Anesthesia. Open J Anesthesiol 2016; (6): 85-90.
[http://dx.doi.org/10.4236/ojanes.2016.66014]

[82]   Fu AD, McDonald HR, Eliott D, *et al.* Complications of general anesthesia using nitrous oxide in eyes with preexisting gas bubbles. Retina 2002; 22(5): 569-74.
[http://dx.doi.org/10.1097/00006982-200210000-00006] [PMID: 12441721]

[83]   Murgatroyd H, Bembridge J. Intraocular pressure. Contin Educ Anaesth Crit Care Pain 2008; 8(3): 100-3.
[http://dx.doi.org/10.1093/bjaceaccp/mkn015]

[84]   Yagan O, Karakahya RH, Tas N, Canakci E, Hanci V, Yurtlu BS. Intraocular pressure changes associated with tracheal extubation: Comparison of sugammadex with conventional reversal of neuromuscular blockade. J Pak Med Assoc 2015; 65(11): 1219-25.
[PMID: 26564297]

[85]   Hristovska AM, Duch P, Allingstrup M, Afshari A. The comparative efficacy and safety of sugammadex and neostigmine in reversing neuromuscular blockade in adults. A Cochrane systematic review with meta-analysis and trial sequential analysis. Anaesthesia 2018; 73(5): 631-41.
[http://dx.doi.org/10.1111/anae.14160] [PMID: 29280475]

[86]   Moore BJ, Stocks C, Owens PL. Trends in Emergency Department Visits, 2006–2014. HCUP Statistical Brief #227. September 2017. Agency for Healthcare Research and Quality, Rockville, MD. www.hcup-us.ahrq.gov/reports/statbriefs/sb227-Emergency-Department-Visit-Trends.pdf

[87]   Kochanek KD, Murphy SL, Xu JQ, Arias E. Deaths: Final data for 2017. National Vital Statistics Reports 2019; 68(9)

[88]   Densmore JC, Lim HJ, Oldham KT, Guice KS. Outcomes and delivery of care in pediatric injury. J Pediatr Surg 2006; 41(1): 92-8.
[http://dx.doi.org/10.1016/j.jpedsurg.2005.10.013] [PMID: 16410115]

[89]   Brantley MD, Lu H, Barfield WD, Holt JB. Visualizing pediatric mass critical care hospital resources by state 2008.http://proceedings.esri.com/library/userconf/health10/docs/esri_hc_2010_op2.pdf

[90]   Notrica DM, Weiss J, Garcia-Filion P, *et al.* Pediatric trauma centers: correlation of ACS-verified trauma centers with CDC statewide pediatric mortality rates. J Trauma Acute Care Surg 2012; 73(3): 566-70.
[http://dx.doi.org/10.1097/TA.0b013e318265ca6f] [PMID: 22929485]

CHAPTER 11

Neonatal Emergency Surgeries

Yue Monica Li[1] and **Michael Schwartz[1]**

[1] *Department of Anesthesiology, Cooper Medical School of Rowan University, Cooper University Health Care, Camden, NJ, USA*

Abstract: Anesthesia for neonatal emergencies can be extremely challenging for the anesthesiologist. Fortunately, with medical advancements, many neonatal emergencies can be treated medically, reducing the need for emergency surgical intervention. Nonetheless, care of sick neonates, especially those who are premature, requires sufficient knowledge, experience, and vigilance. This chapter aims to provide a brief overview of pertinent anatomy and physiology relevant to the care of neonates in emergency cases. Some basic and overarching anesthetic considerations will be addressed, including an essential setup. Finally, this chapter will highlight key aspects of specific neonatal surgical emergencies, including gastrointestinal surgeries, airway surgeries, and neurosurgery.

Keywords: Abdominal wall defect, Anatomy, Anesthesia, Choanal atresia, Congenital diaphragmatic hernia, Emergency surgery, Gastroschisis, Necrotizing enterocolitis, Neonatal, Omphalocele, Physiology, Subglottic stenosis, Tracheoesophageal fistula.

INTRODUCTION

The neonatal period, defined as the first 28 days of life, is an extremely delicate period of life. The United States has one of the highest rates of infant mortality as a developed country, with a rate of 5.87 deaths per 1,000 live births. The neonatal mortality rate is almost twice as high as that of the postneonatal infant mortality rate (3.88 deaths per 1,000 live births *versus* 1.99 deaths per 1,000 live births) [1, 2]. The top two causes of neonatal mortality are 1) prematurity and low birthweight (LBW), and 2) congenital malformations. Despite a slight decline in neonatal mortality from 2007 to 2011, there has been an increase in rates of preterm LBW-associated deaths. Mortality rates are also disproportionately high in infants of non-Hispanic black and American Indian or Alaska Native women (10.93 per 1,000 live births and 7.59 per 1,000 live births, *versus* 4.89 per.

* **Corresponding author Bharathi Gourkanti:** Department of Anesthesiology, Cooper Medical School of Rowan University, Cooper University Health Care, Camden, NJ, USA; E-mail: gourkantibharathi@cooperhealth.edu

Bharathi Gourkanti, Irwin Gratz, Grace Dippo, Nathalie Peiris and Dinesh K. Choudhry (Eds.)
All rights reserved-© 2022 Bentham Science Publishers

1,000 live births in non-Hispanic white women) [2] Despite advances in neonatal care, the relatively high rate of neonatal mortality is still a significant burden that needs to be addressed.

The anesthesiologist is an important part of a multidisciplinary team taking care of the sick neonate for emergent or urgent surgeries. Taking care of the sick neonate is one of the biggest challenges for the anesthesiologist. Thorough knowledge of neonatal anatomy, physiology, and disease processes is crucial. This chapter explores the relevant anatomy and physiology of the neonatal and will describe the anesthetic management of select common neonatal emergency surgeries.

NEONATAL PHYSIOLOGY

Knowledge of neonatal anatomy and physiology is crucial to the care of neonates. In this chapter, we will briefly review the relevant anatomy and physiology as it pertains to anesthetic care for the neonate. For more details on pediatric anatomy and physiology, refer to Chapter I.

Respiratory and Airway Physiology

A neonate's immature development of the lungs, chest wall, and airway, combined with high oxygen consumption, can easily lead to hypoxia under general anesthesia (GA).Table **1 and 2** highlight the differences between neonatal and adult respiratory and airway physiology, respectively.

Table 1. Differences in Respiratory Physiology between Neonate and Adult.

Respiratory	Neonate	Adult
O_2 consumption	6-7 ml/kg/min	3-4 ml/kg/min
Total lung capacity	~50 ml/kg	~80-90 ml/kg
Minute Vent	~200-350 mL/kg/min	~90 ml/kg/min
Alveolar vent (Va)	~200 ml/kg/min	~40 ml/kg/min
FRC	~35 ml/kg (27ml/kg in neonate)	~40 ml/kg (similar to infants)
Va/FRC ratio	5:1	1.5:1
Closing capacity	Larger than FRC	Smaller than FRC
Alveoli	Immature alveoli - 1/10th of adults	Alveoli continue to develop until 18 months, morphologic and physiologic aspects of lung first decade.

(Table 1) cont.....

Respiratory	Neonate	Adult
Rib cage	Extends from the vertebral column horizontally, high cartilage and decreased muscle tone, chest wall compliance decreased	Extends from the vertebral column caudally, chest wall compliance increases throughout childhood and adolescence.
Diaphragm	Increased work due to paradoxical movement of the rib cage; 25% type I slow-twitch fibers	50% type I slow-twitch fibers
Elastic recoil	Decreased	Increase of elastic fibers during childhood

Table 2. Differences in Airway between Neonate and Adult.

Airway	Neonate	Adults
Head	Large occiput requiring shoulder roll or stabilization	Need to be placed in sniffing position
Laryngeal Position	Birth: Larynx C1-2 Cricoid C3	Larynx C5-6 Cricoid top of C7
Tongue	Large, common cause of obstruction	Smaller
Epiglottis	Long, omega-shaped Hyoid bone is right above thyroid cartilage, which makes the epiglottis protrude.	Flatter, more flexible
Vocal folds	Anterior vocal ligaments are more caudal, causing vocal folds to be angled and concave.	Vocal folds perpendicular to trachea
Subglottis	Funnel shaped The cricoid ring is only complete cartilage and is the nonexpandable and narrowest part	Funnel-shaped (classically, the larynx is the smallest portion)

Pulmonary Development

During 17-28 weeks of gestation, the gas-exchange portion and the air-blood barrier of the lungs are formed (canalicular stage). Around 28-36 weeks, air spaces expand and surfactants appear (saccular stage). Beyond week 36, alveoli develop and continue to develop into childhood (alveolar stage). In the premature infant, poor development of the lung parenchyma and the lack of surfactants lead to alveolar collapse and poor gas exchange. As a result, there is an increase in ventilation-perfusion mismatch and intrapulmonary shunting [3].

Oxygen consumption in the neonate is twice as high as that of an adult (6-8 ml/kg/min compared to 3-4 ml/kg/min). The neonate's chest wall is cartilaginous and horizontal instead of angled like in adults. Lung elastic recoil is also high, which draws in a compliant chest wall leading to easy airway collapse and low functional residual capacity (FRC). Tidal volume per kilogram is similar to older children and adults, but respiratory rate, and therefore minute ventilation (MV), is increased. The MV to FRC ratio is high (5:1 compared to 1.5:1 in older children and adults). As a result, the FRC is less efficient at buffer gas exchange during periods of apnea (such as during induction). The closing volume is high, resulting in airway closure and intrapulmonary shunting. These factors, combined with high oxygen consumption, contribute to the rapid desaturation of neonates during periods of apnea. The neonate's diaphragm is also flattened and composed of fewer slow-twitch fibers compared to adults. Combined with a narrow airway that leads to higher resistance and increased work of breathing, the neonate can quickly tire out with spontaneous respiration. This is why endotracheal intubation with controlled ventilation is the preferred method of managing the airway [4].

Airway Anatomy

The neonate's unfavorable airway can lead to difficulty intubating. The larynx is situated at 1-2 cervical levels, *versus* C5-6 in adults. This leads to an anterior airway and difficulty visualizing the vocal cords. Heinrich *et al.* found that 3.2% of neonates were Cormack-Lehane grade III/IV views [5]. The anterior vocal ligaments are more caudal and angled, which can cause difficulty in passing the endotracheal tube. The tongue is also relatively larger in the neonate, which can cause obstruction during ventilation. The anesthesia provider should always have an oral airway nearby during induction and the emergence of anesthesia. The large occiput also tends to flex the neck. Often, a shoulder role is required during intubation. The epiglottis is also long and omega shaped. A Miller blade is generally used during intubation in order to sweep the epiglottis from the view of the vocal cords. The subglottis is the narrowest at the cricoid ring, which is the only complete non-expandable cartilage. Airway edema can result if the endotracheal tube is too large or if the balloon is overinflated. An air leak at 20-30 cmH_2O, which is the approximate capillary pressure of the tracheal mucosa, should be present [6].

Systematic reviews have shown that perioperatively, cuffed endotracheal tubes do not increase the risk of tracheal edema and stridor and may reduce the number of intubation attempts compared to uncuffed endotracheal tubes. Prolonged use of low pressure cuffed endotracheal tubes in the pediatric ICU was also not significantly associated with subglottic stenosis [7]. With uncuffed endotracheal tubes, the work of breathing is reduced, although this benefit is insignificant with controlled ventilation or pressure support. At our institution, we prefer the use of low-pressure high-volume microcuffed endotracheal tubes for neonates.

Availability of proper equipment is crucial prior to the induction of anesthesia, as rapid desaturation means there is very little time for error. As with any pediatric case, the setup should include endotracheal tubes of two to 3 different sizes, several different blades, and several different sized oral airways. An experienced anesthesia provider should perform the intubation, as delay in delivery of oxygen can cause profound hypoxia with associated bradycardia.

Apnea of Prematurity

Apnea of prematurity (AOP) is defined as cessation of breathing for greater than 20 seconds or less if accompanied by bradycardia (30 beats per minute below baseline) or hypoxemia. AOP is both central, mediated by an immature central nervous system, and obstructive. AOP is generally seen in neonates less than 33 weeks post-conceptual age (PCA) and in nearly all infants less than 1000 g weight. Similarly, the respiratory response in premature neonates is diminished to hypercarbia and hypoxia. Generally, apnea is treated with tactile stimulation, caffeine, and airway maneuvers.

Cardiac Physiology

In utero, the main goal of fetal circulation is to deliver oxygenated blood from the placenta to vital organs. As such, circulation through the lung is bypassed from the right to the left side of the heart *via* the ductus arteriosus and foramen ovale and is driven by the high resistance through the pulmonary vasculature. Upon the neonate's first few breaths, due to an increase in oxygen and prostaglandins, pulmonary vascular resistance decreases and systemic vascular resistance increases substantially. The foramen ovale closes functionally with the first few breaths, although it may take years to close anatomically (or never in 25% of patients), while the ductus arteriosus closes in the first 24 hours. In the setting of acute respiratory distress, such as that seen in the premature and those with cardiopulmonary pathologies such as congenital diaphragmatic hernia (CDH) and congenital heart disease, the ductus arteriosus remains patent, and right to left shunting can persist. This leads to persistent pulmonary hypertension (PPHN) of the newborn, which can further exacerbate hypoxia and impair right heart function [3, 4]. Management of PPHN is described in the CDH section of this chapter.

Cardiac myocytes in the neonate are immature and disorganized. Stroke volume is relatively fixed, so cardiac output depends on heart rate. Neonates also have an exaggerated vagal response in which bradycardia occurs with hypoxia, hypercarbia, and laryngoscopy. This becomes important during the induction of anesthesia and is the reason why some clinicians choose to prophylactically administer atropine prior to laryngoscopy and intubation.

Central Nervous System

In adults, cerebral autoregulation occurs over a mean arterial pressure range of

60-160 mmHg. In neonates, however, cerebral autoregulation is not very well delineated. Most likely, autoregulation occurs in a much lower range and may be impaired in the premature, severe hypoxia, and trauma. Blood vessels in the brain are also thin-walled with poor connective tissue support, which can lead to intraventricular hemorrhage (IVH) with large fluctuations in cerebral blood flow. Large swings in blood pressure, hypoxia, and hypercarbia should be avoided [8].

Before the 1980s, the perception was that neonates do not experience pain. However, we have learned since then that neonates do experience a stress response and may even be hypersensitive to pain [9]. This is especially important as neonates have a high parasympathetic response, and inadequately attenuated stress response to pain can cause bronchospasm and pulmonary vasoconstriction, leading to difficulties with ventilation, oxygenation, and cardiac function. Intravenous or regional analgesia must be considered for any neonatal surgery. Prior to any neuraxial anesthesia, the neonate should be evaluated for any vertebral anomalies, such as looking for a sacral dimple or pursuing imaging if the neonate has a known syndrome or anomaly associated with spinal anomalies.

Inhalational Anesthetic

Minimum alveolar concentration (MAC) is highest in the preterm infant and decreases with increasing age. The exception is sevoflurane, in which the highest MAC occurs in infants around 6 months of age. Inhalational induction occurs quicker in the neonate compared to the adult due to an increase in cardiac output to vessel-rich organs and an increase in alveolar ventilation.

A neonate's myocardium is more sensitive to the effects of volatile anesthetic, and hypotension occurs more readily than older children or adults [10]. Opioids, muscle relaxants, and ketamine can be safely used for maintenance of anesthesia in the setting of hypotension.

Renal Physiology

Neonates have higher blood volume than older infants and adults. Term neonate's blood volume is around 80-90 ml/kg, while premature neonates have 90-100 ml/kg. Prior to surgery, the blood volume and allowable blood loss should be calculated. Fluid management should consider fluid deficit and insensible loss. Systolic blood pressure is a good indicator of the fluid status of the neonate, and often hypotension is fluid responsive [4].

Neonates have immature nephrons and glomerular filtration rates (GFR). GFR is 25% that of adults and may affect the metabolism of various drugs such as neuromuscular blocking drugs. The tubular function is also reduced, which can cause decreased excretion of conjugated drugs such as morphine and its active metabolic. Concentrating ability is also reduced, and neonates are at risk of hyper- or hyponatremia [4].

Gastrointestinal Physiology

Neonates have immature livers and inefficient phase I (oxidation-reduction and hydrolysis) and phase II (conjugation) metabolism, leading to a longer duration of action of most anesthetic drugs. Plasma protein levels, such as alpha-1 acid glycoprotein, are low, leading to less protein binding and more free circulating drugs. Glycogen storage is present at birth but is insufficient in producing adequate glucose with prolonged fasting [3].

Glucose needs to be monitored in a neonate undergoing surgery, especially in the premature, as they can become hypoglycemic. Neonates arriving from the NICU generally have running dextrose-containing fluids. If the neonate has been nil per os (NPO) without dextrose maintenance fluids, intraoperative glucose should be checked.

Thermoregulation

Neonates have a large body surface area to mass ratio and thin skin, which can cause them to lose heat rapidly. Their thermogenesis is also less efficient; they utilize non-shivering thermogenesis from brown fat, which consumes more oxygen. Prior to the start of surgery, the room must be warmed. Other measures include under-body warm air convection blankets, overhead heating lamps, and fluid warmers. Heat loss can also occur during the transport of the neonate to the NICU. Warm blankets and gel warmer pads are typically used. Hu *et al.* found that safely wrapping very low birth weight (VLBW) neonates with polyethylene plastic bags decreased the incidence of hypothermia [11].

ANESTHESIA FOR SPECIFIC SURGERIES NECROTIZING ENTEROCOLITIS

Necrotizing enterocolitis (NEC) is a disorder characterized by ischemic necrosis of the intestinal mucosa that can cause sepsis and a severe inflammatory response [12, 13]. It is one of the most common and urgent surgical newborn emergencies and continues to be a source of perinatal and long-term morbidity in affected neonates. NEC encompasses a range of disorders, from classic NEC associated with prematurity to NEC-like disease in term or near-term neonates due to a hypoxic-ischemic event or underlying anomalies. NEC associated with prematurity, which encompasses 90% of NEC cases, is usually late-onset after feeding has been initiated, *versus* early-onset (first few days of life) in NEC-like disease [13]. This section will focus predominantly on NEC associated with prematurity.

Epidemiology

The incidence of NEC in the United States is about 1 to 3 per 1000 live births, with the highest rate amongst non-Hispanic Black neonates [14, 15]. The incidence of NEC and its associated mortality seems to be decreasing, despite the younger age of viability over the years [16]. NEC most commonly affects premature infants less than 32 weeks gestation and very low birth weight (VLBW) infants (less than 1500 g weight). Incidence increases with decreasing gestational age and birth weight. Mortality rates range from 15-30% and, similarly, are inversely related to gestational age and birth weight. For those requiring surgery, in the setting of sepsis or perforated bowel, the mortality rate is as high as 50% [17].

Pathophysiology

Although the pathophysiology is not entirely known, NEC in preterm infants is thought to be a result of a multifactorial process that involves a triggering factor in a susceptible host, leading to an exaggerated inflammatory response mediated by cytokines and chemokines. Premature neonates have an immature intestinal tract with poor immune defenses and barrier function and impaired motility and mesenteric blood flow. Factors leading to mucosal injury or bacterial overgrowth can cause bacterial translocation into the intestinal tissue [18, 19]. Feeding generally precedes 90% of preterm infants who develop NEC, with the risk of disease greater in neonates receiving formula *versus* breast milk [20]. Agents that reduce gastric acidity are also associated with NEC [21, 22]. Impairment in microvascular flow and anemia with subsequent blood transfusions are also thought to contribute to bowel injury [12, 23]. An exaggerated immune response subsequently leads to the activation of cytokines and can cause necrosis [13, 24].

Diagnosis

NEC is generally diagnosed clinically based on abdominal signs and symptoms. The most common signs are feeding intolerance, increase in gastric residuals, abdominal distention, and bloody stools after 8-10 days of age [13, 25]. Non-specific signs include apnea, lethargy, and signs of shock (*e.g.*, hypotension, fever or hypothermia). Abdominal X-rays can show the classic intramural gas, which is indicative of pneumatosis intestinalis, pneumoperitoneum, a dilated loop of bowel, or portal venous air (Fig. **1**) [13]. Radiography is not as sensitive in the extremely premature and cannot be relied on as the sole criteria for diagnosis. Ultrasonography can also be used to detect fluid collections and visualization of bowel quality and vasculature [26]. Laboratory studies may show thrombocytopenia, increased in prolonged prothrombin and partial thromboplastin times, decreased fibrinogen, and increased D-dimer as a sign of disseminated intravascular coagulation (DIC). Hyponatremia, hyperglycemia, and metabolic acidosis are suggestive of sepsis [27]. The Bell staging criteria provides a clinical definition of NEC based on the severity of symptoms and radiographic and laboratory findings (Table 3) [28, 29]. Neonates at high risk for NEC should be monitored closely as the disease course progresses rapidly from mild non-specific signs to sudden onset of gastrointestinal signs, shock, and multiorgan dysfunction [30].

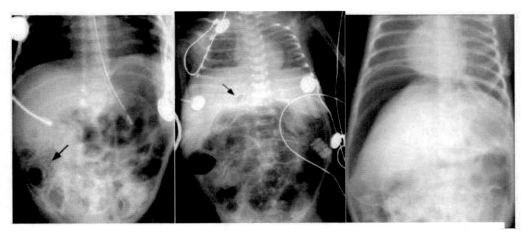

Fig. (1). Radiographic evidence of NEC. Permission: Katz, D. Camden, NJ: Cooper University Hospital.

Table 3. Modified Bell's Criteria for Staging of Necrotizing Enterocolitis.

Stage	Diagnosis of NEC	Gastrointestinal Findings	Other Clinical Findings	Radiographic Findings
Stage I	Suspect	Poor feeding, increased gastric residuals, emesis, abdominal distention, fecal occult blood	Temperature instability, lethargy, apnea, bradycardia	Abdominal distention with mild ileus
Stage IIA	Definite	Above + occult or gross blood in stool, marked abdominal distention	Above	Significant abdominal distention, small bowel separation, persistent bowel loops, focal pneumatosis

(Table 3) cont.....

Stage	Diagnosis of NEC	Gastrointestinal Findings	Other Clinical Findings	Radiographic Findings
Stage IIB	Definite	Diffuse pneumatosis, ascites	Mild metabolic acidosis, thrombocytopenia	Diffuse pneumatosis, portal-venous gas, abdominal wall cellulitis, right lower quadrant mass
Stage IIIA	Advanced	Rigid abdomen	Hypotension, acidosis, apnea, respiratory failure, DIC, neutropenia	Gasless abdomen, tense ascites
Stable IIIB	Advanced	Perforated bowel	Above, with signs of shock	Free air

Adapted from 1) Bell MJ, Ternberg JL, Feigin RD, Keating JP, Marshall R, Barton L *et al*. Neonatal necrotizing enterocolitis; Therapeutic decisions based upon clinical staging; Annals of surgery. 1978;187(1):1-7. 2) Kliegman RM, Fanaroff AA. Necrotizing enterocolitis; The New England journal of medicine; 1984;310(17):1093-103.

Preoperative Management

Because NEC can lead to significant mortality and morbidity, preventive measures should be utilized in premature and low birth weight neonates. Preventive measures include feeding the neonate with breastmilk in small increments, probiotic and prebiotic agents, various growth factors, anti-cytokine agents, and steroids [13].

Once NEC is suspected, the management approach is based on the severity of the disease. For Bell stage I or IIA, medical management is sufficient. For Bell stage III or stage II failing to respond to medical management, surgery is usually performed [31].

The goals of medical management are to discontinue enteral feeds, supportive care, empiric antibiotic therapy, and close monitoring *via* serial exams and imaging. Once NEC is diagnosed, enteral feeds must be discontinued due to ileus associated with NEC. Parenteral nutrition should be initiated *via* central venous catheter, along with a fluid replacement for third space loss. Gastric decompression should also be initiated and continued until the ileus has resolved. Infants in shock may require inotropes or mechanical ventilation for cardiopulmonary support. Metabolic derangements and coagulopathies should also be corrected. Broad-spectrum antibiotics should be initiated in those suspected of having NEC that provides coverage for late-onset sepsis, as well as anaerobes if bowel perforation is suspected. It is important to monitor the clinical status of the neonate with serial exams, laboratory and radiographic studies as the neonate's condition can deteriorate rapidly [12, 13].

Surgery is indicated if there is evidence of bowel perforation or bowel necrosis. The only absolute indication for surgery is pneumoperitoneum on radiography. Neonates who are deteriorating clinically may be considered for surgical intervention, as they may have severe bowel necrosis and are at high risk for perforation. Primary peritoneal drainage is performed to expel air, fluid, and stool. This may be preferred in extremely low birth weight (ELBW) neonates who are too sick to tolerate an exploratory laparotomy. This procedure is predominantly performed by the NICU beside [31].

Laparotomy is performed to resect the area of the affected bowel (*i.e.*, perforated or necrotic), and usually, an enterostomy and distal mucous fistula are placed until reanastomosis at a later date. In cases where the affected bowel segment is short, a primary anastomosis may be performed [31].

Neonates requiring surgery for NEC are often severely ill with signs of shock, metabolic derangements, and coagulopathy. Preoperative assessment of cardiopulmonary status is crucial as these neonates often require mechanical ventilation and blood pressure support. Furthermore, they are usually LBW and extremely premature and may have co-existent lung disease in addition to impaired ventilation due to abdominal distention. If the more sophisticated ICU ventilator, including high-frequency oscillator ventilator (HFOV), is required for the operation, arrangements with the respiratory therapist must be made for its transport. These neonates may also require pulmonary vasodilators, including nitric oxide, as they can have PPHN and may be prone to pulmonary hypertensive crisis. Vasopressor infusions and bolus doses of epinephrine should be available on hand for blood pressure support. Infants with NEC are coagulopathic, and as such, blood products including red blood cells, fresh frozen plasma (FFP), and platelets need to be made readily available. Ideally, a discussion should occur with the family and explain the risk of anesthesia, including death [12, 17].

Intraoperative Management

The neonate is usually being mechanically ventilated on arrival to the OR. Monitors include standard monitors and an arterial line for blood pressure monitoring and blood sampling. However, obtaining an arterial line in an LBW neonate is challenging and may require a surgical cut down. At least two intravenous access should be available for the delivery of fluids and blood products, and considerations can be made for a central line if vasopressors are required. Maintenance of anesthesia should consider hemodynamics. Usually, the neonate does not tolerate much volatile anesthetic, and nitrous oxide should be avoided in the setting of bowel distention. At our institution, we use a combination of fentanyl and rocuronium as a bolus or infusion and low levels of volatile anesthetic as allowed. Care must be taken to warm the neonate given the large area of exposed bowel and infusion of fluids and blood products [17].

Postoperative Management

After laparotomy, neonates almost universally remain on mechanical ventilation and are transported back to the NICU. The mortality rate for NEC is high-- around 10-30%. In neonates who undergo surgical management, Wadhawan *et al.* showed that mortality is as high as 53.5% and neurocognitive impairment is as high as 82.3% [32]. NEC continues to be one of the most devastating diseases for neonates. Despite a lot of progress, further research is needed for preventative strategies.

CONGENITAL ABDOMINAL WALL DEFECTS

Introduction

Gastroschisis and omphalocele are the most common congenital abdominal wall defects [12]. The incidence of gastroschisis is increasing with about 3.7 per 10,000 live births. On the other hand, the incidence of omphalocele has remained steady, with an incidence of about 2 per 10,000 live births [33, 34]. The reason may be because gastroschisis is not genetically linked and is thought to occur due to ischemic injury early in pregnancy, while omphalocele has a greater genetic component [35]. Diagnosis of these defects is often made prenatal *via* ultrasound and maternal α-fetoprotein. Given the complexity of these lesions and the possibility of associated anomalies, delivery of these babies should take place in a tertiary care center with appropriate high-risk obstetrics, NICU care, pediatric surgeons, and pediatric anesthesiologists [36, 37].

Gastroschisis is an abdominal wall defect usually 2-5 cm in diameter, usually to the right of the umbilical cord, with protrusion of the large and small bowel through the defect, and without a covering membrane [12, 37, 38]. Gastroschisis more frequently occurs as isolated lesions, although intestinal atresia can occur in 10% of patients [37].

Omphalocele is a large midline abdominal wall defect greater than 4 cm that occurs between the inner edge of the rectus abdominis [12, 35, 39]. Abdominal contents herniate into the umbilical sac and are covered by an amniotic layer, Wharton's jelly, and the inner peritoneal [12, 37]. Omphaloceles are categorized by size (small or giant), location (epigastric, central, or hypogastric), and the status of the covering membrane (intact or rupture) [40]. In addition to the bowel, other viscera can protrude and be contained in the membrane, including the liver, spleen, stomach, and gonads. Most neonates with omphaloceles have associated congenital anomalies and as such prenatal testing should be instituted [41]. About 30-40% of omphaloceles are associated with Trisomy 21, 18, or 13 [12, 36]. Other associated anomalies occur in 80% of patients with normal karyotypes. The most common anomalies are cardiac in nature, which account for 18-24%. Other anomalies include VACTERL (vertebral, anal, cardiac, TEF, renal, and limb) defects, holoprosencephaly, and anencephalus [37, 42]. Associated syndromes include cloacal exstrophy, Donnai-Barrow syndrome, Pentalogy of Cantrell, and Beckwith-Wiedemann [36, 37]. Patients with giant omphaloceles can have pulmonary hypoplasia due to poor lung development in utero [37, 40].

Preoperative Management

The primary management goals after delivery of neonates with abdominal wall defects are to evaluate and stabilize the cardiopulmonary status of the infant (especially in patients with omphalocele), maintain euvolemia and normothermia, treat sepsis, and correct any electrolyte abnormalities [12, 36, 43]. Subsequent evaluation of associated anomalies should be undertaken prior to surgery. The omphalocele or gastroschisis can be dressed in saline-soaked gauze and impervious dressing in order to minimize losses (Fig. **2**) [12]. Because non-ruptured omphaloceles are covered with a membrane (Fig. **3**), insensible fluid and temperature loss are less than that associated with gastroschisis. An orogastric or nasogastric tube should be inserted to decompress the stomach.

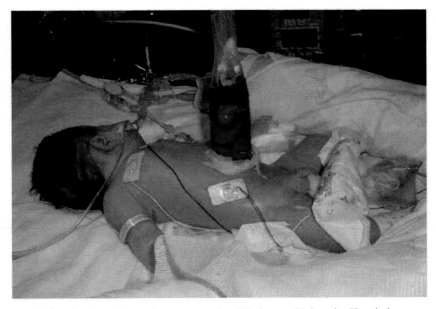

Fig. (2). Gastroschisis in Silo. Permission: Katz, D. Camden, NJ: Cooper University Hospital.

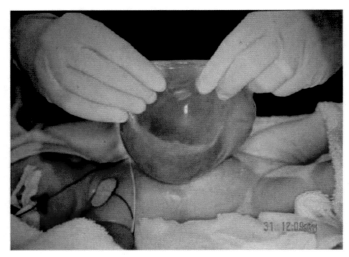

Fig. (3). Omphalocele with bowel encased in a membrane. Permission: Katz, D. Camden, NJ: Cooper University Hospital.

Intraoperative Management

Surgical management includes primary closure of small abdominal defects, silo placement with serial reductions and delayed closure, and serial reduction without fascial closure [37]. The goal of surgery is to repair the abdominal wall defect without causing complications of abdominal compartment syndrome [37]. High intraabdominal pressure can impair respiratory function and cause decreased blood flow to vital organs, including the heart, kidneys, and brain. Primary closure, if feasible in a stable neonate with no known cardiopulmonary issues, is usually performed in the first few hours of life [38]. Delayed closure occurs with larger defects and involves placement of a spring-loaded silo in which reduction of the bowel occurs until the entire contents of the viscera are returned within the abdominal cavity. Only then would fascial closure take place.

Prior to the induction of anesthesia, consider decompressing the stomach *via* an orogastric or nasogastric tube. Anesthesia may be carried out with rapid sequence induction for a general anesthetic with an endotracheal tube in order to avoid abdominal distension. Consider the placement of an epidural catheter for intra- and postoperative pain management, which is associated with a shorter duration of postoperative ventilation [44]. In addition to standard monitors, consider arterial catheters if the patient has cardiopulmonary comorbidities. A central venous catheter may also be used to monitor intra-abdominal pressure and to facilitate postoperative parenteral nutrition. A postductal pulse oximeter placed on the lower extremity can be used to detect poor perfusion of lower extremities as a sign of abdominal compartment syndrome. Maintenance of anesthesia can be performed *via* volatile or intravenous anesthetics, although nitrous oxide should be avoided because it distends the bowel. Neuromuscular blockade is generally used to facilitate abdominal decompression and closure. Given the exposed abdominal viscera, isotonic fluids should be given at 8 to 15 ml/kg per hour for insensible loss. Maintenance fluids should consist of dextrose in order to prevent hypoglycemia [12, 37, 45]. Blood products should be made available in the event of large blood loss.

Postoperative Management

Unless the defect is small, mechanical ventilation is usually required postoperatively until gut edema decreases and respiratory compliance returns to normal [37, 44]. Patients must be monitored for complications of abdominal compartment syndrome, including increased pulmonary peak pressures, decreased urine output, and hypotension. Late complications include malrotation and adhesions causing bowel obstruction.

CONGENITAL DIAPHRAGMATIC HERNIA

Introduction

Congenital diaphragmatic hernia (CDH) is caused by a developmental defect of the diaphragm early in gestation, although 10% can develop later in life. It has an incidence of about 1 in 2,500 to 5,000 live births. The mortality rate is high at 10-23% [46 - 48]. About 40% of the cases are associated with other anomalies, including congenital heart disease and chromosomal abnormalities (Table **4**). CDH with associated anomalies confers an even higher risk of mortality than those with an isolated lesion [49, 50]. Most lesions occur on the left side, with 15% occurring on the right side and 1-2% occurring bilaterally [51].

Table 4. Anomalies Associated with CDH.

Anomaly	-	% (subcategory %)
Cardiovascular	-	50.3
-	Ventricular Septal Defect	(35)
-	Atrial Septal Defect	(29)
-	Coarctation of the Aorta	(7.1)
Gastrointestinal	-	30
-	Meckel Diverticulum	(42)
-	Anal Atresia	(13)

Anomaly		% (subcategory %)
Table 4) cont..... Renal	-	17
-	Hydronephrosis	(35)
-	Hypospadias	(17)
-	Renal agenesis	(14)
Musculoskeletal	-	13
Central Nervous System	-	10
Bronchopulmonary	-	13
Chromosomal/Syndrome	-	20

(Adapted from Zaiss I, Kehl S, Link K, Neff W, Schaible T, Sütterlin M *et al.* Associated malformations in the congenital diaphragmatic hernia. American Journal of Perinatology. 2011;28(3):211-8.)

The pathophysiology of CDH arises from the poor development of the lungs in utero. Early in gestation, abdominal contents herniate into the chest cavity, usually on the left side (Fig. **4**). This leads to lung hypoplasia, reduced pulmonary arterial branching, and increased muscular hyperplasia of the pulmonary arterial tree during this crucial time of pulmonary development. As a result, the neonate develops respiratory distress in the first few hours of life. The transition from fetal circulation may be protracted, and often neonates have persistent pulmonary hypertension of the newborn (PPHN). Because mortality is often associated with cardiopulmonary sequelae of pulmonary hypertension, management of this disease has shifted from immediate surgery to the medical management of pulmonary hypertension and optimization of cardiopulmonary status [52, 53].

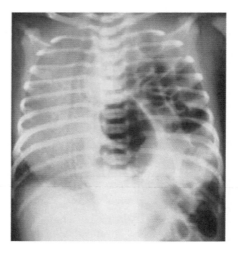

Fig. (4). Left-sided CDH with bowel visible in the left chest cavity. Permission: Katz, D. Camden, NJ: Cooper University Hospital.

CDH is often diagnosed prenatally by ultrasound around 24 weeks of gestation. Once diagnosed, a subsequent detailed evaluation is performed to assess the location of the defect, the position of the liver, the observed/expected lung-t-head (O/E LHR) ratio as a measure of the severity of lung hypoplasia, and any associated anomalies [54, 55]. Neonates with left-sided CDH and an O/E LHR ratio of >50% are thought to have more favorable outcomes.

Fetal endoscopic tracheal occlusion (FETO) is a procedure in which the trachea is occluded to contain lung fluids and promote lung growth. Belfort *et al.* examined the use of FETO at 28 weeks gestation on postnatal outcomes and found that 6 months, 1-year, and 2-year survival rates were significantly higher in those treated with the FETO procedure compared to those not treated [56, 57]. The clinical trial is still underway at the time of writing.

Preoperative Management

A standardized multidisciplinary approach to management, such as that of the CDH EURO Consortium, The Canadian Congenital Diaphragmatic Hernia Collaborative, and various academic institutions, have been shown to improve outcomes [54, 55, 58].

Delivery should occur at a tertiary care center with the capability to place neonates on extracorporeal membrane oxygenation (ECMO), if necessary. Studies have not concluded an optimal time of delivery, but Hutcheon *et al.* showed that mortality decreases with increasing gestational age [59].

Postnatally, the goal of preoperative management is to stabilize the cardiopulmonary status of the neonatal prior to surgery, which has been shown to improve outcomes compared to immediate surgical repair [60]. Goals of management involve the stabilization of the infant's oxygenation and ventilation, pulmonary and systemic perfusion, and acid-base status.

Immediately after delivery in neonates with respiratory distress, intubation should occur to avoid the use of bag-mask ventilation that can result in distension of the abdominal and further compression of the lungs. Delay in intubation can also worsen ventilation and increase acidosis. Preductal saturations should remain between 80-95%. If intravenous access is available, consider medications such as fentanyl to attenuate the stress response to laryngoscopy in order to minimize an increase in pulmonary arterial pressure [61]. Fractional inspired oxygen (FiO_2) should be minimized to achieve this saturation in order to avoid oxygen toxicity. The ventilation goal is to reduce lung injury and decrease pulmonary pressure. As such, low peak pressures <25 cm H_2O are preferred. Permissive hypercapnia, keeping $PaCO_2$ levels between 50 and 70 mmHg, is accepted and shown to improve survival. In the NICU, the initial ventilation strategy should start with conventional ventilation instead of HFOV. The CDH EURO Consortium has shown a shorter duration of ventilation and a lesser need for inhaled nitric oxide (iNO) with initial conventional ventilation is required [54]. If a peak inspiratory pressure (PIP) >28 cmH$_2$O is required, consider HFOV or ECMO.

Sedation should be utilized to reduce the stress response. However, neuromuscular blockade, although enhancing compliance, should be avoided in order to preserve spontaneous ventilation [62].

An echocardiogram is generally obtained without the first hours of life to assess cardiac anomalies, degree of pulmonary hypertension, right heart function, and the presence of right to left heart shunting.

An arterial line should be inserted in order to measure blood gas and to monitor blood pressure. Blood pressure should be kept normotensive in order to avoid right to left shunt. Fluids bolus of normal saline at 10-20 ml/kg can be utilized to maintain blood pressure, although care must be taken to avoid excess fluids. Consider inotropic agents such as dopamine, dobutamine, epinephrine, or norepinephrine if needed to maintain blood pressure.

In a neonate with pulmonary hypertension, which may manifest as low preductal saturations, iNO should be initiated as a first-line therapy as it has been shown to decrease the need for ECMO [63]. If there is no response to iNO, prostacyclin and phosphodiesterase inhibitors can be given [54, 55, 64].

If oxygenation cannot be adequately achieved, ECMO should be considered (Table 5) for criteria.

Table 5. Criteria for ECMO.

Criteria
Inability to maintain preductal sat >85% or postductal sat > 70%
Respiratory acidosis (pH <7.15)
Metabolic acidosis (lactate >5mml/L and pH <7.15)
PIP > 28 cm H$_2$O or mean airway pressure > 17 cm H$_2$O
Hypotension refractory to inotropes
Oxygenation index* > 40 present for at least 3 hours

* Oxygenation index (OI) = [mean airway pressure (MAP) × FiO$_2$ × 100]÷PaO$_2$
Adapted from: Snoek KG, Reiss IK, Greenough A, Capolupo I, Urlesberger B, Wessel L *et al*. Standardized Postnatal Management of Infants with Congenital Diaphragmatic Hernia in Europe: The CDH EURO Consortium Consensus - 2015 Update. Neonatology. 2016;110(1):66-74.

Surgical repair should only be considered when the neonate has been stabilized. Reported survival rates in neonates with delayed surgical repair ranges from 79-92% [60, 65]. Criteria outlined by the CDH EURO Consortium includes: 1) mean arterial pressure normal for gestational age, 2) preductal saturation levels of 85-95% on FiO_2 below 50%, 3) lactate below 3 mmol/L, and 4) urine output more than 1 ml/kg/h [54]. However, surgery may be performed while on ECMO, which may improve survival if done earlier [66].

Intraoperative Management

Repair of the diaphragmatic defect can be done *via* a thoracoscopic approach or a thoracotomy, and the defect itself can be fixed through a primary repair or a patch repair (Fig. **5**). Thoracoscopic repair which may not be feasible in patients with severe pulmonary dysfunction. Single lung ventilation worsens ventilation-perfusion mismatch, decreasing oxygenation. Insufflation of the chest cavity also increases the partial pressure of carbon dioxide ($PaCO_2$), causing further pulmonary vasoconstriction and worsening of pulmonary hypertension. Generally, the thoracoscopic approach is reserved for patients with mild to moderate pulmonary hypertension. Thoracoscopic approach with patch repair was traditionally thought to have an increased rate of recurrence [67], but more recently, Qin *et al.* demonstrated no difference in recurrence and better hemodynamics, shorter surgery, shorter postoperative mechanical ventilation and hospitalization in the thoracoscopic group [68].

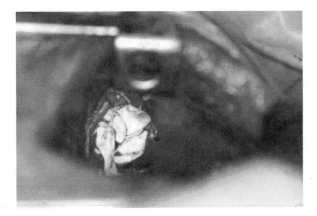

Fig. (5). Patch repair of CDH*via* Thoracotomy. Permission: Katz, D. Camden, NJ: Cooper University Hospital.

Generally, patients with CDH arrive to the operating room intubated or, in those with severe lung hypoplasia who require high ventilatory support or iNO, the surgery can be performed in the NICU. Induction in a non-intubated patient should be done intravenously with rapid sequence intubation in order to avoid insufflation of the stomach. The arterial line and central line should be considered in addition to standard monitoring, especially in a patient with significant pulmonary hypertension or congenital heart disease. The goals of the anesthetic management mirror the goals of NICU management; optimize oxygenation, ventilation, perfusion, and acid-base status. Ventilation should be kept at low pressures, and oxygenation should achieve saturation of 85-95% on the lowest FiO_2 possible. pH should be kept above 7.25. Inhalational agents can be used as it is favorable towards pulmonary vasodilation. However, it decreases systemic vascular resistance and may not be tolerated in sick neonates. Generally, a moderate to high opioid dose is used instead to reduce sympathetic response to surgery. Care must be taken to make sure the infant is warm, as hypothermia can lead to pulmonary vasoconstriction and the worsening of pulmonary hypertension [53].

Postoperative Care and Outcomes

After surgery, neonates generally remain intubated and are taken back to NICU for postoperative care. Respiratory distress and pulmonary hypertension can still persist. Goals of care reflect preoperative management of minimizing lung damage, reducing pulmonary hypertension, and optimizing acid-base status.

The survival rate for CDH is about 70% at 1 year [69]. Neonates with large defects generally have more herniated viscera and subsequently more hypoplastic lungs. Thus, the size of the defect, the presence of the liver in the chest cavity, and the requirement for patch repair are good clinical predictors of mortality. Brindle *et al.* modified the CDH Study Group tool and found that low birth weight, low Apgar, several pulmonary hypertension, major cardiac anomaly, and chromosomal anomaly are predictors of mortality [70, 71]. Postoperatively, Goonasekera *et al.* found that an oxygenation index of >5.4 predicted mortality with 100% sensitivity [72]. Oxygenation index is an assessment of lung function and is defined as:

$$\text{Oxygenation Index} = \frac{FiO_2 \times MAP}{PaO_2}$$

Infants who survive may still have debilitating diseases later in life. About 50-70% of infants have chronic lung disease in the first year of life, and about 28% still require bronchodilators beyond the second year of life [73]. Neurocognitive delay is also a sequela of CDH. About 30-80% of patients have both cognitive and motor delays in the first 3 years of life but do show some improvement with age [74]. Intestinal obstruction and malrotation from adhesions occur in about 10% of postoperative CDH patients [75].

TRACHEOESOPHAGEAL FISTULA AND ESOPHAGEAL ATRESIA

Tracheoesophageal fistula (TEF) is a congenital anomaly that occurs in about 1 in 4,500 live births [76]. The anomaly is caused by a defect in the lateral septation of the foregut into the esophagus and trachea. The fistula tract results from a branch of the embryonic lung bud that fails to undergo branching due to defective epithelial-mesenchymal interactions [77]. The connection between the gastrointestinal tract and trachea leads to aspiration pneumonia postnatally if left untreated. 50% of TEF are associated with other syndromes, including the VACTERL (malformations including vertebral, anal, cardiac, TEF, renal, and limb defects), CHARGE syndrome (coloboma, heart defects, atresia choanae, growth retardation, genital abnormalities, and ear abnormalities), and congenital heart or genitourinary defects [76, 78].

About 95% of TEF have esophageal atresia (EA). 5% are H type TEF or without esophageal atresia. The most common type of TEF is the C type, which involves proximal esophageal atresia and distal TEF. Most fistulas occur above the carina, but about 11% occur below the carina, and 22% occur within 1 cm of the carina, making ventilation difficult [79, 80].

The presence of EA causes polyhydramnios during pregnancy, and sometimes a diagnosis of TEF can be made prenatally on ultrasound. However, a large portion of cases are diagnosed postnatally when the neonate is choking, has respiratory distress or is unable to tolerate feeds. Diagnosis of TEF with EA is confirmed when an orogastric catheter cannot pass farther than 10-15 cm, and a radiograph demonstrates the catheter curled in the upper esophageal pouch. Occasionally, water-soluble contrast can be given under fluoroscopy but must be suctioned immediately to avoid aspiration. This is commonly used to diagnose H-type TEF without EA. The lack of esophageal atresia can delay diagnosis for years and sometimes even up to early adulthood [81, 82].

Preoperative Management

Prior to surgery, the neonate should be worked up for associated anomalies, including those associated with VACTERL. Most importantly, an echocardiogram must be obtained to rule out congenital heart disease prior to surgery. Vertebral anomalies should also be investigated if an epidural catheter is to be placed for analgesia. Surgery, although urgent to prevent aspiration, is not emergent, and the neonate should be stabilized prior to surgery. An orogastric tube should be inserted to intermittently suction secretions and decrease the risk of aspiration. Mechanical ventilation should be avoided if possible due to the difficulty of keeping the endotracheal tube beyond the fistula to avoid insufflation of the stomach [83].

Intraoperative Management

The surgical approach depends on the type of TEF. Prior to the procedure, an endoscopic exam is performed to determine fistula location, size, the presence of other fistulas, and other airway anomalies. For the most common type, Type C, surgery is performed by right thoracotomy or a thoracoscopic approach. Increasingly, thoracoscopy is performed unless the neonate is premature, is of low birth weight, or has cardiac or pulmonary pathology. The fistula is ligated, and the proximal esophagus is connected to the distal esophagus. If the gap between the two ends of the esophagus is large, surgery is performed in a staged repair [83, 84]. In a type H fistula, occlusion can be performed by bronchoscopy and application of tissue adhesive or fibrin glue. Alternatively, surgical ligation *via* a right cervical dissection can be performed [84, 85]. This chapter will focus on the anesthetic management of patients with type C TEF.

Knottenbelt *et al*. found anesthetic techniques for TEF repair vary widely amongst providers. In a neonate without an endotracheal tube (ETT), induction of anesthesia can be performed *via* intravenous or inhalation [86]. The endotracheal tube, preferably a cuffed tube without Murphy's eye, can be inserted proximal to the fistula, distal to the fistula, or into the left mainstem bronchus. Although simple to do, insertion of the ETT proximal to the fistula can cause distension of the stomach and further difficulty with ventilation. This should only be reserved for neonates with good lung compliance. Inserting the ETT distal to the fistula bypasses ventilation of the stomach. However, this technique is difficult to achieve and maintain throughout the case. This technique is best when the fistula to carina distance is long. Left mainstem bronchus intubation bypasses ventilation of the fistula and can facilitate surgery by deflating the right lung. This is often achieved with the aid of a fiberoptic bronchoscope. Occluding the fistula with a bronchial blocker, such as a Fogarty catheter, can also be performed, although this technique is not widely used [79, 86].

Classically, spontaneous ventilation is maintained in order to decrease insufflation of the stomach. Spontaneous ventilation should be maintained during bronchoscopy in the event there are upper airway anomalies [79, 84]. In the absence of such anomalies and if the neonate has good lung compliance, the neonate can be ventilated with low positive pressure. Knottenbelt *et al*. found that all but two patients received neuromuscular blockade during maintenance of anesthesia. High-frequency oscillatory ventilation (HFOV) has also been utilized for better surgical conditions [87].

In addition to standard monitors, an arterial line should be inserted to monitor hemodynamics, especially during a thoracoscopic case. The neonate is usually positioned in a lateral-prone position with the right side elevated approximately 30 degrees [83].

Intravenous opioids are the most popular mode of analgesia. Epidural catheters, paravertebral blocks, and intercostal blocks have also been employed [86].

Postoperative Management

Unless there is good lung compliance and the low tension on the esophageal anastomosis, the neonate is kept intubated postoperatively to avoid complications associated with postoperative laryngoscopy. However, the goal is for early extubation to reduce stress on esophageal anastomosis. Knottenbelt *et al.* found that only about 34% of neonates are extubated within two days, and only 13% were extubated in the operating room.

Mortality continues to fall with advances in NICU care and surgical technique [84]. Generally, neonates with congenital heart disease, prematurity, and low birth weight have the highest risk of morbidity and mortality following repair.

Even with high survival rates, children with a history of repaired TEF often face morbidity associated with esophageal strictures, dysphagia, gastro-esophageal reflux disease, and respiratory problems. They often return to the operating room many times for stricture dilation and to the hospital with bronchitis [84].

AIRWAY EMERGENCIES

General Considerations for Neonatal Airway Surgery

A normal neonate's anatomy makes for a difficult airway. In the presence of an airway anomaly, securing an airway and performing anesthesia can be incredibly challenging.

Airway setup should include endotracheal tubes, laryngoscopes, oral and nasal airways of several different sizes. Supraglottic airways should also be readily available, although they may not seat well in neonates and may be too large for premature and LBW infants. Video laryngoscopy and fiberoptic bronchoscopy should also be made available if a difficult airway is anticipated. Medications for cardiopulmonary resuscitation, including atropine and epinephrine, should be readily available.

Because of the high parasympathetic tone in neonates, the anesthesiologist must prepare for bronchospasm or laryngospasm. Postponement of the procedure should be considered in neonates with signs of upper or lower respiratory tract infection due to a high risk of hypoxemia and respiratory complications. Depth of anesthesia should be maintained to avoid bronchospasm or laryngospasm. Considerations must be made to maintain spontaneous ventilation in neonates with airway anomalies or risk for difficult airways.

Specific Anomalies

Choanal Atresia

Congenital choanal atresia is a bony obstruction of the posterior nasopharynx. Because infants are nose breathers, this obstruction can cause respiratory distress in case of bilateral obstruction or thick nasal discharge in unilateral obstruction. It is a rare anomaly and occurs in 1 in every 5000 live births and is predominantly in females [88]. About one-third of cases are bilateral and about 50% are associated with a congenital syndrome, such as CHARGE syndrome (colobomas, heart defects, atresia choanae, retardation of growth and cognition, genitourinary anomalies, and ear anomalies), Treacher Collins, and cleft lip and/or palate [89]. Choanal atresia is suspected if a catheter cannot be passed through the nasopharynx and is confirmed using fiberoptic nasal endoscopy or CT scan. An echocardiogram should be obtained prior to surgery to evaluate for cardiac defects.

Immediate treatment of respiratory distress includes ensuring airway patency by placing an oral airway or intubation. Surgery of bilateral atresia is usually early, while unilateral atresia can be delayed. Surgery often occurs *via* a transnasal approach to remove the atresia plate [90].

Prior to surgery, the anesthesiologist must conduct a thorough evaluation of the airway, as Yildirim *et al.* found about 22% of patients had difficult airways [91]. In addition, other associated syndromes and anomalies should be determined. Prior to induction, adequate airway equipment should be available and set up in the room, including supraglottic airway and video laryngoscopy and/or fiberoptic bronchoscopy if the patient has features of a difficult airway. An inhalational induction may be preferred in order to preserve spontaneous ventilation.

Pierre Robin Sequence

Neonates with Pierre-Robin sequence (PRS) have characteristic micrognathia (small mandible) and glossoptosis (a downward displacement of the tongue) that causes airway obstruction. These patients also generally have collapse of other airway structures, such as the epiglottis and the base of the tongue. Although usually isolated, neonates with PRS can have associated syndrome such as Stickler, 22q11.2 deletion, fetal alcohol syndrome, and Treacher-Collins syndrome [92]. Incidence of PRS is rare, about 1:8,500 to 1:14,000 live births [93, 94].

Patients with mild PRS may go untreated as micrognathia improves with age. In the delivery room or NICU, immediate treatment includes prone positioning and nasopharyngeal airways. Surgical treatment varies from center to center and includes tongue lip adhesion or mandibular distraction osteogenesis. Tracheostomy can be performed if PRS is severe and the tongue-lip adhesion or mandibular distraction are likely to fail. Severe PRS is seen more commonly in children with associated syndromes, central apnea, or in VLBW neonates [95].

Thorough evaluation of the patient is crucial for airway management. Infants should obtain a sleep study, craniofacial CT, and swallowing study. Factors such as desaturation while supine, feeding difficulties, sternal and intercostal retractions, apneic spells may indicate severe obstruction. Nasal endoscopy may be used to determine the degree of airway collapse and the presence of laryngeal abnormalities.

Induction of anesthesia should maintain spontaneous ventilation. Intubation can be achieved by various techniques utilizing fiberoptic bronchoscopes through a supraglottic airway or video laryngoscopy. When the obstruction is severe, a supraglottic airway may be placed without any sedation [96]. Often, assistance such as a jaw thrust or pulling the tongue forward is required to visualize the larynx or advance the endotracheal tube during fiberoptic intubation. If intubation still fails, the surgeon may attempt a rigid bronchoscope. Emergent tracheostomy and extracorporeal membrane oxygenation (ECMO) are the last options if an airway cannot be secured.

Patients with PRS can have central apnea and may be sensitive to opioids. Postoperatively, a decision must be made whether to keep the infant intubated based on preoperative severity of PRS, intraoperative opioid use, and airway edema. In a patient who is vigorous postoperatively and whose airway edema is minimal, extubation may be attempted. However, emergently reintubating a neonate is more challenging than planned intubation. The anesthesiologist must be

prepared for reintubation, including ensuring that surgeons are available and equipment is on hand for tracheostomy and ECMO.

Subglottic stenosis

Subglottic stenosis is a narrowing of the subglottis commonly at the level of the cricoid, the only complete ring in the subglottis (Fig. **6**). The subglottis is considered stenotic if it is 4 mm or less in a term neonate or 3mm or less in a preterm neonate. Subglottic stenosis can be congenital or acquired. Congenital subglottic stenosis is thought to be due to the failure of the airway to recanalize during embryonic development. It is commonly associated with other anomalies such as trisomy 21, CHARGE, and 22q11 deletion. Acquired subglottic stenosis occurs in the setting of trauma such as tracheal intubation. Neonates present with stridor or croup, feeding difficulties, cyanosis, or respiratory distress [97]. The severity of the stenosis is graded according to the Myer-Cotton grading system; grade I is a 50% stenosis, grade II is a 51-70% stenosis, grade III is a 71 to 90% stenosis, and grade IV is complete stenosis [98].

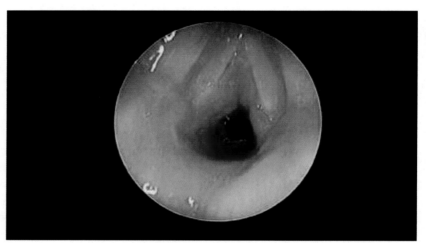

Fig (6). A video image of Subglottic Stenosis. Permission: Solomon, D. Camden, NJ: Cooper University Hospital.

Patients with suspicion for subglottic stenosis arrive to the operating room for rigid bronchoscopy under general anesthesia for diagnosis and evaluation of other potential airway abnormalities. Rigid bronchoscopy involves a shared airway between the surgical and the anesthesia team. The surgeon may require intermittent bag-mask ventilation or intubation in order to maintain oxygenation. Neonates with grade II stenosis with respiratory distress may undergo endoscopic dilation or CO_2 laser treatment. Patients with higher-grade lesions may require tracheostomy and laryngotracheoplasty, utilizing cartilage graft for tracheal reconstruction [97, 99].

Neonates with subglottic stenosis can have tenuous airways, which can lead to dangerous intraoperative hypoxia with airway instrumentation. Furthermore, surgical procedures often require a shared and sometimes unsecured airway. Planning and communication are paramount for these airway procedures.

Preoperative evaluation of neonates with subglottic stenosis should include evaluation of associated anomalies. Pulmonary status should be optimized in children undergoing the airway procedure to minimize laryngospasm, bronchospasm, or hypoxia intraoperatively. For rigid bronchoscopies, surgeons generally require the patient to be breathing spontaneously without an endotracheal tube. Sometimes, the anesthesia circuit can be connected to the side port of their bronchoscopy for oxygenation. Because end-tidal CO_2 may not be reliable, it is important to observe chest rise for adequate ventilation. Induction of anesthesia can be accomplished intravenously or *via* inhalation. Maintenance of anesthesia is performed intravenously due to unreliable delivery of inhalational agents without a secured airway. It is important to maintain the depth of anesthesia to avoid coughing, laryngospasm, or bronchospasm associated with light anesthesia. Propofol, along with a short-acting opioid such as remifentanil, are good choices to reduce the stress response to rigid bronchoscopy while maintaining the ability for a fast wakeup at the end of the procedure. An antisialogogue can decrease secretions that may hinder the view and cause laryngospasm or bronchospasm. Steroids should also be given to reduce postoperative airway edema. The surgeon generally injects lidocaine through the vocal cords to minimize coughing. At the conclusion of the procedure, an endotracheal tube can be inserted, or the neonate can be masked with or without oral airway during the emergence of anesthesia. At our institution, we prefer spontaneous ventilation *via* mask until the neonate is sufficiently awake and responsive. Postoperatively, these patients should be observed in the intensive care unit for potential postoperative respiratory distress caused by airway edema.

CONCLUSION

Although many neonatal emergencies can now be treated medically, term and premature neonates still frequently require emergent surgical procedures. These are extremely challenging cases for anesthesiologists, even for those who have formal pediatric training. Familiarity with a safe and comprehensive operating room setup can be life-saving. The care of these patients requires experience, vigilance, familiarity with the key features of the child's illness and unique physiology, and knowledge of specific aspects of the proposed procedure.

CONSENT FOR PUBLICATION

Not applicable.

CONFLICT OF INTEREST

The author declares no conflict of interest, financial or otherwise.

ACKNOWLEDGEMENTS

Declared none.

REFERENCES

[1]   Ely DM, Driscoll AK, Matthews TJ. Infant Mortality by Age at Death in the United States, 2016. NCHS Data Brief 2018; (326): 1-8.
[PMID: 30475688]

[2]   Mathews TJ, Driscoll AK. Trends in Infant Mortality in the United States, 2005-2014. NCHS Data Brief 2017; (279): 1-8.
[PMID: 28437240]

[3]   Smith's Anesthesia for Infants and Children. Philadelphia: Elsevier 2011.

[4]   Gormley SMCCP. Basic principles of anaesthesia for neonates and infants. Br J Anaesth 2001; 1(5): 130-3.

[5]   Heinrich S, Birkholz T, Ihmsen H, Irouschek A, Ackermann A, Schmidt J. Incidence and predictors of difficult laryngoscopy in 11,219 pediatric anesthesia procedures. Paediatr Anaesth 2012; 22(8): 729-36.
[http://dx.doi.org/10.1111/j.1460-9592.2012.03813.x] [PMID: 22340664]

[6]   Vijayasekaran S, Lioy J, Maschhoff K. Airway disorders of the fetus and neonate: An overview. Semin Fetal Neonatal Med 2016; 21(4): 220-9.
[http://dx.doi.org/10.1016/j.siny.2016.03.004] [PMID: 27039115]

[7]   Greaney D, Russell J, Dawkins I, Healy M. A retrospective observational study of acquired subglottic stenosis using low-pressure, high-volume cuffed endotracheal tubes. Paediatr Anaesth 2018; 28(12): 1136-41.
[http://dx.doi.org/10.1111/pan.13519] [PMID: 30375105]

[8]   Rhee CJ, da Costa CS, Austin T, Brady KM, Czosnyka M, Lee JK. Neonatal cerebrovascular autoregulation. Pediatr Res 2018; 84(5): 602-10.
[http://dx.doi.org/10.1038/s41390-018-0141-6] [PMID: 30196311]

[9]   Perry M, Tan Z, Chen J, Weidig T, Xu W, Cong XS. Neonatal Pain: Perceptions and Current Practice. Crit Care Nurs Clin North Am 2018; 30(4): 549-61.
[http://dx.doi.org/10.1016/j.cnc.2018.07.013] [PMID: 30447813]

[10]   Friesen RH, Henry DB. Cardiovascular changes in preterm neonates receiving isoflurane, halothane, fentanyl, and ketamine. Anesthesiology 1986; 64(2): 238-42.
[http://dx.doi.org/10.1097/00000542-198602000-00018] [PMID: 3946810]

[11]   Hu XJ, Wang L, Zheng RY, Lv TC, Zhang YX, Cao Y, *et al.* Using polyethylene plastic bag to prevent moderate hypothermia during transport in very low birth weight infants: a randomized trial. Journal of perinatology : official journal of the California Perinatal Association 2018; 38(4): 332-6.
[http://dx.doi.org/10.1038/s41372-017-0028-0]

[12]   Brett CMaD, Peter J. Anesthesia for General Surgery in the Neonate. In: Davis PJaC, Franklyn P, Eds. Smith's Anesthesia for Infants and Children Ninth ed. Philadelphia, PA: Elsevier Inc 2017; pp. 517-616.

[13]   Neu J, Walker WA. Necrotizing enterocolitis. N Engl J Med 2011; 364(3): 255-64.
[http://dx.doi.org/10.1056/NEJMra1005408] [PMID: 21247316]

[14]   Stoll BJ, Hansen NI, Bell EF, *et al.* Trends in Care Practices, Morbidity, and Mortality of Extremely
        Preterm Neonates, 1993-2012. JAMA 2015; 314(10): 1039-51.
        [http://dx.doi.org/10.1001/jama.2015.10244] [PMID: 26348753]

[15]   Holman RC, Stoll BJ, Curns AT, Yorita KL, Steiner CA, Schonberger LB. Necrotising enterocolitis
        hospitalisations among neonates in the United States. Paediatr Perinat Epidemiol 2006; 20(6): 498-
        506.
        [http://dx.doi.org/10.1111/j.1365-3016.2006.00756.x] [PMID: 17052286]

[16]   Horbar JD, Edwards EM, Greenberg LT, *et al.* Variation in Performance of Neonatal Intensive Care
        Units in the United States. JAMA Pediatr 2017; 171(3): e164396.
        [http://dx.doi.org/10.1001/jamapediatrics.2016.4396] [PMID: 28068438]

[17]   Brusseau R, McCann ME. Anaesthesia for urgent and emergency surgery. Early Hum Dev 2010;
        86(11): 703-14.
        [http://dx.doi.org/10.1016/j.earlhumdev.2010.08.008] [PMID: 20952136]

[18]   Hsueh W, Caplan MS, Qu XW, Tan XD, De Plaen IG, Gonzalez-Crussi F. Neonatal necrotizing
        enterocolitis: clinical considerations and pathogenetic concepts. Pediatr Dev Pathol 2003; 6(1): 6-23.
        [http://dx.doi.org/10.1007/s10024-002-0602-z] [PMID: 12424605]

[19]   Hunter CJ, Upperman JS, Ford HR, Camerini V. Understanding the susceptibility of the premature
        infant to necrotizing enterocolitis (NEC). Pediatr Res 2008; 63(2): 117-23.
        [http://dx.doi.org/10.1203/PDR.0b013e31815ed64c] [PMID: 18091350]

[20]   Berseth CL. Feeding strategies and necrotizing enterocolitis. Curr Opin Pediatr 2005; 17(2): 170-3.
        [http://dx.doi.org/10.1097/01.mop.0000150566.50580.26] [PMID: 15800406]

[21]   Terrin G, Passariello A, De Curtis M, *et al.* Ranitidine is associated with infections, necrotizing
        enterocolitis, and fatal outcome in newborns. Pediatrics 2012; 129(1): e40-5.
        [http://dx.doi.org/10.1542/peds.2011-0796] [PMID: 22157140]

[22]   Guillet R, Stoll BJ, Cotten CM, *et al.* Association of H2-blocker therapy and higher incidence of
        necrotizing enterocolitis in very low birth weight infants. Pediatrics 2006; 117(2): e137-42.
        [http://dx.doi.org/10.1542/peds.2005-1543] [PMID: 16390920]

[23]   Wan-Huen P, Bateman D, Shapiro DM, Parravicini E. Packed red blood cell transfusion is an
        independent risk factor for necrotizing enterocolitis in premature infants. Journal of perinatology :
        official journal of the California Perinatal Association 2013; 33(10): 786-90.
        [http://dx.doi.org/10.1038/jp.2013.60]

[24]   Sharma R, Tepas JJ III, Hudak ML, *et al.* Neonatal gut barrier and multiple organ failure: role of
        endotoxin and proinflammatory cytokines in sepsis and necrotizing enterocolitis. J Pediatr Surg 2007;
        42(3): 454-61.
        [http://dx.doi.org/10.1016/j.jpedsurg.2006.10.038] [PMID: 17336180]

[25]   Parker LA, Weaver M, Murgas Torrazza RJ, *et al.* Effect of Gastric Residual Evaluation on Enteral
        Intake in Extremely Preterm Infants: A Randomized Clinical Trial. JAMA Pediatr 2019; 173(6): 534-
        43.
        [http://dx.doi.org/10.1001/jamapediatrics.2019.0800] [PMID: 31034045]

[26]   Silva CT, Daneman A, Navarro OM, *et al.* Correlation of sonographic findings and outcome in
        necrotizing enterocolitis. Pediatr Radiol 2007; 37(3): 274-82.
        [http://dx.doi.org/10.1007/s00247-006-0393-x] [PMID: 17225155]

[27]   Hällström M, Koivisto AM, Janas M, Tammela O. Laboratory parameters predictive of developing
        necrotizing enterocolitis in infants born before 33 weeks of gestation. J Pediatr Surg 2006; 41(4): 792-
        8.2006;
        [http://dx.doi.org/10.1016/j.jpedsurg.2005.12.034]

[28]   Bell MJ, Ternberg JL, Feigin RD, *et al.* Neonatal necrotizing enterocolitis. Therapeutic decisions
        based upon clinical staging. Ann Surg 1978; 187(1): 1-7.

[http://dx.doi.org/10.1097/00000658-197801000-00001] [PMID: 413500]

[29]   Kliegman RM, Fanaroff AA. Necrotizing enterocolitis. N Engl J Med 1984; 310(17): 1093-103.
[http://dx.doi.org/10.1056/NEJM198404263101707] [PMID: 6369134]

[30]   Wang K, Tao G, Sylvester KG. Recent Advances in Prevention and Therapies for Clinical or Experimental Necrotizing Enterocolitis. Dig Dis Sci 2019; 64(11): 3078-85.
[http://dx.doi.org/10.1007/s10620-019-05618-2] [PMID: 30989465]

[31]   Robinson JR, Rellinger EJ, Hatch LD, *et al.* Surgical necrotizing enterocolitis. Semin Perinatol 2017; 41(1): 70-9.
[http://dx.doi.org/10.1053/j.semperi.2016.09.020] [PMID: 27836422]

[32]   Wadhawan R, Oh W, Hintz SR, Blakely ML, Das A, Bell EF, *et al.* Neurodevelopmental outcomes of extremely low birth weight infants with spontaneous intestinal perforation or surgical necrotizing enterocolitis. Journal of perinatology : official journal of the California Perinatal Association 2014; 34(1): 64-70.
[http://dx.doi.org/10.1038/jp.2013.128]

[33]   Wilson RD, Johnson MP. Congenital abdominal wall defects: an update. Fetal Diagn Ther 2004; 19(5): 385-98.
[http://dx.doi.org/10.1159/000078990] [PMID: 15305094]

[34]   Alvarez SM, Burd RS. Increasing prevalence of gastroschisis repairs in the United States: 1996-2003. J Pediatr Surg 2007; 42(6): 943-6.
[http://dx.doi.org/10.1016/j.jpedsurg.2007.01.026] [PMID: 17560199]

[35]   Frolov P, Alali J, Klein MD. Clinical risk factors for gastroschisis and omphalocele in humans: a review of the literature. Pediatr Surg Int 2010; 26(12): 1135-48.
[http://dx.doi.org/10.1007/s00383-010-2701-7] [PMID: 20809116]

[36]   Gamba P, Midrio P. Abdominal wall defects: prenatal diagnosis, newborn management, and long-term outcomes. Semin Pediatr Surg 2014; 23(5): 283-90.
[http://dx.doi.org/10.1053/j.sempedsurg.2014.09.009] [PMID: 25459013]

[37]   Christison-Lagay ER, Kelleher CM, Langer JC. Neonatal abdominal wall defects. Semin Fetal Neonatal Med 2011; 16(3): 164-72.
[http://dx.doi.org/10.1016/j.siny.2011.02.003] [PMID: 21474399]

[38]   Skarsgard ED. Management of gastroschisis. Curr Opin Pediatr 2016; 28(3): 363-9.
[http://dx.doi.org/10.1097/MOP.0000000000000336] [PMID: 26974976]

[39]   Ionescu S, Mocanu M, Andrei B, *et al.* Differential diagnosis of abdominal wall defects - omphalocele *versus* gastroschisis. Chirurgia (Bucur) 2014; 109(1): 7-14.
[PMID: 24524464]

[40]   Gonzalez KW, Chandler NM. Ruptured omphalocele: Diagnosis and management. Semin Pediatr Surg 2019; 28(2): 101-5.
[http://dx.doi.org/10.1053/j.sempedsurg.2019.04.009] [PMID: 31072456]

[41]   Cohen-Overbeek TE, Tong WH, Hatzmann TR, *et al.* Omphalocele: comparison of outcome following prenatal or postnatal diagnosis. Ultrasound Obstet Gynecol 2010; 36(6): 687-92.
[http://dx.doi.org/10.1002/uog.7698] [PMID: 20509138]

[42]   Baird PA, MacDonald EC. An epidemiologic study of congenital malformations of the anterior abdominal wall in more than half a million consecutive live births. Am J Hum Genet 1981; 33(3): 470-8.

[43]   Verla MA, Style CC, Olutoye OO. Prenatal diagnosis and management of omphalocele. Semin Pediatr Surg 2019; 28(2): 84-8.
[http://dx.doi.org/10.1053/j.sempedsurg.2019.04.007] [PMID: 31072463]

[44]   Raghavan M, Montgomerie J. Anesthetic management of gastrochisis--a review of our practice over

the past 5 years. Paediatr Anaesth 2008; 18(11): 1055-9.
[http://dx.doi.org/10.1111/j.1460-9592.2008.02762.x] [PMID: 18950329]

[45]   Mhamane R, Dave N, Garasia M. Delayed primary repair of giant omphalocele: anesthesia challenges. Paediatr Anaesth 2012; 22(9): 935-6.
[http://dx.doi.org/10.1111/j.1460-9592.2012.03907.x] [PMID: 22834470]

[46]   Goonasekera C, Ali K, Hickey A, *et al.* Mortality following congenital diaphragmatic hernia repair: the role of anesthesia. Paediatr Anaesth 2016; 26(12): 1197-201.
[http://dx.doi.org/10.1111/pan.13008] [PMID: 27779353]

[47]   Kotecha S, Barbato A, Bush A, *et al.* Congenital diaphragmatic hernia. Eur Respir J 2012; 39(4): 820-9.
[http://dx.doi.org/10.1183/09031936.00066511] [PMID: 22034651]

[48]   Mah VK, Zamakhshary M, Mah DY, *et al.* Absolute *vs* relative improvements in congenital diaphragmatic hernia survival: what happened to "hidden mortality". J Pediatr Surg 2009; 44(5): 877-82.
[http://dx.doi.org/10.1016/j.jpedsurg.2009.01.046] [PMID: 19433161]

[49]   Montalva L, Lauriti G, Zani A. Congenital heart disease associated with congenital diaphragmatic hernia: A systematic review on incidence, prenatal diagnosis, management, and outcome. J Pediatr Surg 2019; 54(5): 909-19.
[http://dx.doi.org/10.1016/j.jpedsurg.2019.01.018] [PMID: 30826117]

[50]   Zaiss I, Kehl S, Link K, *et al.* Associated malformations in congenital diaphragmatic hernia. Am J Perinatol 2011; 28(3): 211-8.
[http://dx.doi.org/10.1055/s-0030-1268235] [PMID: 20979012]

[51]   Partridge EA, Peranteau WH, Herkert L, *et al.* Right- *versus* left-sided congenital diaphragmatic hernia: a comparative outcomes analysis. J Pediatr Surg 2016; 51(6): 900-2.
[http://dx.doi.org/10.1016/j.jpedsurg.2016.02.049] [PMID: 27342009]

[52]   Bloss RS, Aranda JV, Beardmore HE. Congenital diaphragmatic hernia: pathophysiology and pharmacologic support. Surgery 1981; 89(4): 518-24.
[PMID: 7209799]

[53]   Fennessy P, Crowe S, Lenihan M, Healy M. Anesthesia consensus on clinical parameters for the timing of surgical repair in congenital diaphragmatic hernia. Paediatr Anaesth 2018; 28(8): 751-2.
[http://dx.doi.org/10.1111/pan.13459] [PMID: 30144230]

[54]   Snoek KG, Reiss IK, Greenough A, *et al.* Standardized Postnatal Management of Infants with Congenital Diaphragmatic Hernia in Europe: The CDH EURO Consortium Consensus - 2015 Update. Neonatology 2016; 110(1): 66-74.
[http://dx.doi.org/10.1159/000444210] [PMID: 27077664]

[55]   Puligandla PS, Skarsgard ED, Offringa M, *et al.* Diagnosis and management of congenital diaphragmatic hernia: a clinical practice guideline. CMAJ : Canadian Medical Association journal = journal de l'Association medicale canadienne 2018; 190(4): E103-2.

[56]   Belfort MA, Olutoye OO, Cass DL, *et al.* Feasibility and Outcomes of Fetoscopic Tracheal Occlusion for Severe Left Diaphragmatic Hernia. Obstet Gynecol 2017; 129(1): 20-9.
[http://dx.doi.org/10.1097/AOG.0000000000001749] [PMID: 27926636]

[57]   Style CC, Olutoye OO, Belfort MA, *et al.* Fetal endoscopic tracheal occlusion reduces pulmonary hypertension in severe congenital diaphragmatic hernia. Ultrasound Obstet Gynecol 2019; 54(6): 752-8.
[http://dx.doi.org/10.1002/uog.20216]

[58]   Jancelewicz T, Brindle ME, Guner YS, Lally PA, Lally KP, Harting MT. Toward Standardized Management of Congenital Diaphragmatic Hernia: An Analysis of Practice Guidelines. J Surg Res 2019; 243: 229-35.

[http://dx.doi.org/10.1016/j.jss.2019.05.007] [PMID: 31226462]

[59] Hutcheon JA, Butler B, Lisonkova S, *et al*. Timing of delivery for pregnancies with congenital diaphragmatic hernia. BJOG 2010; 117(13): 1658-62. 010.02738.x].
[http://dx.doi.org/10.1111/j.1471-0528.2010.02738.x] [PMID: 21125710]

[60] Frenckner B, Ehrén H, Granholm T, Lindén V, Palmér K. Improved results in patients who have congenital diaphragmatic hernia using preoperative stabilization, extracorporeal membrane oxygenation, and delayed surgery. J Pediatr Surg 1997; 32(8): 1185-9.
[http://dx.doi.org/10.1016/S0022-3468(97)90679-5] [PMID: 9269967]

[61] Caldwell CD, Watterberg KL. Effect of premedication regimen on infant pain and stress response to endotracheal intubation. Journal of perinatology : official journal of the California Perinatal Association 2015; 35(6): 415-8.
[http://dx.doi.org/10.1038/jp.2014.227]

[62] Wung JT, Sahni R, Moffitt ST, Lipsitz E, Stolar CJ. Congenital diaphragmatic hernia: survival treated with very delayed surgery, spontaneous respiration, and no chest tube. J Pediatr Surg 1995; 30(3): 406-9.
[http://dx.doi.org/10.1016/0022-3468(95)90042-X] [PMID: 7760230]

[63] Konduri GG, Solimano A, Sokol GM, *et al*. A randomized trial of early *versus* standard inhaled nitric oxide therapy in term and near-term newborn infants with hypoxic respiratory failure. Pediatrics 2004; 113(3 Pt 1): 559-64.
[http://dx.doi.org/10.1542/peds.113.3.559] [PMID: 14993550]

[64] Abman SH, Hansmann G, Archer SL, *et al*. Pediatric Pulmonary Hypertension: Guidelines From the American Heart Association and American Thoracic Society. Circulation 2015; 132(21): 2037-99.
[http://dx.doi.org/10.1161/CIR.0000000000000329] [PMID: 26534956]

[65] Downard CD, Jaksic T, Garza JJ, *et al*. Analysis of an improved survival rate for congenital diaphragmatic hernia. J Pediatr Surg 2003; 38(5): 729-32.
[http://dx.doi.org/10.1016/jpsu.2003.50194] [PMID: 12720181]

[66] Fallon SC, Cass DL, Olutoye OO, *et al*. Repair of congenital diaphragmatic hernias on Extracorporeal Membrane Oxygenation (ECMO): does early repair improve patient survival? J Pediatr Surg 2013; 48(6): 1172-6.
[http://dx.doi.org/10.1016/j.jpedsurg.2013.03.008] [PMID: 23845603]

[67] Costerus S, Zahn K, van de Ven K, Vlot J, Wessel L, Wijnen R. Thoracoscopic *versus* open repair of CDH in cardiovascular stable neonates. Surg Endosc 2016; 30(7): 2818-24.
[http://dx.doi.org/10.1007/s00464-015-4560-8] [PMID: 26490767]

[68] Qin J, Ren Y, Ma D. A comparative study of thoracoscopic and open surgery of congenital diaphragmatic hernia in neonates. J Cardiothorac Surg 2019; 14(1): 118.
[http://dx.doi.org/10.1186/s13019-019-0938-3] [PMID: 31242917]

[69] Grizelj R, Bojanić K, Vuković J, *et al*. Epidemiology and Outcomes of Congenital Diaphragmatic Hernia in Croatia: A Population-Based Study. Paediatr Perinat Epidemiol 2016; 30(4): 336-45.
[http://dx.doi.org/10.1111/ppe.12289] [PMID: 27016030]

[70] Brindle ME, Cook EF, Tibboel D, Lally PA, Lally KP. A clinical prediction rule for the severity of congenital diaphragmatic hernias in newborns. Pediatrics 2014; 134(2): e413-9.
[http://dx.doi.org/10.1542/peds.2013-3367] [PMID: 25022745]

[71] Congenital Diaphragmatic Hernia Study Group. Estimating disease severity of congenital diaphragmatic hernia in the first 5 minutes of life. J Pediatr Surg 2001; 36(1): 141-5.
[http://dx.doi.org/10.1053/jpsu.2001.20032]

[72] Aggarwal A, Lohani R, Suresh V. Case series on anesthesia for video-assisted thoracoscopic surgery for congenital diaphragmatic hernia in children. Anesth Essays Res 2016; 10(1): 128-31.
[http://dx.doi.org/10.4103/0259-1162.164736] [PMID: 26957707]

[73]   Muratore CS, Kharasch V, Lund DP, *et al.* Pulmonary morbidity in 100 survivors of congenital diaphragmatic hernia monitored in a multidisciplinary clinic. J Pediatr Surg 2001; 36(1): 133-40.
[http://dx.doi.org/10.1053/jpsu.2001.20031] [PMID: 11150452]

[74]   Danzer E, Gerdes M, Bernbaum J, *et al.* Neurodevelopmental outcome of infants with congenital diaphragmatic hernia prospectively enrolled in an interdisciplinary follow-up program. J Pediatr Surg 2010; 45(9): 1759-66.
[http://dx.doi.org/10.1016/j.jpedsurg.2010.03.011] [PMID: 20850617]

[75]   Lund DP, Mitchell J, Kharasch V, Quigley S, Kuehn M, Wilson JM. Congenital diaphragmatic hernia: the hidden morbidity. J Pediatr Surg 1994; 29(2): 258-62.
[http://dx.doi.org/10.1016/0022-3468(94)90329-8] [PMID: 8176602]

[76]   Lupo PJ, Isenburg JL, Salemi JL, *et al.* Population-based birth defects data in the United States, 2010-2014: A focus on gastrointestinal defects. Birth Defects Res 2017; 109(18): 1504-14.
[http://dx.doi.org/10.1002/bdr2.1145] [PMID: 29152924]

[77]   Crisera CA, Grau JB, Maldonado TS, Kadison AS, Longaker MT, Gittes GK. Defective epithelial-mesenchymal interactions dictate the organogenesis of tracheoesophageal fistula. Pediatr Surg Int 2000; 16(4): 256-61.
[http://dx.doi.org/10.1007/s003830050740] [PMID: 10898225]

[78]   Shaw-Smith C. Oesophageal atresia, tracheo-oesophageal fistula, and the VACTERL association: review of genetics and epidemiology. J Med Genet 2006; 43(7): 545-54.
[http://dx.doi.org/10.1136/jmg.2005.038158] [PMID: 16299066]

[79]   Ho AM, Dion JM, Wong JC. Airway and Ventilatory Management Options in Congenital Tracheoesophageal Fistula Repair. J Cardiothorac Vasc Anesth 2016; 30(2): 515-20.
[http://dx.doi.org/10.1053/j.jvca.2015.04.005] [PMID: 26154573]

[80]   Fischer J, Balleisen J, Holzki J, Cernaianu G, Alejandre Alcàzar M, Dübbers M. Tracheoscopic Findings and Their Impact on Respiratory Symptoms in Children with Esophageal Atresia. European journal of pediatric surgery: official journal of Austrian Association of Pediatric Surgery [*et al*] =. Z Kinderchir 2019.

[81]   Fallon SC, Langer JC, St Peter SD, *et al.* Congenital H-type tracheoesophageal fistula: A multicenter review of outcomes in a rare disease. J Pediatr Surg 2017; 52(11): 1711-4.
[http://dx.doi.org/10.1016/j.jpedsurg.2017.05.002] [PMID: 28528013]

[82]   Edelman B, Selvaraj BJ, Joshi M, Patil U, Yarmush J. Anesthesia Practice: Review of Perioperative Management of H-Type Tracheoesophageal Fistula. Anesthesiol Res Pract 2019; 2019: 8621801.
[http://dx.doi.org/10.1155/2019/8621801] [PMID: 31781201]

[83]   Slater BJ, Rothenberg SS. Tracheoesophageal fistula. Semin Pediatr Surg 2016; 25(3): 176-8.
[http://dx.doi.org/10.1053/j.sempedsurg.2016.02.010] [PMID: 27301604]

[84]   Broemling N, Campbell F. Anesthetic management of congenital tracheoesophageal fistula. Paediatr Anaesth 2011; 21(11): 1092-9.
[http://dx.doi.org/10.1111/j.1460-9592.2010.03377.x] [PMID: 20723095]

[85]   Richter GT, Ryckman F, Brown RL, Rutter MJ. Endoscopic management of recurrent tracheoesophageal fistula. J Pediatr Surg 2008; 43(1): 238-45.
[http://dx.doi.org/10.1016/j.jpedsurg.2007.08.062] [PMID: 18206490]

[86]   Knottenbelt G, Costi D, Stephens P, Beringer R, Davidson A. An audit of anesthetic management and complications of tracheo-esophageal fistula and esophageal atresia repair. Paediatr Anaesth 2012; 22(3): 268-74.
[http://dx.doi.org/10.1111/j.1460-9592.2011.03738.x]

[87]   Mortellaro VE, Fike FB, Adibe OO, *et al.* The use of high-frequency oscillating ventilation to facilitate stability during neonatal thoracoscopic operations. J Laparoendosc Adv Surg Tech A 2011; 21(9): 877-9.

[http://dx.doi.org/10.1089/lap.2011.0134] [PMID: 21859342]

[88] Kwong KM. Current Updates on Choanal Atresia. Front Pediatr 2015; 3: 52.
[http://dx.doi.org/10.3389/fped.2015.00052] [PMID: 26106591]

[89] Rajan R, Tunkel DE. Choanal Atresia and Other Neonatal Nasal Anomalies. Clin Perinatol 2018; 45(4): 751-67.
[http://dx.doi.org/10.1016/j.clp.2018.07.011] [PMID: 30396416]

[90] Cedin AC, Atallah AN, Andriolo RB, Cruz OL, Pignatari SN. Surgery for congenital choanal atresia. Cochrane Database Syst Rev 2012; (2): CD008993.
[PMID: 22336856]

[91] Yildirim ZB, Akdağ M, Çelik F, Baysal E. Anesthesia Management in Patients With Choanal Atresia. J Craniofac Surg 2016; 27(8): 1991-4.
[http://dx.doi.org/10.1097/SCS.0000000000003086] [PMID: 28005740]

[92] Cladis F, Kumar A, Grunwaldt L, Otteson T, Ford M, Losee JE. Pierre Robin Sequence: a perioperative review. Anesth Analg 2014; 119(2): 400-12.
[http://dx.doi.org/10.1213/ANE.0000000000000301] [PMID: 25046788]

[93] Printzlau A, Andersen M. Pierre Robin sequence in Denmark: a retrospective population-based epidemiological study. Cleft Palate Craniofac J 2004; 41(1): 47-52.
[http://dx.doi.org/10.1597/02-055] [PMID: 14697070]

[94] Gangopadhyay N, Mendonca DA, Woo AS. Pierre robin sequence. Semin Plast Surg 2012; 26(2): 76-82.
[http://dx.doi.org/10.1055/s-0032-1320065] [PMID: 23633934]

[95] Smith MC, Senders CW. Prognosis of airway obstruction and feeding difficulty in the Robin sequence. Int J Pediatr Otorhinolaryngol 2006; 70(2): 319-24.
[http://dx.doi.org/10.1016/j.ijporl.2005.07.003] [PMID: 16112206]

[96] Stricker PA, Budac S, Fiadjoe JE, Rehman MA. Awake laryngeal mask insertion followed by induction of anesthesia in infants with the Pierre Robin sequence. Acta Anaesthesiol Scand 2008; 52(9): 1307-8.
[http://dx.doi.org/10.1111/j.1399-6576.2008.01751.x] [PMID: 18823480]

[97] Marston AP, White DR. Subglottic Stenosis. Clin Perinatol 2018; 45(4): 787-804. 7.013].
[http://dx.doi.org/10.1016/j.clp.2018.07.013] [PMID: 30396418]

[98] Myer CM III, O'Connor DM, Cotton RT. Proposed grading system for subglottic stenosis based on endotracheal tube sizes. Ann Otol Rhinol Laryngol 1994; 103(4 Pt 1): 319-23.
[http://dx.doi.org/10.1177/000348949410300410] [PMID: 8154776]

[99] Eid EA. Anesthesia for subglottic stenosis in pediatrics. Saudi J Anaesth 2009; 3(2): 77-82.
[http://dx.doi.org/10.4103/1658-354X.57882] [PMID: 20532108]

CHAPTER 12

Pediatric Ambulatory Anesthesia

Abraham G. Oommen¹, Mark A. Dobish² and Manish Purohit¹

¹ Department of Anesthesiology and Perioperative Medicine, Nemours A.I. duPont Hospital for Children, Sidney Kimmel Medical College at Thomas Jefferson University, Wilmington, DE, USA

² Department of Anesthesiology, MedStar Georgetown University Hospital, Washington, D.C., USA

Abstract: Over the past five decades, there has been a marked increase in the number of pediatric procedures performed at ambulatory surgical centers (ASCs). This is the result of multiple factors such as new anesthetic and analgesic agents, new surgical techniques, and advances in technology. As our health care economics continue to evolve, it is almost certain that the perioperative landscape will shift even further towards ambulatory care. The advantages of outpatient surgery include reduced separation from parents, decreased risk of hospital-acquired infections, less dietary and nutritional disruption, improved parental satisfaction, and reduced cost. However, the care of children having ambulatory surgery presents a specific set of challenges. A hallmark of ambulatory surgery is the overall efficiency of the process from the time of anesthetic induction until discharge from the hospital. Many factors can delay discharge procedures, such as preoperative anxiolytics, which can linger for hours, not amenable to regional anesthetics requiring narcotics, postoperative emergence delirium (ED), and postoperative nausea and vomiting (PONV). The purpose of this chapter is to describe preoperative patient evaluation, patient selection criteria, suitable anesthetic techniques, modes of postoperative analgesia highlighting non-opioid techniques, and the various challenges that outpatient surgery presents to pediatric anesthesia providers. Issues relating to postoperative ED and PONV that frequently delay discharge will also be discussed.

Keywords: Ambulatory anesthesia, Apnea, Deep extubation, Emergence delirium, Health care economics, Non-opioid surgery, Obstructive sleep apnea, Opioid-free surgery, Outpatient surgery, PACU nursing economics, Postoperative nausea and vomiting, Premature, Regional anesthesia, Same-day surgery.

INTRODUCTION

Ambulatory anesthesia is becoming more commonplace in pediatric surgery. This has been the result of multiple factors such as newer anesthetic and analgesic

* **Corresponding author Bharathi Gourkanti:** Department of Anesthesiology, Cooper Medical School of Rowan University, Cooper University Health Care, Camden NJ, United States; E-mail: gourkantibharathi@cooperhealth.edu

Bharathi Gourkanti, Irwin Gratz, Grace Dippo, Nathalie Peiris and Dinesh K. Choudhry (Eds.)
All rights reserved-© 2022 Bentham Science Publishers

agents, non-invasive and more advanced surgical techniques, and new developments in technology. In 2010, there were an estimated 2,916,000 ambulatory surgical procedures performed on children under the age of 15 years. The most common cases performed in children were myringotomy tube placement (699,000), tonsillectomy with or without adenoidectomy (289,000), and adenoidectomy alone (89,000) [1]. There were 228,000 miscellaneous procedures performed due to technological advances in diagnostic and therapeutic modalities. Orthopedic procedures came in third with over 173,000 procedures performed in 2010 [1]. Many children are excellent candidates for outpatient surgery, given the simple nature of many procedures and the lack of any pertinent medical history. Some of the advantages of outpatient surgery include reduced separation time from parents, decreased risk of hospital-acquired infections, less dietary and nutritional disruption, improved parental satisfaction, and reduced cost. These advantages are especially useful in infants and preschool-aged children who benefit from decreased separation from parents. In addition, the decreased risk of infection has never been more important than at the time of writing this chapter during the coronavirus 2019 (COVID-19) pandemic. Providing safe anesthesia in an ambulatory surgery center (ASC) is not without specific challenges.

Appropriate patient selection is the foremost challenge. Children that are appropriate for ASCs should have few or no chronic health conditions, all of which should be well controlled. Procedures should be brief in duration (time restrictions vary by state), cause minimal fluid shifts, minimize end-organ stress and have a minimal risk of blood loss since there is no on-site blood bank required. Furthermore, each patient should be appropriately evaluated on the day of surgery and assessed for any current upper respiratory infection, which may necessitate a delay in the procedure. Exacerbations of chronic medical conditions such as asthma or gastroesophageal reflux disease should also prompt clinicians to ensure adequate control of the disease processes prior to proceeding with elective surgery. Lastly, certain pre-existing health conditions such as congenital heart disease, end-stage renal disease, and infants with a history of prematurity are inappropriate for ambulatory surgery.

The hallmark of ASCs is expedited throughput and large turnover volume. Many dated facilities may find it impossible to maintain social distancing between patients, families, and caregivers during the COVID-19 pandemic and future pandemics because of a lack of space in the preoperative and PACU areas.

Therefore, future ASC construction should plan for adequate social distancing without sacrificing efficiency.

Common Outpatient Procedures

Otolaryngologic procedures account for the majority of ambulatory surgeries performed in pediatric patients. However, many other surgeries performed by general surgeons, urologists, orthopedists, and ophthalmologists are suitable for outpatient care, as outlined in Table 1. The procedures share common features that make them ideal choices for the ASC setting. They involve a small surgical incision, minimal fluid shifts, little blood loss, and limited organ stress.

Table 1. Common outpatient procedures organized by specialty.

General Surgery	Hernia, Hydrocele, Orchiopexy
Otolaryngology	Tonsillectomy with or without adenoidectomy, Myringotomy Tubes, Frenulectomy, Sinus Surgery
Urology	Circumcision, Hypospadias, Cystoscopy
Ophthalmology	Strabismus Repair, Nasolacrimal Duct Probing, Trabeculectomy, Chalazion Excision
Plastic Surgery	Simple Tissue Transfers, Rhinoplasty, Otoplasty
Gastroenterology	Colonoscopy, EGD
Radiology	PICC Line Placement, MRI/CT Studies, Drain Placement
Dentistry	Oral Rehabilitation (Crowns, fillings, extractions, *etc.*)

ENT surgery is regarded as having the highest risk in the pediatric ambulatory setting with many unique postoperative complications that warrant special consideration [2]. An appropriate choice of anesthetic is important during ENT surgery since certain agents delay PACU discharge and negate any benefits gained by performing the procedure in an outpatient setting. The cost associated with a lengthy PACU stay may exceed that of planned overnight admission [3].

Tonsillectomy with or without adenoidectomy (T&A) poses unique considerations related to the underlying disease pathology. The procedure has two primary indications, obstructive sleep apnea (OSA) or chronic tonsillar infections. Children presenting the former indication may or may not present with a sleep study to quantify the severity of their OSA (Table 2). Increased sensitivity to opioids is well documented in this patient population and narcotics should be used judiciously. Non-opioid analgesic techniques are discussed later in this chapter. Furthermore, children with OSA will continue to have obstructive apneic events for several weeks to months after the removal of tonsillar and/or adenoid tissue. Many institutions advocate an extended observation period in the recovery room of a minimum of 90 minutes, devoid of any significant apneic episodes or desaturations. At the author's institution, patients are admitted for observation after T&A for OSA if any of the following criteria are met: under the age of 3, sleep study showing an apnea-hypopnea index (AHI) greater than 10, obesity, or any underlying syndromic pathology. If any of the preceding criteria are met, the patient is not a candidate for ambulatory care.

Table 2. Pediatric polysomnography testing for OSA.

Apnea Hypopnea Index (AHI)
Mild 1 – 5
Moderate 6 – 10
Severe > 10

Immediate and delayed postoperative complications following T&A are varied. Significant vascular injury is the most feared complication from T&A. Arterial bleeds are usually apparent immediately after surgery in the PACU and arise from injury to significant arterial branches of the external carotid artery. Branches of the facial or maxillary artery may be damaged during an adenoidectomy. In contrast, venous bleeding can also occur following T&A but most commonly, presents 5-10 days following surgery as a result of sloughing of eschar from the wound bed. Presentation is typically more indolent and maybe first noticed as blood in one's sputum or hematemesis. Nonetheless, significant amounts of blood loss can occur before returning to the emergency department for evaluation. Standard PACU discharge criteria, such as the absence of nausea or vomiting and the ability to tolerate oral intake, also pose more of a challenge in these patients compared to others.

NPO GUIDELINES

NPO times (Table **3**) are based on gastric emptying times after patients have consumed each of the above food groups with radioactive tracers. Meals with high fat or protein content may prolong the fasting period. Neonates and infants should be encouraged to continue oral intake until the required cutoff time. This may decrease a child's irritability in the holding area and expedite intravenous line placement following an inhalational induction. Since nonhuman milk is similar to solids in gastric emptying time, consider the amount ingested when determining an appropriate fasting period [4]. A brief telehealth check in the evening before surgery can optimize NPO times and avoid unanticipated delays or cancellations.

Table 3. Perioperative fasting guidelines recommended by the American Society of Anesthesiology [4].

Clear Liquids*	2 hours
Breast Milk	4 hours
Infant Formula, Non-human Milk Light Meal⁺	6 hours
Full Meal	8 hours

*Clear liquids include water, juices (without pulp), coffee without cream, clear tea, and carbonated beverages
⁺Light meal includes toast with clear liquids

Preoperative Evaluation

The appropriate evaluation of incoming patients is vital to the success of an ambulatory surgery program. The process begins in the surgeon's office with an initial evaluation and discussion of expectations. An anesthesiologist should also review all cases to prevent any unexpected cancellations or delays. Furthermore, many institutions utilize nursing staff to call and screen patients the day before surgery to review and reinforce NPO guidelines and verify the appropriate state of health. Logistical details such as time to arrive, parking, and the exact location of the surgery check-in area can also be reviewed at this time. See Chapter 4 "Preoperative Evaluation and Planning" for a more extensive discussion on this topic.

Upper Respiratory Infections

One of the most common issues encountered in pediatric anesthesiology is the presence of an upper respiratory infection (URI). Children under the age of four years experience an average of eight URIs per year, with symptoms lasting up to 3 weeks [5]. Therefore, URI is the most common cause for procedural cancellation [6]. All children presenting signs of a URI such as runny nose, fever, cough, and general irritability should be evaluated to determine the etiology. Some conditions, such as vasomotor or seasonal rhinitis, are non-infectious in etiology and do not warrant cancellation. In contrast, similar symptoms may be indicative of an underlying viral or bacterial process that can significantly increase the risk of adverse respiratory events such as bronchospasm, laryngospasm, and desaturation [7]. Symptoms of infection include persistent fevers, thick purulent sputum, and a wet cough. If the decision is made to delay surgery, there is no overall consensus on the most appropriate time to reschedule. One study of over 9,000 patients found a statistically significant decrease in respiratory events in patients presenting <2 weeks after cancellation *vs.* 2-4 weeks following cancellation (29% *vs.* 8%) [5].

Asthma & Reactive Airway Disease

A history of reactive airway disease (RAD) or asthma should be assessed and classified by level of control (Table **4**) through symptomatology and medication compliance [8]. It is a common practice to administer bronchodilating medications in the preoperative area if clinically warranted. In addition, it is wise to tailor an anesthetic to minimize complications from RAD, most notably through the use of bronchodilating medications such as volatile anesthetics (sevoflurane or isoflurane) or ketamine. If appropriate, avoidance of intubation decreases the risk of exacerbating RAD.

Table 4. Evaluation of control of asthma/reactive airway symptoms [8].

Component	Level of Control			
-	Complete	Good	Partial	None
Daytime symptoms	None	<2x/week	>2x/week	Continuous
Nighttime symptoms	None	<1x/month	>1x/month	Weekly
Need for rescue med	None	<2x/week	>2x/week	Daily
Activity limited	None	None	Some	Extreme
Exacerbation risk	0	1	2	3

The most common complication of asthma/RAD is bronchospasm which can present as desaturation, laryngospasm, and/or increased airway secretions. Emergency medications including albuterol and epinephrine should be available before the induction of any general anesthetic, especially if the trachea will be intubated. Patients are commonly extubated deep to prevent bronchospasm from noxious stimuli during emergence. Classification of diagnosed asthma in the pediatric population is based on the level of control exhibited by signs and symptoms. Patients with only partial or poor control of asthma should not be cared for in an ambulatory setting, given the potential for respiratory complications. The term reactive airway disease is not an actual diagnosis and is reserved for those patients who present signs and symptoms of bronchoconstriction but may be too young to be fully evaluated for asthma [8].

Postoperative Apnea Risk Factors

Postoperative apnea in premature and term infants is a unique and common issue in pediatric anesthesiology. Apnea is defined as the cessation of breathing for 20 seconds or longer. Prematurity is defined as being born prior to 37 weeks' estimated gestational age. Premature infants are at a higher risk and not suitable candidates for ambulatory surgical procedures due to immature respiratory centers, inadequate temperature regulation, and immature gag reflexes. Other risk factors, besides a history of prematurity that are known to cause postoperative apnea include anemia, hypoxia, hypothermia, and hypocalcemia. It is commonly believed that sedative medications and general anesthetics increase this risk. At the author's institution, it is required to observe all premature infants who are less than 55 weeks post-conceptional age (PCA) for 24 hours. For infants born at term, this time period is shortened and only required until an infant has reached 45 weeks PCA.

Obstructive Sleep Apnea

Sleep apnea must be appropriately screened for when considering outpatient surgical care. The American Academy of otolaryngologists defines severe OSA as an apnea-hypopnea index greater than or equal to 10 obstructive events/hour, oxygen saturation less than 80%, or both [9]. Patients fitting into this criteria have a higher risk of perioperative respiratory complications, and care at an ambulatory facility should be avoided.

Premedication

Premedication (premed) is a useful adjunct in the pediatric population allowing for easier separation of the patient from the parent. Separation anxiety is present in nearly all children beginning at 6-10 months of age and lasting through to grade school. As coping mechanisms develop, some patients and families may opt to forego the premed with the hope of less postoperative sedation. It should be noted that removing a young child from their parents without appropriate anxiolysis, whether by medication or distraction therapy, has been associated with emergence delirium and regression of development up to 2-3 weeks postoperatively.

Midazolam

The most commonly used medication is midazolam. Midazolam can be given in a number of ways, but when used for elective cases, it is usually administered either nasally or orally. Intranasal dosing ranges from 0.2 mg/kg - 0.25 mg/kg and requires a concentrated formulation of midazolam usually 5 mg/ml. This allows its use in patients up to 20 kg, after which the volume of injectate needed becomes an issue. The onset of action is quicker than by mouth due to the rich vascular supply in the nasal mucosa.

Oral midazolam is usually given as a liquid at a dose of 0.5 mg/kg not to exceed a total dose of 15 mg at the authors' institution. Special care should be given when administering this medication, as young patients may spit out part of the dose due to its undesirable taste. Coaching parents and allowing them to administer the medication to the child has been successful but should be supervised by preoperative staff. Experienced preoperative nurses are able to successfully administer premedication under almost any circumstance.

Occasionally, some children with severe behavioral issues or autism may have unanticipated responses after oral midazolam, such as lack of response or paradoxical extreme disinhibition. Approximately 14% of children are "non-responders" to oral midazolam and may require secondary dosing, increased dosing, or use of another medication [10].

Dexmedetomidine and Ketamine

Although oral midazolam is the most common preoperative anxiolytic, other options do exist, such as intranasal dexmedetomidine dose of 1-2 µg/kg. Dexmedetomidine is a highly selective α2 agonist.

Ketamine is the most commonly used IM agent for difficult and aggressive children. Fig. (1) illustrates common doses and medications used in a ketamine injection, frequently referred to as a ketamine dart. A high concentration ketamine (100 mg/ml) preparation should be used to limit the overall administered volume [11].

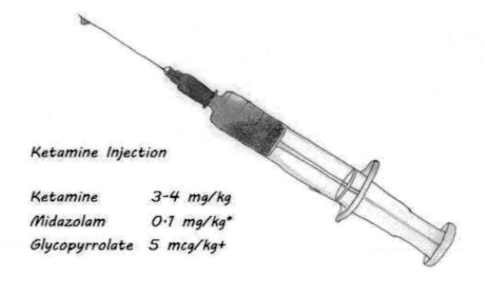

Ketamine Injection

Ketamine	3-4 mg/kg
Midazolam	0·1 mg/kg*
Glycopyrrolate	5 mcg/kg+

Illustration by Neha Barkat

Fig. (1). Commonly used cocktail of medications for the aggressive patient.* Limited to 2 mg usually + Limited to 200 mcg to limit overall volume.

Narcotic use for premedication has largely been abandoned due to a lack of amnestic and anxiolytic properties and an increased incidence of postoperative nausea and vomiting.

Parental Presence on Induction

An alternative to premedication that has gained recent popularity is parental presence on induction (PP). This refers to the presence of one parent present during induction and provides several advantages. One advantage of PP is the ability to avoid premedication, particularly in myringotomy tube placement, as it may delay discharge due to lingering sedative effects. Disadvantages of PP include an increased burden on the anesthesiologist and staff to control a parent who is not familiar with the operating room environment, unpredictable reactions by a parent upon seeing their child anesthetized, and parents who are overly anxious themselves. Despite these disadvantages, several studies have shown that many parents prefer to be present during induction [12, 13]. PP has not been shown to be any more effective than oral midazolam [12].

In the COVID-19 era, at this author's institution, parental presence has been virtually eliminated to maintain social distancing, conserve personal protective equipment, and limit OR traffic.

Anesthetic Approach

The goal of an ambulatory care plan is to provide high-level anesthetic care tailored to the patient and surgical needs while focusing on safe and rapid discharge. The ideal anesthetic maintenance agent should be easily titratable, wear off quickly, and have minimal residual side effects [11].

Induction

Most patients presenting to ASCs will not have IV access prior to induction. An inhalational induction is routinely performed in pediatric care, but methodologies vary. Premedication helps ensure a calm patient and decreases combativeness, separation anxiety, and secretions that may lead to physical injury and/or laryngospasm. Scenting the mask with flavored lip balm is routine practice to mitigate the odor of inhaled agents and foster mask acceptance.

Common complications of an inhalational induction include cough, periods of breath-holding, apnea, laryngospasm, and cardiovascular effects such as bradycardia. A variety of techniques exist utilizing nitrous oxide and sevoflurane. A study in 2000 looked at a comparison of inhalation induction with 2%, 4%, 6%, and 8% sevoflurane in nitrous oxide for pediatric patients, and it showed that coughing, laryngospasm, and breath holding was the highest in the 8% group [14]. A meta-analysis from 2016 provided low-quality evidence suggesting that the high initial concentration sevoflurane technique probably results in a shorter time to induction of anesthesia with a difference between 24 to 82 seconds [15].

Complications in the high and low initial concentration induction groups were comparable except for apnea, which appeared more commonly in the high initial concentration group [15].

The anesthesiologist must be ready to deal with the potential complications of an inhalational induction. This ranges from something as mild as coughing to potential hypoxic cardiac arrest from ongoing laryngospasm. See Fig. (**2**) for the appropriate treatment algorithm of laryngospasm. Any practitioner routinely caring for pediatric patients should calculate intramuscular rescue doses and be prepared with the correct equipment for rapid administration of medications. The deltoid muscle is the preferred site for IM injections due to its high vascular supply and proximity to the airway.

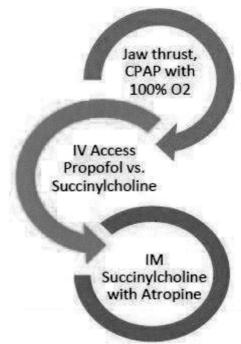

Fig. (2). Treatment of laryngospasm during an inhalational induction *IV succinylcholine dosing 1 mg/kg; IM succinylcholine dosing 4 mg/kg; IV/IM atropine 20 mcg/kg.

Airway Utilization

Delivering a safe anesthetic while minimizing risk is the goal of every anesthesiologist, and this process occurs many times a day in the ASC. Choice of airway device includes a simple mask, a laryngeal mask airway (LMA) or endotracheal tube (ETT). One advantage of an LMA over an ETT is reduced laryngeal and airway irritation [16]. Studies have shown that reducing stimulation to the larynx and trachea decreases adverse respiratory events. ETTs are more stimulating than LMAs and LMAs are more stimulating than simple masks [17]. Given a patient with a recent URI or an asthmatic with an irritable airway, one should take these factors into consideration when choosing the appropriate airway to utilize.

Appropriate sizing of the simple mask, LMA and ETT is an important consideration for the pediatric provider. A simple mask should provide a seal around the nose and chin of the patient to facilitate positive pressure ventilation. LMA sizing is generally based on patient weight and packaging recommendations should be followed. It is generally better to use a smaller LMA when deciding between two sizes. Larger than appropriate LMAs can cause oropharyngeal trauma and bleeding, whereas a smaller LMA is easily swapped out, if needed, due to the presence of an air leak. A standard formula for cuffed ETT sizing is given below. There should be an air leak with the cuff deflated to 18-20 cm H_2O or below to prevent croup and ischemia to the tracheal mucosa with lengthy procedures.

$$[{}^{Age}/_4] + 4 = \text{Size of cuffed ETT}$$

Appropriate depth of anesthesia is achieved for tracheal intubation *via* a combination of propofol and inhaled sevoflurane. Paralytic agents are generally avoided as they are not routinely needed for successful intubation.

Tracheal Extubation

Extubation can be performed deep or awake. Deep extubation is preferred to improve turnover time and minimize irritating stimuli. Patients must be spontaneously breathing and well anesthetized for deep extubation to be successful. Immediately upon extubation, the patient should be assessed for airway patency. Fogging in the mask, adequate chest rise, lack of upper airway obstruction and end-tidal CO_2 capnography should all be observed in quick succession to confirm airway patency. If any of these indicators are missing, bag-mask ventilation should be gently attempted to assess for airway patency prior to initiating the laryngospasm treatment algorithm in Fig. (**2**). It is imperative to have seasoned PACU staff assume care of a deeply extubated patient as blood or secretions in the oropharynx may trigger vocal cord spasms requiring prompt recognition and intervention. A study of 900 patients showed no difference in the incidence of perioperative respiratory complications in children undergoing an adenotonsillectomy following an awake *vs.* deep extubation [18].

Anesthetic Management of Common Procedures

Myringotomy and Ventilating Tubes

Myringotomy and tube placement are used for the treatment of otitis media. If left untreated, otitis media has the potential to cause hearing loss. A myringotomy refers to the incision of the tympanic membrane usually accompanied by the placement of a ventilating tube. The two common types of otitis media are acute otitis media and otitis media with effusion.

Preoperative management involves appropriate premedication. Nasal midazolam 0.25 mg/kg can generally be administered up to 20 kg or a max dose of 5 mg (volume limited). This intranasal administration should be split evenly between each nostril to maximize absorption. Following premedication, acetaminophen suspension 15 mg/kg is given orally for pain control. Oral acetaminophen is rapidly absorbed, achieving therapeutic levels within minutes, making it the preferred route over rectal administration [19].

Induction of general anesthesia is accomplished *via* an inhalational technique using a combination of nitrous oxide and sevoflurane. An IV should be ready for insertion at all times, but due to the brevity of the procedure, it is usually unnecessary. Children with more recent URIs may benefit from IV placement due to increased airway reactivity. It is not uncommon for a pediatric anesthesiologist to survey a patient's extremities to scout out a desirable IV location should the situation devolve quickly.

Maintenance of anesthesia is achieved by mask ventilation using sevoflurane. The concentration of sevoflurane is turned down from 8% after an adequate plane of anesthesia is achieved and titrated to avoid the side effects of high-dose sevoflurane. The patient's head is turned from side to side to allow surgical exposure. This can result in airway obstruction necessitating an oral airway or repositioning. The myringotomy is generally the most stimulating aspect of the case. The surgeon alerts the room that there is a "knife in the ear" in close proximity to the tympanic membrane. This alerts the room that the bed should not be moved or accidentally jostled and informs the anesthesiologist to keep the patient's head still. Movement is greatly magnified under the presence of the surgical microscope. Patients without an IV are given IM ketorolac 0.5 mg/kg (max 15 mg) in the deltoid for additional pain control. Of note, a study of 100 children undergoing myringotomy and ear tube placement using only sevoflurane without any premedication found an unacceptably high risk (67%) of postoperative agitation [20]. Nasal dexmedetomidine or fentanyl may be used to minimize emergence delirium and pain.

Adenotonsillectomy (T&A)

As mentioned above, T&A is the second most common outpatient procedure. Refer to Chapter 14, "Common Pediatric Surgical Procedures," for a more extensive discussion of the procedure and anesthetic management. Most tonsillectomies with or without adenoidectomy are performed at ASCs. However, the frequency of perioperative respiratory issues in children under 3 years old is elevated, and ambulatory surgery should be avoided [21].

For T&A in the otherwise healthy child, a combination of sevoflurane, dexamethasone, NSAIDs, acetaminophen and morphine/fentanyl can be used for perioperative anesthetic and analgesic management. Dexamethasone is routinely used for PONV, pain and airway edema control. In one study, the minimum morphine sparing dose of dexamethasone is reported to be 0.5 mg/kg [22] and this dose is most frequently administered. At this authors' institution, the maximum dose used is 0.5 mg/kg up to 10 mg. A Cochrane meta-analysis including 955 pediatric patients found no increased risk of bleeding, requiring surgical control with the use of NSAIDs after tonsillectomy [23]; however, surgical preference still prevails. It is the general practice of many surgeons to allow NSAID use in the PACU after adequate hemostasis for intracapsular tonsillectomies but to avoid NSAID use with total traditional tonsillectomies.

Herniorrhaphy, Umbilical Hernia, and Circumcision

Below is a summary of the anesthetic management of these common outpatient procedures which are detailed further in Chapter 14 "Common Pediatric Surgical Procedures."

Inguinal Hernia

- More common in premature infants and males
- Accomplished *via* spinal or general anesthetic (GA)
- Supplemental caudal block for a bilateral procedure under GA
- Supplemental transversus abdominis plane block, ilioinguinal block or local infiltration for a unilateral procedure under GA

Umbilical Hernia

- More common in premature and low birth weight infants
- LMA or ETT depending on surgical request for muscle relaxation
- Rectus sheath block bilaterally *vs.* local infiltration

Circumcision

- Parental preference and foreskin pathology are common indications
- Spinal or GA
- Supplemental dorsal penile nerve block has been shown to be as effective as a caudal block with fewer side effects [24]

Endoscopy

Outpatient endoscopies are performed for a variety of gastrointestinal concerns. An inhalation induction followed by IV placement with a subsequent propofol bolus allows for an adequate depth of anesthesia for LMA placement. Maintenance of anesthesia is achieved *via* sevoflurane. An LMA is routinely placed at the author's institution. Propofol sedation without an advanced airway is another option that is widely used in adult practice and other pediatric institutions. A jaw thrust is given to aid in passing the endoscope into the esophagus, which is the most stimulating part of the procedure.

For colonoscopy, pediatric patients are in either a frog leg or lateral decubitus position based on proceduralist preference. Once the procedure is complete, the LMA can be removed deep as long as the patient is spontaneously ventilating, allowing for rapid turnover.

Airway choice must be carefully planned when anesthetizing an infant or neonate for endoscopy. It is not uncommon for the endoscope to cause tracheal compression resulting in difficulty with gas exchange. Depending on proceduralist experience and length of the procedure, intubation may be warranted.

Imaging

As imaging technologies evolve, more procedures and MRIs can be performed safely in ASCs. Moderate to deep sedation using the sequence of midazolam and/or inhaled nitrous oxide, IV placement, propofol bolus and infusion is commonly employed. Propofol bolus is usually $1 - 2$ mg/kg and an infusion is started at 200 mcg/kg/min and titrated to effect. Propofol has been referred to as an excellent and perhaps ideal agent for use in imaging or radiation treatment procedures [25]. Patients with craniofacial or airway anatomic abnormalities should be scheduled at tertiary centers if sedation or anesthesia is required. Please refer to Chapter 13, "Non-operating Room Pediatric Anesthesia," for further discussion on the anesthetic management for radiological procedures and various imaging modalities.

Non-opioid Techniques

Since the rise of the opioid epidemic, there has been a concerted effort to change prescribing patterns and incorporate a multimodal analgesic regimen limiting opioid use. Fig. (**3**) shows a variety of medications from different classes that allow perioperative care to progress with non-narcotic techniques. Refer to Part 2, Chapter 6 "Pediatric Pain Management and Regional Anesthesia," for a more extensive discussion on pain management and ultrasound-guided regional anesthetics.

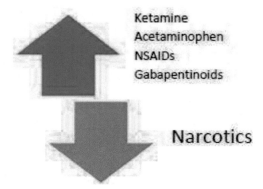

Ketamine
Acetaminophen
NSAIDs
Gabapentinoids

Narcotics

Fig. (3). Multimodal agents utilized in an opioid-free anesthetic.

Postoperative Ambulatory Considerations

Pediatric ambulatory anesthesia has many of the same concerns and complications of inpatient anesthesia even though the patients are generally healthier based upon selection criteria. In light of the increased turnover at ASCs, factors that affect and delay discharge times require appropriate planning. Anticipation and prevention of common complications using a multimodal approach to the anesthetic are paramount. This approach can decrease nursing workload allowing for a better distribution of resources as well as reducing parental anxiety.

Deep Extubation

Deep extubation improves overall efficiency and may be indicated for certain procedures. As a solo provider, it is difficult to respond to a desaturating patient with laryngospasm in the PACU while in the midst of an inhalation induction with the next case. Alternatively, a patient can be extubated deep for indications such as RAD, but the anesthesiologist should not induce the next patient until the prior patient shows an adequate return of airway protective reflexes in the PACU.

PONV

The most common complication in pediatric ambulatory anesthesia is postoperative nausea and vomiting (PONV), affecting 8-42% of patients and delaying discharge [26]. Causes of PONV are multifactorial, with certain patients at greater risk than others. Eberhart noted an increased likelihood of PONV based upon multiple criteria. In practice, however, multiple practitioners have modified these factors specifically in terms of age and type of surgery [27]. PONV has been noted in children younger than 3 years of age, therefore, many practitioners consider two years of age as a risk factor. Similarly, others have noted that other surgeries are as emetogenic as strabismus surgery and now consider these procedures as risk factors (Table **5**). With the presence of each factor, the risk of nausea and vomiting increases to 10%, 30%, 55% up to 70% with all four risk factors as noted below.

Table 5. Risk factors for PONV.

Risk Factor	Eberhart's Criteria [27]	Smith's Anesthesia for Infants and Children modified from Table 42-1 [11]
Surgery type	Strabismus repair	Strabismus repair, Adenotonsillectomy Laparoscopic surgery, Hernia repair Orchiopexy, Penile surgery
Age	Older than 3 years	Older than 2 years
History	Personal or family hx	Personal or family hx
Surgical time	Greater than 30 min	Greater than 30 min

Prophylaxis consists of 5-HT3 antagonists and corticosteroids given in the operating room prior to extubation. Most commonly, ondansetron (0.1 mg/kg, max 4 mg) and dexamethasone (0.1 mg/kg, max 4 mg) act synergistically to decrease the incidence of nausea and vomiting [28]. Other prophylactic measures include transdermal scopolamine patch and propofol as a background infusion. Additionally, a single propofol bolus (0.5-1 mg/kg) at the end of the case has shown to be effective in decreasing the incidence of PONV in the PACU [29]. As a last resort, a total intravenous technique (TIVA) can be substituted for inhaled anesthetics agents.

Intraoperative fluid management has been shown to play a role in the development of PONV. Dehydration secondary to NPO requirements may predispose patients to PONV and may be prevented with the administration of 30 ml/kg of isotonic fluid when compared to 10 ml/kg [30].

Despite PONV prophylaxis, some patients have nausea that is triggered by oral intake given too soon post-procedure in the PACU [31]. The Baxter Animated Retching Faces Nausea Scale (BARF) scale was initially used as an assessment for oncology patients but has been shown by Watcha in 2019 to be an effective tool in pediatric postoperative care. In children 6 years of age or older, a self-assessment score of 4, as noted below, was associated with a need for intervention [32].

Management consists of holding oral intake and re-dosing ondansetron if possible based on previous dosing and time [33]. Fluid rehydration may be of value depending upon the case and the intraoperative management. Diphenhydramine 0.5 mg/kg IV (max 25 mg) may be given but can cause sedation and delay discharge further. Intravenous metoclopramide (0.25 mg/kg, max 10 mg) is another option but may cause extrapyramidal side effects. Propofol boluses (0.5-1 mg/kg) have been used as prophylaxis, as noted above, but also serve as a rescue medication. Care must be used when giving propofol boluses, and the patient must be monitored for sedation and apnea.

Pain Management

Pain management is an essential aspect of pediatric ambulatory anesthesia requiring a multimodal approach to ensure efficient care and timely discharge. Appropriate use of systemic medication along with directed regional techniques will prevent the need for excessive opioid medication, thus minimizing respiratory depression and sedation in the PACU. Regional techniques in ASCs range from neuraxial to peripheral blocks depending on the comfort of the practitioner.

Several pain scoring systems based on patient age may be used to assess the severity of pain and guide treatment. For infants and younger children, the Face Legs Activity Cry and Consolability (FLACC) score allows PACU staff to make clinical judgments on the severity of the pain (Table **6**). Mild pain is scored as 1-3 points. Moderate pain and severe pain have scores of 4-6 and 7-10, respectively. The FLACC score may also be used in older patients who are non-verbal and unable to express themselves. As older patients recover, the scoring system may be changed to the Visual Analog Scale (VAS) or Numeric scale.

Table 6. FLACC Scoring System.

FLACC	0	1	2
Face	No expression	Occasional grimace or frown, withdrawn, disinterested	Chin quivering, clenched jaw
Legs	Normal position or relaxed	Uneasy, restless, tense	Kicking, legs drawn up

(Table 6) cont.....

FLACC	0	1	2
Activity	Lying quietly, normal position, moves easily	Squirming, shifting back and forth, tense	Arched, rigid, or jerking
Cry	No cry (asleep or awake)	Moans or whimpers, the occasional complaint	Crying steadily, screams or sobs, frequent complaints
Consolability	Content, relaxed	Reassured by occasional touching, hugging, or being talked to, distractible	Difficult to console or comfort

In the PACU, analgesic options can be separated into opioid *versus* non-opioid medications. Acetaminophen is the most common medication given in the recovery room. It is available in multiple forms allowing for administration in a variety of situations. Dosing for both the intravenous and oral form is 10-15 mg/kg. Rectal dosing of acetaminophen has shown to be extremely variable from patient to patient; however, if a facility lacks acetaminophen in suspension form, rectal acetaminophen may be used. An initial dose of 40 mg/kg was most consistent in obtaining the needed plasma level [34]. Cutting or splitting the suppository is not recommended.

Nonsteroidal anti-inflammatory medications are another choice for toddlers and older children. Oral ibuprofen dosed at 10 mg/kg (max 400 mg) or ketorolac 0.5 mg/kg (max 15mg) IV are excellent options for acute postoperative pain management for a wide variety of procedures [35].

Opioid medications should be available in the event of severe and uncontrolled pain as part of the multimodal regimen. In most ASCs, both morphine (0.05-0.1 mg/kg) and fentanyl (0.5-1 mcg/kg) are safely used in toddlers and older children. Nalbuphine 0.1 mg/kg IV has been shown to have a good analgesic effect while decreasing the risk of respiratory depression [36].

Alpha 2 agonists such as dexmedetomidine have had a tremendous impact in pediatric anesthesia with a predictable hemodynamic profile in multiple settings such as a pre-procedural anxiolytic and as a treatment for emergence delirium. As an intraprocedural adjunct, it has been shown to be an efficacious alternative to opioids [37].

Oxygen Desaturation

Oxygen desaturation in the ambulatory surgery setting has potentially disastrous consequences with few available resources. Desaturation can occur secondary to multiple causes but can be separated into upper *versus* lower respiratory tract obstruction.

In many cases, practitioners choose to extubate the patient in a deep plane of anesthesia. In this state, airway protective reflexes and muscle tone are diminished, leading to potential obstruction of the upper airway by the tongue. Obstruction can be relieved by placing an oral or nasal airway as well as by placing the patient in a lateral or recovery position.

Laryngospasm can occur in the operating room as well as in the recovery period [38, 39]. As patients desaturate quickly, leading to bradycardia, early recognition and management are essential, with the incidence indirectly correlated with the pediatric experience of the practitioner [40]. Many practitioners deepen the anesthetic plane of the patient with a bolus of propofol [41]. However, as propofol also acts as a cardiac depressant, it may hasten the onset of bradycardia, requiring further intervention. Succinylcholine (1mg/kg) IV or (3-4mg/kg) IM is considered the definitive treatment in an emergency, (Fig. **2**) [42].

As the patient attempts spontaneous inspiration against a closed glottis, negative pressure pulmonary edema (NPPE) may occur from increased interstitial pressure pulling fluid into the pulmonary tissue [43]. NPPE may require further management, including oxygen, diuretic therapy, and possible admission to an inpatient facility.

Bronchospasm, usually associated with asthmatic patients, may occur in patients of any age with bronchial hyperreactivity secondary to illness or external factors such as secondhand smoke [44, 45]. Over 80% of episodes of bronchospasm occur during induction and maintenance, but a flare can present at any time during the perioperative course [46]. Intubation and extubation increase the risk through airway stimulation, causing reflex spasm of the bronchial smooth muscle though this may be blunted through deep extubation [47]. The resulting respiratory difficulty is manifested as wheezing, accessory muscle use, and nasal flaring, resulting in oxygen desaturation. Once the diagnosis of bronchospasm is confirmed, continuous positive airway pressure with 100% oxygen *via* a tight-fitting mask should be initiated. Treatment consists of intravenous or subcutaneous terbutaline (0.01 mg/kg, max 0.4 mg) if available. IV or subcutaneous epinephrine (1 mcg/kg) is another option if terbutaline is unavailable. Inhaled beta 2 agonists such as albuterol may not be effective if bronchospasm is severe but should be initiated once air entry and exit are auscultated. An airway cart should be nearby as emergent intubation may be required.

Emergence Delirium

Emergence delirium, in the DSM-5, is characterized as an agitation without awareness of surroundings, thus creating the impression of a child in extreme and unconsolable distress [48]. The nursing staff is also placed under duress during these events as multiple providers are required to prevent injury to the patient, provide emotional support to the parents, and protect surgical sites or peripheral intravenous lines from injury or loss. An episode of emergence delirium may last up to 45 minutes and thus delay discharge significantly if pharmacologic intervention is needed while potentially traumatizing unprepared family members [49].

Children aged 2-5 years are the primary patient population who experience emergence delirium. The use of volatile anesthetics has been noted as a risk factor, with some claiming that rapid recovery associated with sevoflurane *versus* halothane may be to blame [50]. Preoperative anxiety is also a known risk factor [51]. See Table **7** below for a list of risk factors for emergence delirium. See Chapter 6, "PACU Management and Emergence Delirium," for a more extensive discussion on emergence delirium.

Table 7. Risk Factors of Emergence Delirium [52].

Risk factors for Emergence Delirium [52]
Rapid emergence from anesthesia
Short-acting volatile agents
Postoperative pain
Surgery type - tonsils, thyroid, middle ear, eye
Ages 2-5 years
Preoperative Anxiety
Child temperament - more emotional, more impulsive, less social

Unplanned Admission

Many ASCs are now stand-alone facilities with only an affiliation or partnership with a hospital. Therefore, while patients are screened for co-morbid conditions to minimize the risk of perioperative issues, the potential for adverse events remains. It is, therefore, necessary to have in place policies and protocols delineating procedures for the transfer of patients to emergency rooms or inpatient floors. Additionally, it may be necessary for the anesthesiologist to accompany the patient requiring plans for another provider to continue care for the patients remaining in the ASC. Contingency plans should be devised for such a scenario.

CONCLUSION

ASCs are an integral part of pediatric surgical care. These centers are especially adept at ensuring patient and parent satisfaction by providing excellent medical care. In the pre-COVID-19 era, ASCs saw steady growth year after year as new boundaries and standards of care were set. In the future, it is possible that with appropriate social distancing measures, ASCs will play an even larger role in the care of pediatric patients, limiting the exposure of patients and their families to pathogens in large tertiary care centers.

CONSENT FOR PUBLICATION

Not applicable.

CONFLICT OF INTEREST

The author declares no conflict of interest, financial or otherwise.

ACKNOWLEDGEMENTS

Declared none.

REFERENCES

[1]   Hall MJ, Schwartzman A, Zhang J, Liu X. Ambulatory Surgery Data From Hospitals and Ambulatory Surgery Centers: United States, 2010. Natl Health Stat Rep 2017; (102): 1-15.

[2]   Murat I, Constant I, Maud'huy H. Perioperative anaesthetic morbidity in children: a database of 24,165 anaesthetics over a 30-month period. Paediatr Anaesth 2004; 14(2): 158-66.
[http://dx.doi.org/10.1111/j.1460-9592.2004.01167.x] [PMID: 14962332]

[3]   Shapiro NL, Seid AB, Pransky SM, Kearns DB, Magit AE, Silva P. Adenotonsillectomy in the very young patient: cost analysis of two methods of postoperative care. Int J Pediatr Otorhinolaryngol 1999; 48(2): 109-15.
[http://dx.doi.org/10.1016/S0165-5876(99)00011-7] [PMID: 10375035]

[4]   Practice Guidelines for Preoperative Fasting and the Use of Pharmacologic Agents to Reduce the Risk of Pulmonary Aspiration: Application to Healthy Patients Undergoing Elective Procedures: An Updated Report by the American Society of Anesthesiologists Task Force on Preoperative Fasting and the Use of Pharmacologic Agents to Reduce the Risk of Pulmonary Aspiration. Anesthesiology 2017; 126(3): 376-93.
[http://dx.doi.org/10.1097/ALN.0000000000001452] [PMID: 28045707]

[5]   von Ungern-Sternberg BS, Boda K, Chambers NA, *et al.* Risk assessment for respiratory complications in paediatric anaesthesia: a prospective cohort study. Lancet 2010; 376(9743): 773-83.
[http://dx.doi.org/10.1016/S0140-6736(10)61193-2] [PMID: 20816545]

[6]   Elwood T, Morris W, Martin LD, *et al.* Bronchodilator premedication does not decrease respiratory adverse events in pediatric general anesthesia. Can J Anaesth 2003; 50(3): 277-84.
[http://dx.doi.org/10.1007/BF03017798] [PMID: 12620952]

[7]   Cohen MM, Cameron CB. Should you cancel the operation when a child has an upper respiratory tract infection? Anesth Analg 1991; 72(3): 282-8.

[8] Expert Panel Report 3 (EPR-3): Guidelines for the Diagnosis and Management of Asthma-Summary Report 2007. J Allergy Clin Immunol 2007; 120(5) (Suppl.): S94-S138.
[http://dx.doi.org/10.1016/j.jaci.2007.09.029] [PMID: 17983880]

[9] Mitchell RB, Archer SM, Ishman SL, *et al.* Clinical Practice Guideline: Tonsillectomy in Children (Update). Otolaryngol Head Neck Surg 2019; 160(1_suppl) (Suppl.): S1-S42.2019;

[10] Kain ZN, MacLaren J, McClain BC, *et al.* Effects of age and emotionality on the effectiveness of midazolam administered preoperatively to children. Anesthesiology 2007; 107(4): 545-52.
[http://dx.doi.org/10.1097/01.anes.0000281895.81168.c3] [PMID: 17893449]

[11] Davis PJ, Cladis FP, Motoyama EK. Smith's anesthesia for infants and children St. Louis: Mo : Mosby 2011.

[12] Braude N, Ridley SA, Sumner E. Parents and paediatric anaesthesia: a prospective survey of parental attitudes to their presence at induction. Ann R Coll Surg Engl 1990; 72(1): 41-4.
[PMID: 2301901]

[13] Caldwell-Andrews AA, Blount RL, Mayes LC, Kain ZN. Behavioral interactions in the perioperative environment: a new conceptual framework and the development of the perioperative child-adult medical procedure interaction scale. Anesthesiology 2005; 103(6): 1130-5.
[http://dx.doi.org/10.1097/00000542-200512000-00005] [PMID: 16306723]

[14] Hsu YW, Pan MH, Huang CJ, Cheng CR, Wu KH, Wei TT. Comparison of inhalation induction with 2%, 4%, 6%, and 8% sevoflurane in nitrous oxide for pediatric patients. Ma Tsui Hsueh Tsa Chi 2000; 38(2): 73-8.
[PMID: 11000669]

[15] Boonmak P, Boonmak S, Pattanittum P. High initial concentration *versus* low initial concentration sevoflurane for inhalational induction of anaesthesia. Cochrane Database Syst Rev 2016; (6): CD006837
[http://dx.doi.org/10.1002/14651858.CD006837.pub3] [PMID: 27356171]

[16] Brimacombe J. The advantages of the LMA over the tracheal tube or facemask: a meta-analysis. Can J Anaesth 1995; 42(11): 1017-23.
[http://dx.doi.org/10.1007/BF03011075] [PMID: 8590490]

[17] Tait AR, Pandit UA, Voepel-Lewis T, Munro HM, Malviya S. Use of the laryngeal mask airway in children with upper respiratory tract infections: a comparison with endotracheal intubation. Anesth Analg 1998; 86(4): 706-11.
[http://dx.doi.org/10.1213/00000539-199804000-00006] [PMID: 9539588]

[18] Baijal RG, Bidani SA, Minard CG, Watcha MF. Perioperative respiratory complications following awake and deep extubation in children undergoing adenotonsillectomy. Paediatr Anaesth 2015; 25(4): 392-9.
[http://dx.doi.org/10.1111/pan.12561] [PMID: 25370474]

[19] Anderson BJ, Holford NH, Woollard GA, Kanagasundaram S, Mahadevan M. Perioperative pharmacodynamics of acetaminophen analgesia in children. Anesthesiology 1999; 90(2): 411-21.
[http://dx.doi.org/10.1097/00000542-199902000-00014] [PMID: 9952146]

[20] Lapin SL, Auden SM, Goldsmith LJ, Reynolds AM. Effects of sevoflurane anaesthesia on recovery in children: a comparison with halothane. Paediatr Anaesth 1999; 9(4): 299-304.
[http://dx.doi.org/10.1046/j.1460-9592.1999.00351.x] [PMID: 10411764]

[21] Berkowitz RG, Zalzal GH. Tonsillectomy in children under 3 years of age. Arch Otolaryngol Head Neck Surg 1990; 116(6): 685-6.
[http://dx.doi.org/10.1001/archotol.1990.01870060043006] [PMID: 2340121]

[22] Elhakim M, Ali NM, Rashed I, Riad MK, Refat M. Dexamethasone reduces postoperative vomiting and pain after pediatric tonsillectomy. Can J Anaesth 2003; 50(4): 392-7.
[http://dx.doi.org/10.1007/BF03021038] [PMID: 12670818]

[23]   Cardwell M, Siviter G, Smith A. Non-steroidal anti-inflammatory drugs and perioperative bleeding in paediatric tonsillectomy. Cochrane Database Syst Rev 2005; (2): CD003591
[PMID: 15846670]

[24]   August DA, Everett LL. Pediatric ambulatory anesthesia. Anesthesiol Clin 2014; 32(2): 411-29.
[http://dx.doi.org/10.1016/j.anclin.2014.02.002] [PMID: 24882128]

[25]   Heard C, Harutunians M, Houck J, Joshi P, Johnson K, Lerman J. Propofol anesthesia for children undergoing magnetic resonance imaging: a comparison with isoflurane, nitrous oxide, and a laryngeal mask airway. Anesth Analg 2015; 120(1): 157-64.
[http://dx.doi.org/10.1213/ANE.0000000000000504] [PMID: 25625260]

[26]   Kovac AL. Management of postoperative nausea and vomiting in children. Paediatr Drugs 2007; 9(1): 47-69.
[http://dx.doi.org/10.2165/00148581-200709010-00005] [PMID: 17291136]

[27]   Eberhart LHJ, Geldner G, Kranke P, *et al.* The development and validation of a risk score to predict the probability of postoperative vomiting in pediatric patients. Anesth Analg 2004; 99(6): 1630-7.
[http://dx.doi.org/10.1213/01.ANE.0000135639.57715.6C] [PMID: 15562045]

[28]   Bolton CM, Myles PS, Nolan T, Sterne JA. Prophylaxis of postoperative vomiting in children undergoing tonsillectomy: a systematic review and meta-analysis. Br J Anaesth 2006; 97(5): 593-604.
[http://dx.doi.org/10.1093/bja/ael256] [PMID: 17005507]

[29]   Kim EG, Park HJ, Kang H, Choi J, Lee HJ. Antiemetic effect of propofol administered at the end of surgery in laparoscopic assisted vaginal hysterectomy. Korean J Anesthesiol 2014; 66(3): 210-5.
[http://dx.doi.org/10.4097/kjae.2014.66.3.210] [PMID: 24729843]

[30]   Ashok V, Bala I, Bharti N, Jain D, Samujh R. Effects of intraoperative liberal fluid therapy on postoperative nausea and vomiting in children-A randomized controlled trial. Paediatr Anaesth 2017; 27(8): 810-5.
[http://dx.doi.org/10.1111/pan.13179] [PMID: 28585750]

[31]   Schreiner MS, Nicolson SC, Martin T, Whitney L. Should children drink before discharge from day surgery? Anesthesiology 1992; 76(4): 528-33.
[http://dx.doi.org/10.1097/00000542-199204000-00007] [PMID: 1550277]

[32]   Watcha MF, Lee AD, Medellin E, Felberg MT, Bidani SA. Clinical Use of the Pictorial Baxter Retching Faces Scale for the Measurement of Postoperative Nausea in Children. Anesth Analg 2019; 128(6): 1249-55.
[http://dx.doi.org/10.1213/ANE.0000000000003850] [PMID: 31094795]

[33]   Gan TJ, Diemunsch P, Habib AS, *et al.* Consensus guidelines for the management of postoperative nausea and vomiting. Anesth Analg 2014; 118(1): 85-113.
[http://dx.doi.org/10.1213/ANE.0000000000000002] [PMID: 24356162]

[34]   Birmingham PK, Tobin MJ, Fisher DM, Henthorn TK, Hall SC, Coté CJ. Initial and subsequent dosing of rectal acetaminophen in children: a 24-hour pharmacokinetic study of new dose recommendations. Anesthesiology 2001; 94(3): 385-9.
[http://dx.doi.org/10.1097/00000542-200103000-00005] [PMID: 11374595]

[35]   Motov S, Yasavolian M, Likourezos A, *et al.* Comparison of Intravenous Ketorolac at Three Single-Dose Regimens for Treating Acute Pain in the Emergency Department: A Randomized Controlled Trial. Ann Emerg Med 2017; 70(2): 177-84.
[http://dx.doi.org/10.1016/j.annemergmed.2016.10.014] [PMID: 27993418]

[36]   Schnabel A, Reichl SU, Zahn PK, Pogatzki-Zahn E. Nalbuphine for postoperative pain treatment in children. Cochrane Database Syst Rev 2014; (7): CD009583.
[http://dx.doi.org/10.1002/14651858.CD009583.pub2]

[37]   He XY, Cao JP, Shi XY, Zhang H. Dexmedetomidine *versus* morphine or fentanyl in the management of children after tonsillectomy and adenoidectomy: a meta-analysis of randomized controlled trials.

Ann Otol Rhinol Laryngol 2013; 122(2): 114-20.
[http://dx.doi.org/10.1177/000348941312200207] [PMID: 23534126]

[38] Mamie C, Habre W, Delhumeau C, Argiroffo CB, Morabia A. Incidence and risk factors of perioperative respiratory adverse events in children undergoing elective surgery. Paediatr Anaesth 2004; 14(3): 218-24.
[http://dx.doi.org/10.1111/j.1460-9592.2004.01169.x] [PMID: 14996260]

[39] Hampson-Evans D, Morgan P, Farrar M. Pediatric laryngospasm. Paediatr Anaesth 2008; 18(4): 303-7.
[http://dx.doi.org/10.1111/j.1460-9592.2008.02446.x] [PMID: 18315635]

[40] Schreiner MS, O'Hara I, Markakis DA, Politis GD. Do children who experience laryngospasm have an increased risk of upper respiratory tract infection? Anesthesiology 1996; 85(3): 475-80.
[http://dx.doi.org/10.1097/00000542-199609000-00005] [PMID: 8853076]

[41] Batra YK, Ivanova M, Ali SS, Shamsah M, Al Qattan AR, Belani KG. The efficacy of a subhypnotic dose of propofol in preventing laryngospasm following tonsillectomy and adenoidectomy in children. Paediatr Anaesth 2005; 15(12): 1094-7.
[http://dx.doi.org/10.1111/j.1460-9592.2005.01633.x] [PMID: 16324030]

[42] Walker RW, Sutton RS. Which port in a storm? Use of suxamethonium without intravenous access for severe laryngospasm. Anaesthesia 2007; 62(8): 757-9.
[http://dx.doi.org/10.1111/j.1365-2044.2007.05226.x] [PMID: 17635421]

[43] Bolaji BO, Oyedepo OO, Dunmade AD, Afolabi OA. Negative pressure pulmonary oedema following adenoidectomy under general anaesthesia: a case series. West Afr J Med 2011; 30(2): 121-4.
[PMID: 21984461]

[44] Lauer R, Vadi M, Mason L. Anaesthetic management of the child with co-existing pulmonary disease. Br J Anaesth 2012; 109 (Suppl. 1): i47-59.
[http://dx.doi.org/10.1093/bja/aes392] [PMID: 23242751]

[45] Skolnick ET, Vomvolakis MA, Buck KA, Mannino SF, Sun LS. Exposure to environmental tobacco smoke and the risk of adverse respiratory events in children receiving general anesthesia. Anesthesiology 1998; 88(5): 1144-53.
[http://dx.doi.org/10.1097/00000542-199805000-00003] [PMID: 9605672]

[46] Westhorpe RN, Ludbrook GL, Helps SC. Crisis management during anaesthesia: bronchospasm. Qual Saf Health Care 2005; 14(3)e7
[http://dx.doi.org/10.1136/qshc.2002.004457] [PMID: 15933304]

[47] Woods BD, Sladen RN. Perioperative considerations for the patient with asthma and bronchospasm. Br J Anaesth 2009; 103 (Suppl. 1): i57-65.
[http://dx.doi.org/10.1093/bja/aep271] [PMID: 20007991]

[48] First MB. Diagnostic and statistical manual of mental disorders 5th edition, and clinical utility. J Nerv Ment Dis. 2013; 201: pp. (9)727-9.

[49] Voepel-Lewis T, Malviya S, Tait AR. A prospective cohort study of emergence agitation in the pediatric postanesthesia care unit. Anesth Analg 2003; 96(6): 1625-30.
[http://dx.doi.org/10.1213/01.ANE.0000062522.21048.61] [PMID: 12760985]

[50] Cravero JP, Beach M, Dodge CP, Whalen K. Emergence characteristics of sevoflurane compared to halothane in pediatric patients undergoing bilateral pressure equalization tube insertion. J Clin Anesth 2000; 12(5): 397-401.
[http://dx.doi.org/10.1016/S0952-8180(00)00180-X] [PMID: 11025242]

[51] Kain ZN, Caldwell-Andrews AA, Mayes LC, *et al.* Family-centered preparation for surgery improves perioperative outcomes in children: a randomized controlled trial. Anesthesiology 2007; 106(1): 65-74.
[http://dx.doi.org/10.1097/00000542-200701000-00013] [PMID: 17197846]

[52]   Vlajkovic GP, Sindjelic RP. Emergence delirium in children: many questions, few answers. Anesth Analg 2007; 104(1): 84-91.
[http://dx.doi.org/10.1213/01.ane.0000250914.91881.a8] [PMID: 17179249]

CHAPTER 13

Non-operating Room Pediatric Anesthesia

Ian Brotman[1] and **Sindhu Samba[1]**

[1] Department of Anesthesiology, Cooper Medical School of Rowan University, Cooper University Health Care, Camden, NJ, USA

Abstract: Non-operating room anesthesia (NORA) is becoming increasingly popular for pediatric patients and comes with its own unique challenges that warrant consideration in order to provide safe anesthetic care. This chapter is organized by location and discusses considerations for locations such as the radiology suite, interventional radiology, gastroenterology, and oncology sites. Agent selection and anesthetic type can vary even within each locale, and different techniques are presented to help guide the practitioner on what may be expected with each site and procedure. Checklists are provided as cognitive aids for the safe preparation. The postanesthesia recovery period for these patients is also summarized, and discharge criteria are provided.

Keywords: Anaphylaxis, CT scan, Endoscopy, Gastroenterology, Interventional Radiology, Nonoperating Room Anesthesia, MRI, NORA, Nuclear Medicine, PACU, Pediatric, Pediatric Anesthesia, Pediatric Emergency, Radiology.

INTRODUCTION

Non-operating room anesthesia (NORA) is becoming increasingly more common as a higher number of procedures are done outside the operating suite on sicker patients [1]. The increasing volume, along with the complexity of both procedures and patients, has placed more importance on having dedicated anesthesia providers to ensure safe care. Pediatrics is following the trend, similar to that in adults, with procedures occurring throughout the hospital and each location posing unique challenges. This chapter will discuss the anesthetic considerations for many of the commonly encountered NORA locations, such as the radiology, endoscopy, and oncology suites, along with interventional and neurointerventional radiology. While each of these sites is different in the procedures performed, some universal principles can be followed for safe and smooth anesthetic care.

---

* **Corresponding author Bharathi Gourkanti:** Department of Anesthesiology, Cooper Medical School of Rowan University, Cooper University Health Care, Camden, NJ, USA; E-mail: gourkantibharathi@cooperhealth.edu

Bharathi Gourkanti, Irwin Gratz, Grace Dippo, Nathalie Peiris and Dinesh K. Choudhry (Eds.)
All rights reserved-© 2022 Bentham Science Publishers

Preoperative, intraoperative, and postoperative concerns will be addressed. As more procedures are performed outside the operating room on sicker patients, non-operating room anesthesia (NORA) is becoming more complex and more common [1]. The increasing volume, along with the complexity of both cases and patients, has placed more importance on having dedicated anesthesia providers to ensure safe sedation care. Pediatrics is following the same adult trend, with procedures occurring throughout the hospital and each location offering unique challenges. This chapter will discuss the anesthetic considerations for many of the commonly encountered NORA locations, such as the radiology, endoscopy, and oncology suite, along with interventional and neurointerventional radiology. While each of these sites is different in the procedures performed, some universal principles can be followed for a safe and smooth anesthetic. Preoperative, intraoperative, and postoperative considerations will be discussed below, along with commonly encountered difficulties and complications.

GENERAL DIFFICULTIES

Anesthesia outside of the operating room offers several challenges, which only become compounded while dealing with pediatric patients. In areas with limited pediatrics exposure, staff will often have little familiarity with the intricacies of caring for this unique population. This inexperience may extend to the post-anesthesia care recovery nurses, and transport may be required to take the patient from the procedure area to an appropriate recovery destination.

The anesthesia equipment in a NORA location may be unfamiliar or even expired, and appropriate pediatric sizes may be unavailable, making potentially challenging situations even more stressful. The procedure room may also not accommodate the anesthesia setup that would fit in an operating room, or, as in MRI, the equipment may not be compatible with the magnet. Along with equipment, it may be unsafe for an anesthesia provider to remain in the room, and monitoring may be required from a remote location. All of these factors need to be considered when formulating an off-site anesthetic treatment plan and room setup.

Many off-site locations, particularly the radiology suite, may not be accustomed to caring for a patient receiving deep sedation or general anesthesia and may be unfamiliar with recommended nil per os (NPO) guidelines. While an aspiration is an infrequent event and NPO status has not been found to be an independent predictor, the ASA guidelines for NPO status should still be followed in elective procedures [2, 3]. Again, although it may not help prevent an aspiration event, theoretically, the event would be less catastrophic. With that in mind, scheduling of the cases should take into consideration that many pediatric patients and families will have a difficult time following NPO guidelines into the afternoon, and ideally, these cases should be started early in the day [4].

NORA SETUP

Studies comparing the outcomes of the sedation strategy for pediatric NORA anesthesia are lacking, given the small number of participants and the small number of complications [5]. It is difficult to give specific recommendations on specific anesthetics, and the mentioned anesthetic techniques should tailor to patient comorbidities. However, there are recommendations on minimal required location setup, based on a statement provided by the American Society of Anesthesia (ASA) in 2018 on out-of-operating room anesthesia [6]. Many of these practice parameters apply to all NORA procedures and are not unique to the pediatric population (Table 1). Before anesthetic induction, there should be a source of oxygen with enough reserve to supply the entire duration of the procedure.

Table 1. NORA case setup.

Equipment and Monitoring	Airway
Electrical outlet access	Oxygen Source
3-lead EKG	Self-inflating bag valve with age appropriate mask
Sized blood pressure cuff	Age appropriate cuffed endotracheal tube with pediatric stylet
Pulse Oximetry	Laryngoscope and blades
Suction and suction catheter	Laryngeal mask airway sized by patient weight
End-tidal CO2	Nasal and oral airways
Temperature and warming device	Facemask or nasal cannula with end-tidal CO2 monitoring port
Medications	**Miscellaneous**
Infusion pump	Transport Monitor
Emergency Medication Cart	Transport Oxygen
If performing sedation, confirm medications available for emergency conversion to general anesthesia	Recognize emergency help providers available
	Confirm defibrillator location
	Verify patient recovery area

The length of the oxygen delivery apparatus should be long enough to accommodate a large amount of movement, especially in the radiology suite. A backup oxygen source should also be available. Suction should be prepared and double-checked to ensure that it can reach the patient. Emergency equipment is discussed in greater detail below. Regardless of how brief the procedure is, providers should have a self-inflating bag capable of delivering positive pressure ventilation with high oxygen concentration, emergency medications, and a defibrillator immediately available. A dedicated resuscitation space should be established if it is deemed unsafe to provide advanced life support in the procedure area. Adequate space to accommodate the necessary anesthesia equipment should be delineated, with attention to identifying electrical outlet locations. Finally, if inhalational anesthetic gasses are being used, a waste scavenging system should be confirmed for the safety of the providers. The specific setup for the pediatric patient includes having appropriately sized equipment, such as airway devices, suction ends, and intravenous cannulas. Having a pediatric equipment cart with variable sizes of different items that are easy to transport to a NORA site is a convenient way to accommodate the pediatric equipment variability. This cart, much like the code cart, should be checked daily to verify proper stock. An infusion device to titrate both sedative medications and fluid must be available in order to help prevent accidental over administration. It is critically important to ensure that all appropriate equipment is available before initiating an anesthetic, as locating an item after induction may be difficult and dangerous.

NORA SITE CONSIDERATIONS

Radiology Suite: CT and MRI

The most common noninvasive setting requiring anesthesia is the radiology suite, including magnetic resonance imaging (MRI) and computed tomography (CT). CT imaging is rapid, less sensitive to patient movement, and can be completed in minutes, while the duration of MRI scans can be hours long. MRI can be exquisitely sensitive to patient movement and cooperation is required for a viable scan. The ability of a child to participate in the scan is dependent on their age, and cognitive and emotional development. There is no absolute age where a child should tolerate an MRI, and a pre-anesthesia discussion should occur with the parent, child, and MRI technician. Distraction techniques with audio and video technology, positive reinforcement, and dedicated child coping specialists may help avoid pharmacologic sedation [7]. Children with anxiety not abated with a nonpharmacologic approach may require sedation under monitored anesthesia care (MAC). Patient factors such as NPO time and medical comorbidities, such as obstructive sleep apnea, aspiration risk, or airway abnormalities, may necessitate general anesthesia [8].

Anesthetic Considerations for MRI

The magnetic field of the MRI scanner creates a unique environment for the administration of anesthesia. The MRI area is divided into four safety zones as defined by the American College of Radiology, which corresponds to increasing levels of magnetic field exposure [9]. Zones I and II are accessible public areas, with the latter serving as the screening checkpoint by medical staff. Zone III is an area near the magnet, such as the control room, and can be a physical hazard to unscreened patients and personnel. Zone IV is the scanner room and has the highest magnetic field, and, with the magnet always on, is the most significantly hazardous. It is recommended that all ferromagnetic objects be removed in zone III and avoided in zone IV. These include pagers, phones, keys, stethoscopes, pens, and needles. Medical devices and implants such as some pacemakers, aneurysm clips, and epidurals may not be MRI compatible, which is why patient screening is essential before transporting them to the higher magnetic zones.

Due to the limitations of the magnetic fields in zones III and IV, a separate, dedicated induction space creates an environment where all traditional equipment and supplies can be made available for safe induction of anesthesia. In this space, an anesthesia machine and cart are present with standard laryngoscopes and airway equipment. If an induction space is unavailable, then induction can occur in the scanner space, but compatible airway equipment must be verified prior to medication administration. Children can be safely sedated with a carefully titrated propofol infusion, as detailed elsewhere in this book; however, even a small amount of obstruction can lead to small body movements that interfere with image acquisition. For children over the age of two or greater than ten kilograms, a laryngeal mask airway (LMA) can provide adequate support for oxygenation and ventilation. However, it may have difficulty seating properly in smaller infants and neonates. Improper LMA placement can lead to inadequate tidal volumes, worsening obstruction, or ventilator dyssynchrony. In these patients, securing the airway with an endotracheal tube can provide a safe approach to airway management.

ASA guidelines have been updated to reflect the expansion of anesthesia care, and they maintain the use of standard monitoring equipment measuring circulation, oxygenation, ventilation, and temperature at regular intervals [10]. The Pediatric Sedation Research Consortium database examined over 30,000 records related to sedation techniques and outcomes and found that 1 in 400 procedures was associated with respiratory adverse effects such as stridor, laryngospasm, apnea, or wheezing [5]. 1 in 200 sedations required some airway interventions ranging from simple oral airway placement to emergent intubation. This highlights the importance of proper monitoring and familiarity with challenging pediatric patients [11].

Monitoring in the MRI suite can be particularly challenging. MRI compatible monitors include non-ferromagnetic EKG leads, pulse oximeter, blood pressure cuff, end-tidal CO_2, and temperature probe. These are usually portable and can be applied outside the scanner area to ensure continuous monitoring during transport to the magnet. Once the patient is moved to the scanner, all monitors should be rechecked to ensure that they are functioning correctly. Earplugs should be applied to the patient for noise reduction. Circuit extensions will likely be necessary to connect the anesthesia machine to the endotracheal tube or LMA if such is required. Electromagnetic conduction can generate heat within monitor wires, and care should be taken to pad patients to avoid direct contact with wires. Since the airway is not easily accessible, end-tidal CO_2 monitoring and oxygen delivery should be confirmed prior to leaving the room and beginning the scan. The anesthesia provider should be positioned with a clear view of the patient and monitors. Due to changing magnetic fields, there may be interference with monitors resulting in artifacts. Thus, the anesthesia provider should remain vigilant in the frequent assessment of vitals, ventilation, and anesthetic depth.

Anesthesia maintenance can consist of either volatile anesthetic with an oxygen-air mixture or total intravenous anesthesia with propofol. Some infusion pumps are not MRI compatible, and extension tubing may be needed to keep the pump outside of the MRI suite. Since imaging is essentially a painless procedure, the role of opioids is limited. Adjuncts such as dexmedetomidine can be utilized to facilitate a smooth emergence or reduce the requirement of volatile anesthetic. However, undesirable effects such as bradycardia, prolonged recovery, and PACU stay necessitate its utilization on a case-by-case basis.

Interventional Radiology

Interventional radiology is a specialized field that performs minimally invasive procedures utilizing imaging such as fluoroscopy, ultrasound, or CT guidance. Common procedures include vascular access, placement or revision of gastric or gastro-jejunal tubes, needle biopsies, fluid sampling or drainage, lumbar punctures, and treatment of various blood vessel malformations.

Anesthetic techniques can range from local anesthesia to deep sedation or general anesthesia and are based on the procedure, patients' condition, positioning, and resources. Midazolam, propofol, opioids, ketamine, and dexmedetomidine are common medications employed, and all have been used successfully in pediatric sedation. Achieving the appropriate anesthetic depth is challenging, and a thorough understanding of appropriate dosage and side effects is vital. The anesthesia provider should be able to recognize complications and convert to general anesthesia quickly.

General anesthesia with inhalational or intravenous technique is indicated for procedures that are painful, prolonged or require neuromuscular blockade. Airway management can be complicated by an unanticipated difficult airway in a remote location. With limited aid, staff that can offer assistance should be identified prior to induction and called early in the event of a complication. Size-appropriate LMAs should be stocked and, if possible, a video laryngoscope should be accessible. Per standard practice of general anesthesia, routine monitors should be applied and measured at regular intervals. Patient or procedural factors may warrant invasive monitoring *via* an arterial line or central venous line, and a foley catheter is also useful for lengthy procedures to better monitor urine output and fluid balance. Active warming devices should be utilized to prevent hypothermia.

Setup in the radiology suite should be identical to the operating room. However, as previously mentioned, conditions are often suboptimal due to the large area occupied by the fluoroscopy device. The anesthesia machine, cart with supplies, and monitors should be positioned in a way that is accessible but not obstructive to the flow of the fluoroscopy and procedure team. Arms are usually tucked at the side of the patient, making access during the procedure quite difficult. Extension tubing may be necessary, keeping in mind that a drug will take longer to reach the patient with these additions.

Specific Considerations for Neuro-interventional Radiology

Neuro-interventional radiology involves endovascular access for procedures such as diagnostic angiograms, embolization of vascular malformations, cerebral aneurysm coiling, and thrombolysis. There are unique challenges related to cerebral perfusion pressure and controlling intracranial pressure to reduce the risk of stroke or bleeding. Depth of anesthesia must be balanced with preservation of cerebral perfusion pressure. Frequent breath holding may be requested by the interventionalist during the procedure, and general anesthesia with endotracheal intubation with controlled ventilation is recommended. This is particularly useful when there is a risk of vasospasm as controlled ventilation with permissive hypercapnia can promote cerebral vasodilation. Hemodynamic instabilities must be rapidly addressed with vasoactive or vasodilating agents, and invasive blood pressure monitoring *via* an arterial line should be considered for patients requiring close monitoring or with anticipated blood loss. Normothermia should be maintained, and hyperthermia should be avoided, with the typical warming measures such as forced-air warming blankets, room temperature, and fluids [12].

Endovascular access by the femoral route requires a prolonged period of immobility and lying supine "flat time" of approximately six hours to prevent the formation of a hematoma. The interventionalist will hold pressure at the completion of the procedure for several minutes. The anesthesia provider plays a vital role in facilitating a smooth emergence and minimizing coughing and bucking. If an awake patient is unable to cooperate with the position, a pharmacologic agent, such as dexmedetomidine, can be administered to provide sedation while preserving airway reflexes in order to minimize the risk of agitation.

Nuclear Medicine

Nuclear medicine is the administration of radiotracers that emit small amounts of ionizing radiation, which is captured by the scanning device to explore tissue function and blood flow [13, 14]. It is a commonly employed imaging technique in pediatric urology, oncology, and neonatal endocrinology and may have further use in evaluating some gastrointestinal dysmotility and seizure foci [13, 15]. Much like the other procedures in the radiology suite, nuclear medicine scans are not painful, and the involvement of anesthesia is more for patient cooperation for optimal image acquisition.

Because motion degrades the image quality, any anesthetic technique that keeps the child still will be appropriate for a nuclear medicine scan. If intravenous access can be obtained prior to induction, then a propofol-based intravenous sedation with a natural airway can be an appropriate option. Sometimes with the natural airway, a small amount of obstruction can lead to tiny movements of the head, much like with an MRI, with each breath causing motion artifact. An oral or nasal airway may relieve this obstruction, however, it may be necessary to escalate airway management if the patient continues to obstruct and interfere with picture quality. No specific anesthetic agent will interact with the radioactive tracer, and the choice of volatile or intravenous drug can be based on the provider's comfort and the patient's condition. However, with some scans, especially bone, although the procedure itself is not painful, the condition which warrants the imaging may be painful, and some analgesia may be necessary in the postoperative period.

Providers should be aware of radiation safety prior to caring for a nuclear medicine patient. Ionizing radiation is carcinogenic at high doses or chronic long-term exposure [16]. Anesthesia providers should not take breaks around radiation storage sites. It is safe to be in the room with the patient while they are undergoing their scan. Meticulous care should therefore be taken when placing an IV or foley for long scans as many tracers are in the blood and shed in the urine. Finally, no eating or drinking should occur in the scanning area.

Oncology Suite

Pediatric oncology patients often undergo many anesthetics for both diagnosis and treatment. For children undergoing radiation therapy, numerous sedations sessions may be required. Challenges for radiation treatment include the short procedure time, patient isolation requiring remote monitoring, child anxiety from numerous procedures, and consistency with airway management [17].

There have been a variety of anesthetic medications used for pediatric radiation therapy, ranging from inhalational agents, intramuscular or oral sedatives, and intravenous hypnotics [18]. Intravenous anesthesia with propofol has become the technique of choice at many institutions because of its ease in titration to preserve spontaneous ventilation and short duration of action [18 - 20]. In patients who have painful sequela either from their disease or treatment, opioids or ketamine may be used as an adjuvant to their anesthetic.

Prior to initiating therapy, patients are scanned to accurately map the area of radiation treatment [18]. Inaccurate immobilization can cause healthy tissue injury and treatment failure, and as such, casts may be made to ensure that the patient will not move or greatly change position between treatments. If an oral airway device is used for these initial scans, the cast may be altered in such a way that further treatments will require the same airway device utilized. For example, if a child obstructs during the initial sedation and simulation scan requiring a laryngeal mask airway, then each subsequent anesthetic may require a laryngeal mask airway to ensure accurate cast fit. This does not make advanced airway management a contraindication but should be considered when planning future anesthetics.

The patient is monitored remotely to protect the safety of the treatment team. Sometimes visualization of the patient is not possible, as it is in other areas such as MRI. A remote monitor utilizing EKG, blood pressure, pulse oximetry, and capnography is essential to provide safe care. Although the treatment itself may be very short, it is still important to ensure that the patient is ventilating adequately and anesthetic depth is appropriate prior to leaving the treatment area.

Endoscopy Suite

Endoscopic procedures have been increasing in the adult and pediatric population [3]. While the adult patient may tolerate an endoscopic procedure with opioids and benzodiazepine and still have a quick recovery, the uncooperative pediatric patient requires a deeper level of sedation or anesthesia, which is typically achieved with propofol [21, 22].

No optimal anesthetic regimen has been found, and there are many different combinations of opioids, benzodiazepine, and hypnotics used for endoscopies [23]. Three phases of anesthesia must be considered when formulating the treatment plan include induction, maintenance, and recovery.

For induction, intravenous access may not be easily achieved on an awake uncooperative child, and one can attempt oral midazolam followed by intravenous access if they become cooperative following premedication. Alternatively, an inhalational induction followed by IV placement can be accomplished in the procedure room. Oral midazolam has not been shown to increase PACU recovery time even in short outpatient procedures, and its ability to facilitate cooperation in the child should not be overlooked in assisting with a safe and controlled induction [24].

A spontaneously breathing child with a natural airway is an acceptable technique assuming the patient is not an aspiration risk based on his presentation for the procedure or other comorbidities [25]. A laryngeal mask airway may be placed assuming the endoscopist is comfortable with maneuvering the scope around the airway device, and an endotracheal tube is frequently used in smaller children.

Again, there is no absolute maintenance medication during these gastrointestinal procedures. The anesthesia provider should be aware that once the case is completed, there is minimal discomfort, and the use of short-acting agents would facilitate quick PACU discharge. While dexmedetomidine is an effective hypnotic with minimal respiratory side effects, the prolonged PACU stay may make it unsuitable in many endoscopy centers [26 - 28].

Many of the complications seen in the endoscopy suite occur during EGD and are mostly respiratory [29]. Bronchospasm, laryngospasm, airway obstruction, and apnea are likely complications, and the anesthetic provider should be prepared to manage any adverse respiratory event prior to beginning the procedure.

RECOVERY

Postanesthesia care for the NORA patient follows the same standards set by the operating room recovery area [6]. A member of the anesthesia team should transport the child to the recovery area, and a report should be given to the receiving provider, including information on the patient's preoperative condition and intraprocedural course. Monitoring of oxygenation, ventilation, circulation, level of consciousness, and temperature should occur at regular intervals, and pulse oximetry is highly recommended during the initial phases of recovery. Respiratory depression is the most common adverse event of anesthesia, and the adequacy of ventilation should be monitored not only with pulse oximetry but with continuous observation [1]. If feasible, capnography can be employed, although this is usually impractical in the recovery setting. Suction and equipment able to provide positive pressure ventilation should be made easily available in case of respiratory complications [30].

Each procedure will come with its own unique recovery considerations. Arterial puncture, as mentioned, may require the patient to remain still for hours, which may be difficult to accomplish with an irritated or delirious child [29]. Head and neck embolization of tumors or lymph malformations may result in swelling and airway compromise. While many postoperative complications are discussed elsewhere, postoperative nausea and vomiting is the most common complication of anesthesia in infants and children, leading to delayed discharge and possibly unanticipated admission [31].

Discharge criteria such as the Aldrete score, which looks at factors such as respiration, circulation, oxygenation, and activity to determine discharge readiness, were validated in the adult population [32]. Varying ages having differing levels of physical and cognitive development makes a single scale for all pediatric patients difficult to develop. A modified version of the post-anesthesia discharge score system (Ped-PADSS), which examines much of the same values as the Aldrete has been used with success for pediatric ambulatory surgery, is given in Table **2** and is a good guide to help evaluate patient discharge readiness [32, 33]. Regardless of the criteria used, a physician should evaluate the patient prior to discharge from the recovery area.

Table 2. Peds-PADSS discharge criteria.

Pediatric Post-Anesthesia Discharge Scoring System (Peds-PADSS)	
Vital Signs	2 = Variation <20% with preoperative values 1 = Variation between 20 – 40% of preoperative value 0 = Variation > 40% preoperative value
Activity Level	2 = Constant gait without imbalance or baseline activity level 1= Ambulates with assistance or reduced activity from baseline 0 = Cannot walk or hypotonic
Pain	2 = Yes (Painless or acceptable control by oral analgesia) 1 = No (Pain not well controlled)
Bleeding	2 = Minimal 1 = Moderate 0 = Severe
Nausea and Vomiting	2 = Absent to minimal (no treatment needed) 1 = Moderate (controlled with IV medication) 0 = Severe (persistent nausea and vomiting)

A Ped-PADSS score ≥9 at 1-h intervals was needed to allow discharge from the hospital or PACU

NORA EMERGENCIES

Emergencies are inevitable in the medical field, and each off-site anesthesia location presents its own challenge for resuscitation. It is imperative that prior to inducing anesthesia, emergency supplies should be readily available such as airway supplies and mediations. A code cart stocked and regularly checked to contain a defibrillator, advanced life support medications, and airway equipment should be easily accessible by either the anesthetist or off-site staff. A self-inflating bag with size-appropriate masks and suction should also be available. In accordance with the Malignant Hyperthermia Association of US (MHAUS) recommendations, dantrolene should be available at all anesthetizing locations where malignant hyperthermia triggers are used [34]. Ideally, all staff should have pediatric advanced life support training, although this is not always feasible, especially in sites with limited pediatric case volume. Mock codes in each site should also be performed periodically to educate clinical staff and identify areas of deficiency in the emergency workflow [29]. Easily accessible electronic or paper cognitive aids are recommended, as these are highly useful in providing guidance during acute events. A weight-based drug reference manual containing both the milligram dosage and milliliters to draw up said dosage could be attached to the code cart to make medication preparation easier in times of crisis. If a manual is unavailable, then a printout of the current patient's weight and emergency medication dosage should be available.

Anaphylactic reactions during contrast administration are possible even in patients without previous contrast exposure and should be high on the differential diagnosis in patients with unexplained hypotension, with or without other symptoms [35]. Treatment should include discontinuation of the contrast injection along with epinephrine administration (Fig. **1**). The exact route of epinephrine administration is debated, as many emergency medicine texts recommend intramuscular dosing given the rapid plasma rise without arrhythmias or other cardiac complications [36]. In the emergency room, intravenous access is not always reliably obtained, and intramuscular epinephrine allows early resuscitation. In the radiology suite, IV access has already been established to give contrast, and the risk of cardiac complications from appropriate epinephrine dosing is rare in pediatric patients. The recommended epinephrine dosing is 1 mcg/kg IV and repeated as necessary [37]. If multiple boluses of epinephrine are needed, an infusion can be started at 0.05-.1 mcg/kg/min. Fluid boluses up to 60 ml/kg may be required, and hydrocortisone, diphenhydramine, ranitidine, and albuterol can be considered based on clinical assessment. In patients with a history of reaction to contrast media, many institutions are pre-medicating with steroids and antihistamines [38].

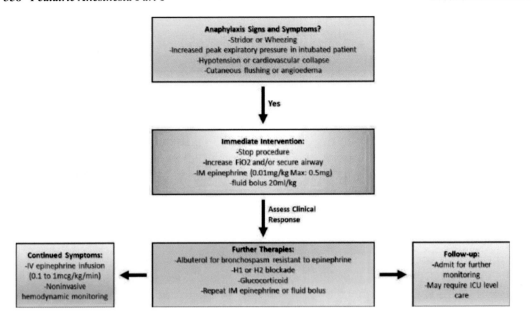

Fig. (1). Anaphylaxis Treatment Algorithm.

Emergencies in the MRI machine also require special considerations. The first step of any code in the MRI should be to remove the patient from the scanner room to an area safe for resuscitation equipment usage. Ferrous material on the emergency equipment and personnel responding to the emergency may become a projectile from the magnet causing further injury to the patient and staff. Quenching of the magnet requires three minutes to remove the magnetic field, and exhaust during the process can cause a hypoxic air mixture within the room [29]. A dedicated emergency area outside the scanner should be established prior to initiating anesthesia, and all the above-mentioned emergency equipment should be accessible.

CONCLUSION

Non-operating room anesthesia is fraught with challenges, including an unfamiliar environment with limited supplies, logistics that can make monitoring difficult, and poor staff awareness of anesthetic dangers. Proper preparation prior to anesthetic induction, including room setup and organization, increases the safety in this unique environment, and the usual anesthesia care standards should not be abandoned. Situation planning should also be reviewed with the entire team, focusing on the commonly encountered emergencies seen at the site. Finally, a dedicated post-anesthesia recovery area should be available to recover the patient.

With these measures in place, pediatric non-operating room anesthesia can be practiced safely.

CONSENT FOR PUBLICATION

Not applicable.

CONFLICT OF INTEREST

The author declares no conflict of interest, financial or otherwise.

ACKNOWLEDGEMENTS

Declared none.

REFERENCES

[1]   Metzner J, Domino KB. Risks of anesthesia or sedation outside the operating room: the role of the anesthesia care provider. Curr Opin Anaesthesiol 2010; 23(4): 523-31.
        [http://dx.doi.org/10.1097/ACO.0b013e32833b7d7c] [PMID: 20531171]

[2]   Beach ML, Cohen DM, Gallagher SM, Cravero JP. Major Adverse Events and Relationship to Nil per Os Status in Pediatric Sedation/Anesthesia Outside the Operating Room: A Report of the Pediatric Sedation Research Consortium. Anesthesiology 2016; 124(1): 80-8.
        [http://dx.doi.org/10.1097/ALN.0000000000000933] [PMID: 26551974]

[3]   Cohen LB, Wecsler JS, Gaetano JN, *et al.* Endoscopic sedation in the United States: results from a nationwide survey. Am J Gastroenterol 2006; 101(5): 967-74.
        [http://dx.doi.org/10.1111/j.1572-0241.2006.00500.x] [PMID: 16573781]

[4]   Brady MC, Kinn S, Ness V, O'Rourke K, Randhawa N, Stuart P. Preoperative fasting for preventing perioperative complications in children. Cochrane Database of Systematic Reviews 2009; 4.
        [http://dx.doi.org/10.1002/14651858.CD005285.pub2]

[5]   Cravero JP, Blike GT. Pediatric anesthesia in the nonoperating room setting. Curr Opin Anaesthesiol 2006; 19(4): 443-9.
        [http://dx.doi.org/10.1097/01.aco.0000236147.83364.99] [PMID: 16829729]

[6]   American Society of Anesthesiologists Committee on Standards and Practice Parameters. Statement on nonoperating room anesthetizing locations 2018.https://www.asahq.org/standards-an- -guidelines/statement-on-nonoperating-room-anesthetizing-locations

[7]   Belani KG. Pediatric Non-OR Anesthesia (NORA)–The Essentials. ASA Newsl 2019; 83(11): 10-3.

[8]   Maddirala S, Theagrajan A. Non-operating room anaesthesia in children. Indian J Anaesth 2019; 63(9): 754-62.
        [http://dx.doi.org/10.4103/ija.IJA_486_19] [PMID: 31571689]

[9]   Kanal E, Barkovich AJ, Bell C, *et al.* ACR guidance document on MR safe practices: 2013. J Magn Reson Imaging 2013; 37(3): 501-30.
        [http://dx.doi.org/10.1002/jmri.24011] [PMID: 23345200]

[10]   American Society of Anesthesiologists Committee on Standards and Practice Parameters. Standards of basic anesthetic monitoring 2015.https://www.asahq.org/standards-and-guidelines/standards-for-b-

[11]   Walls JD, Weiss MS. Safety in non-operating room anesthesia (NORA). APSF Newsletter 2019; 341: 3-4.

[12]   Youn AM, Ko YK, Kim YH. Anesthesia and sedation outside of the operating room. Korean J Anesthesiol 2015; 68(4): 323-31.
[http://dx.doi.org/10.4097/kjae.2015.68.4.323] [PMID: 26257843]

[13]   Biassoni L, Easty M. Paediatric nuclear medicine imaging. Br Med Bull 2017; 123(1): 127-48.
[http://dx.doi.org/10.1093/bmb/ldx025] [PMID: 28910997]

[14]   Fahey FH, Treves ST, Adelstein SJ. Minimizing and communicating radiation risk in pediatric nuclear medicine. J Nucl Med 2011; 52(8): 1240-51.
[http://dx.doi.org/10.2967/jnumed.109.069609] [PMID: 21764783]

[15]   Veitch TA. Pediatric nuclear medicine, Part II: Common procedures and considerations. J Nucl Med Technol 2000; 28(2): 69-75.
[PMID: 10824616]

[16]   Bolus NE. Review of common occupational hazards and safety concerns for nuclear medicine technologists. J Nucl Med Technol 2008; 36(1): 11-7.
[http://dx.doi.org/10.2967/jnmt.107.043869] [PMID: 18287195]

[17]   Twite MD, Friesen RH. Pediatric sedation outside the operating room: the year in review. Curr Opin Anaesthesiol 2005; 18(4): 442-6.
[http://dx.doi.org/10.1097/01.aco.0000168331.11853.03] [PMID: 16534273]

[18]   Anghelescu DL, Burgoyne LL, Liu W, Hankins GM, Cheng C, Beckham PA, *et al.* Safe anesthesia for radiotherapy in pediatric oncology: St. Jude Children's Research Hospital Experience, 2004–2006. Internal Journal of Radiation Oncology * Biology * Physics 2008; 71(2): 491-7.

[19]   Harris EA. Sedation and anesthesia options for pediatric patients in the radiation oncology suite. Int J Pediatr 2010; 2010: 870921.
[http://dx.doi.org/10.1155/2010/870921] [PMID: 20490268]

[20]   Khurmi N, Patel P, Koushik S, Daniels T, Kraus M. Anesthesia practice in pediatric radiation oncology: Mayo Clinic Arizona's Experience 2014–2016. Paediatr Drugs 2018; 20(1): 89-95.
[http://dx.doi.org/10.1007/s40272-017-0259-8] [PMID: 28786083]

[21]   Faigel DO, Baron TH, Goldstein JL, *et al.* Guidelines for the use of deep sedation and anesthesia for GI endoscopy. Gastrointest Endosc 2002; 56(5): 613-7.
[http://dx.doi.org/10.1016/S0016-5107(02)70104-1] [PMID: 12397263]

[22]   Abu-Shahwan I, Mack D. Propofol and remifentanil for deep sedation in children undergoing gastrointestinal endoscopy. Paediatr Anaesth 2007; 17(5): 460-3.
[http://dx.doi.org/10.1111/j.1460-9592.2006.02132.x] [PMID: 17474953]

[23]   Lightdale JR, Mahoney LB, Schwarz SM, Liacouras CA. Methods of sedation in pediatric endoscopy: a survey of NASPGHAN members. J Pediatr Gastroenterol Nutr 2007; 45(4): 500-2.
[http://dx.doi.org/10.1097/MPG.0b013e3180691168] [PMID: 18030225]

[24]   Horgesheimer JJ, Pribble CG, Lugo RA. The effect of midazolam premedication on discharge time in pediatric patients undergoing general anesthesia for dental restorations. Pediatr Dent 2001; 23(6): 491-4.
[PMID: 11800449]

[25]   Koh JL, Black DD, Leatherman IK, Harrison RD, Schmitz ML. Experience with an anesthesiologist interventional model for endoscopy in a pediatric hospital. J Pediatr Gastroenterol Nutr 2001; 33(3): 314-8.]
[http://dx.doi.org/10.1097/00005176-200109000-00016] [PMID: 11593128]

[26]   Edokpolo LU, Mastriano DJ, Serafin J, Weedon JC, Siddiqui MT, Dimaculangan DP. Discharge Readiness after Propofol with or without Dexmedetomidine for Colonoscopy: A Randomized Controlled Trial. Anesthesiology 2019; 131(2): 279-86.
[http://dx.doi.org/10.1097/ALN.0000000000002809]

[27]   Ding L, Zhang H, Mi W, *et al.* Effects of dexmedetomidine on anesthesia recovery period and postoperative cognitive function of patients after robot-assisted laparoscopic radical cystectomy. Int J Clin Exp Med 2015; 8(7): 11388-95.
[PMID: 26379954]

[28]   Candiotti KA, Bergese SD, Bokesch PM, Feldman MA, Wisemandle W, Bekker AY. Monitored anesthesia care with dexmedetomidine: a prospective, randomized, double-blind, multicenter trial. Anesth Analg 2010; 110(1): 47-56.
[http://dx.doi.org/10.1213/ane.0b013e3181ae0856] [PMID: 19713256]

[29]   Mahmoud M, Mason KP. Anesthesia and Sedation for Pediatric Procedures Outside the Operating Room. Smith's Anesthesia for Infants and Children. 9th ed., St. Louis, MO: Elsevier 2017.

[30]   Deutsch N, *et al.* Induction, Maintenance, and Recovery. Smith's Anesthesia for Infants and Children. 9th ed., St. Louis, MO: Elsevier 2017.

[31]   Murat I, Constant I, Maud'huy H. Perioperative anaesthetic morbidity in children: a database of 24,165 anaesthetics over a 30-month period. Paediatr Anaesth 2004; 14(2): 158-66.
[http://dx.doi.org/10.1111/j.1460-9592.2004.01167.x] [PMID: 14962332]

[32]   Moncel JB, Nardi N, Wodey E, Pouvreau A, Ecoffey C. Evaluation of the pediatric post anesthesia discharge scoring system in an ambulatory surgery unit. Paediatr Anaesth 2015; 25(6): 636-41.
[http://dx.doi.org/10.1111/pan.12612] [PMID: 25581378]

[33]   Armstrong J, Forrest H, Crawford MW. A prospective observational study comparing a physiological scoring system with time-based discharge criteria in pediatric ambulatory surgical patients. Can J Anaesth 2015; 62(10): 1082-8.
[http://dx.doi.org/10.1007/s12630-015-0428-6] [PMID: 26149598]

[34]   Larach MG, Gronert GA, Allen GC, Brandom BW, Lehman EB. Clinical presentation, treatment, and complications of malignant hyperthermia in North America from 1987 to 2006. Anesth Analg 2010; 110(2): 498-507.
[http://dx.doi.org/10.1213/ANE.0b013e3181c6b9b2] [PMID: 20081135]

[35]   Kim MH, Lee SY, Lee SE, *et al.* Anaphylaxis to iodinated contrast media: clinical characteristics related with development of anaphylactic shock. PLoS One 2014; 9(6): e100154.
[http://dx.doi.org/10.1371/journal.pone.0100154] [PMID: 24932635]

[36]   Campbell RL, Bellolio MF, Knutson BD, *et al.* Epinephrine in anaphylaxis: higher risk of cardiovascular complications and overdose after administration of intravenous bolus epinephrine compared with intramuscular epinephrine. J Allergy Clin Immunol Pract 2015; 3(1): 76-80.
[http://dx.doi.org/10.1016/j.jaip.2014.06.007] [PMID: 25577622]

[37]   Wittkugel EP, Samol NB. Special Pediatric Disorders. Smith's Anesthesia for Infants and Children. 9th ed., St. Louis, MO: Elsevier 2017.

[38]   Mervak BM, Davenport MS, Ellis JH, Cohan RH. Breakthrough reaction rates in high-risk inpatients premedicated before contrast-enhanced CT. AJR Am J Roentgenol 2015; 205(1): 77-84.
[http://dx.doi.org/10.2214/AJR.14.13810] [PMID: 26102383]

CHAPTER 14

Anesthesia For Common Pediatric Surgical Procedures

Sabina DiCindio[1] and **Mary Theroux**[1]

[1] *Department of Anesthesiology and Perioperative Medicine, Nemours A.I. duPont Hospital for Children, Sidney Kimmel Medical College at Thomas Jefferson University, Wilmington, DE, USA*

Abstract: Anesthesia for pediatric patients begins with a complete history and physical examination, and a review of family history and the patient's medical chart. Since most surgeries performed in the pediatric population are planned, preoperative preparation is essential. Some of the more common pediatric surgeries include strabismus correction, tonsillectomy and adenoidectomy, pyloromyotomy, appendectomy, circumcision, and hernia repair. This chapter will review the anesthetic management of the aforementioned surgeries.

Keywords: Adenoidectomy, Antiemetic, Anxiety, Appendectomy, Aspiration, Electrolytes, Herniorraphy, Hypercarbia, Hypoxia, Insufflation, Laparoscopic, Laryngospasm, Nausea, Oculocardiac reflex, Pneumoperitoneum, Premedication, Pyloromyotomy, Sleep disordered breathing, Strabismus, Tonsillectomy.

INTRODUCTION

Anesthesia for pediatric patients, as with adults, begins with a complete history and physical along with a review of the family history and the patient's medical chart. Preoperative fear and anxiety are present in up to 75% of children prior to surgery [1]. Preoperative distress is associated with increased postoperative pain, nightmares, separation anxiety and bedwetting [2 - 4]. Psychological preparation for the child is essential and is influenced by the child's developmental and mental state, parental anxiety and cultural biases [5].

Both non-pharmacologic and pharmacologic interventions are available and may be used individually or in combination.

Non-Pharmacological Interventions

The anesthesiologist should try to develop rapport with the child as well as help

---

* **Corresponding author Bharathi Gourkanti:** Department of Anesthesiology, Cooper Medical School of Rowan University, Cooper University Health Care, Camden, NJ, United States; E-mail: gourkantibharathi@cooperhealth.edu

Bharathi Gourkanti, Irwin Gratz, Grace Dippo, Nathalie Peiris and Dinesh K. Choudhry (Eds.)
All rights reserved-© 2022 Bentham Science Publishers

calm parental concerns. Non-pharmacologic options include tours of the preoperative area prior to the day of surgery, interactions with child life specialists, hand held video games or tablets and/or parental presence with induction of anesthesia. Parental presence has not been proven to change the stress of the child nor the postoperative negative behavioral changes; however, parental satisfaction is high [6]. If the parents are allowed to be present for induction, the parents(s) should be educated about what to expect. This discussion can describe the application of the monitors, introduction of the mask, eye rolling, and movement of arms and legs. It is important to mention that the parent must leave when requested and will be escorted out of the room after their child is asleep.

Pharmacologic interventions

Pharmacologic interventions can include, but are not limited to, midazolam, ketamine, dexmedetomidine or subanesthetic dose(s) of propofol in the preoperative area. The objective of preanesthetic medication(s) is to allay anxiety with or without inducing amnesia with a subsequent decrease in the incidence of postoperative negative behaviors. Factors to consider when selecting a premedication include the child's age, allergies, and comorbidities. Routes of administration can be intranasal, oral, intramuscular, intravenous, buccal, sublingual, or rectal. Buccal may not be practical in young children, while the rectal route may be unpopular in older children and is rarely used. The oral route followed by intranasal are the most common routes used, and the intravenous route is used in patients who have intravenous access. A discussion with the parent(s) or caregiver and anesthesiologist determines the need for premedication. Children younger than 6 months may not need any premedication at all, considering that separation anxiety develops approximately around 6-8 months of age. Table **1** lists common agents and their dosing guidelines used for preoperative sedation.

Table I. Preoperative Sedation Medications.

Route	Midazolam (mg/Kg)	Ketamine (mg/Kg)	Dexmedetomidine (mcg/Kg)
Nasal	0.2-0.3 Max 10 mg	3-6 (half dose/nostril)	0.5-1 [7]
Intravenous	0.025-0.1 Max 6-10 mg	1-2[8]	0.33-0.67 [9]
Intramuscular	0.05-0.15 Max 10 mg	2-6	2.5 [9]

(Table 1) cont.....

Route	Midazolam (mg/Kg)	Ketamine (mg/Kg)	Dexmedetomidine (mcg/Kg)
Oral	0.25-0.5 Max 20 mg	6-8	2

SURGERIES

Strabismus

Strabismus repair is performed to realign the visual axes of the eyes by repositioning one or more of the six external ocular muscles. Children presenting for strabismus surgery require a general anesthetic.

Induction of anesthesia can be by the inhalation or intravenous (IV) route. Children and adolescents, until roughly teenage years, commonly prefer having an inhalation induction and an IV placed after they are asleep. Whatever the patient's preference may be, an IV is needed for the case. After the adequate depth of anesthesia is achieved, either an endotracheal (ETT) or laryngeal mask airway (LMA) may be used for ventilation and oxygenation. Most commonly, a volatile anesthetic is used for maintenance of anesthesia; however, if the patient has a significant history of PONV, then a total intravenous anesthetic with propofol may be considered [11]. Communication with the surgeon will ascertain the need for neuromuscular (NM) blockade. There is a 70-79% incidence of the oculo-cardiac (OCR) reflex with strabismus surgery due to traction on the extraocular muscles or pressure on the globe. The afferent pathway is transmitted *via* the long and short ciliary nerves to the ophthalmic division of the trigeminal nerve to the Gasserian ganglion, finally terminating in the ophthalmic division of cranial nerve V in the brainstem. The efferent pathway of this reflex is *via* the nucleus of the vagus nerve (cranial nerve X), which when activated, releases the neurotransmitter, acetylcholine, at the sinoatrial node. The reflex is important during strabismus surgery due to its ability to cause bradycardia, or less commonly atrioventricular block, ventricular ectopy, and asystole. The reflex is often transient and easily treated. Bradycardia can be attenuated by administration of anticholinergics, atropine [10-20 mcg/Kg) or glycopyrrolate [10-20 mcg/Kg) [12]. If bradycardia persists, the anesthesia provider should ask the surgeon to release pressure on the eye muscle or the globe. Other anesthetic related factors that contribute to the occulo-cardiac reflex are light anesthesia, acidosis, hypercarbia, and hypoxia which may need to be attended to and resolved. Sevoflurane and desflurane have a lower incidence of bradycardia during strabismus surgery compared with propofol or remifentanil [13]. Sevoflurane decreases vagal activity, and desflurane increases sympathetic activity as well as causes vagal inhibition at a steady state [12, 14 - 16]. Strabismus surgery has an approximately 80% incidence of nausea and vomiting postoperatively and warrants prophylactic administration of antiemetics such as a 5HT3 antagonist, ondansetron 0.1mg/Kg, with or without dexamethasone, 0.25 mg/Kg [17, 18]. Also, IV hydration with 10-20 ml/Kg can help mitigate postoperative nausea and vomiting (PONV). Postoperative analgesia is best accomplished *via* a multimodal approach minimizing the use of narcotics and using non-opioid analgesics, *i.e.*, non-steroidal anti-inflammatory medications (NSAIDs) and acetaminophen.

Herniorrhaphy

A hernia is an opening in the abdominal wall leading to the protrusion of organs or tissue. Inguinal hernias are due to incomplete development of the processus vaginalis. The incidence is 0.8-4.4%, with 60% occurring on the right and more commonly in males [19, 20]. Hernias are also more common in infants born prematurely compared to term birth [21]. Surgical repair is elective unless the bowel is incarcerated or strangulated. Anesthetic care depends on if the repair is emergent or electively scheduled. If emergent, precautions against aspiration should be taken. General anesthesia is most commonly used with a supplemental caudal or peripheral nerve block (ilioinguinal-iliohypogastric). Some centers use spinal anesthesia in premature infants to decrease the risk of postoperative apnea and in infants to address concerns of potential neurotoxicity of anesthetics. [22] If sedation is added to the spine, the risk of apnea in premature infants is similar to that of a general anesthetic. Spinal anesthetic with bupivacaine 0.5%, 0.2 ml/Kg, lasts for 60-90 minutes, and if the surgery is expected to be longer, a general anesthetic will be needed [23].

For electively scheduled hernia repair, an inhalation or IV induction may be performed. Choice of the airway (an ETT or LMA) often depends on the child's age and associated comorbid conditions. During surgery, if using an LMA, traction on the hernia may result in laryngospasm if the patient is in a light plane of anesthesia. Increasing the inspired concentration of inhaled anesthetic or a bolus of propofol may resolve the laryngospasm. Multimodal analgesia with non-opioid medications and regional anesthesia are preferred reserving narcotics for the occasional patient who may need it. Regional anesthesia aimed at providing postoperative pain relief can include any of the following: caudal block, trans*versus* abdominis plane block, ilioinguinal-iliohypogastric nerve block, or infiltrating the surgical wound with a local anesthetic.

A change in the anesthetic plan is necessary when the surgeon performs either a laparoscopic repair or a laparoscopic examination of the contralateral side. Both will need a secured airway using an ETT and the anesthetic may then include NM relaxation as well.

Umbilical Hernia

Incomplete closure of the fascia of the umbilical ring results in an umbilical hernia. It is more commonly seen in premature and low birth weight infants [24]. Small hernias (less than 1-1.5 cm) will spontaneously close and do not require surgery [25]. At any point, if the bowel becomes incarcerated or strangulated, then surgery is necessary. If the case is emergent, precautions against aspiration should be taken. Anesthetic care includes an inhalation induction with an ETT or LMA for airway maintenance. The size of the defect and surgeon preference will dictate the need for NM relaxation. Again, choices of providing postoperative analgesia include injection of local anesthetic at the surgical site, a rectus sheath block or a neuraxial block (caudal) [26, 27].

Circumcision

Phimosis, recurrent balanitis, religious beliefs or parental preference are some of the indications for circumcision in children. In pediatrics, an inhalation anesthetic with additional regional analgesia (either a penile or a caudal block) is preferred. The surgery itself is about an hour, and airway management can be by ETT or LMA (depending on the age of the child and associated comorbid conditions). In addition to regional anesthesia, acetaminophen or opioid analgesia may be used as part of a multimodal approach to pain. A Cochrane review found no difference in the need for rescue analgesia between a caudal block, a dorsal penile nerve block (DNPB), and the use of parenteral medications. However, greater motor block or leg weakness, which were transient in duration, were observed with the caudal block. At our institution, the surgeon performs a DPNB prior to sterile preparation and draping.

Laparoscopic Surgery

Laparoscopic surgery in the pediatric population can be performed for thoracic and abdominal procedures for all ages, including newborns. Laparoscopic abdominal procedures can be performed for appendectomy and pyloromyotomy. Generally, laparoscopic procedures are associated with early ambulation, rapid return to a normal diet, earlier discharge, less pain, and a decrease in anesthesia and operative time [28 - 32]. Intra-abdominal pressures (IAP) of 6-15 mmHg are maintained for surgery with carbon dioxide (CO_2) [33]. CO_2 is the preferred gas because it does not support combustion, is rapidly absorbed from the peritoneal cavity, and does not expand into bubbles or spaces. However, insufflation of the abdominal cavity has multiple side effects. Hypercapnia is more likely in pediatric patients because insufflated CO_2 is more readily absorbed across the peritoneum. Absorption is increased because of the shorter distance between capillaries and peritoneum as well as an increased absorptive area of peritoneum in relation to body weight [34]. This results in increased pressure of arterial CO_2 with a resultant increase in systemic and pulmonary vascular resistance as well as heart rate. In addition, restricted lung excursion causes a decrease in functional residual capacity, intrapulmonary shunting and atelectasis. Also, cephalad displacement of the diaphragm can result in endobronchial intubation secondary to an upward shift of the carina. All of this results in 60% of patients needing an increase in minute ventilation to restore end tidal CO_2 to baseline [34]. Increased IAP and patient positioning may also cause a decrease in cardiac output secondary to decreased venous return as well as compression of the inferior vena cava. Excess pressure may also result in subcutaneous emphysema, pneumomediastinum or pneumothorax. Other side effects include a decrease in renal blood flow with the potential for a decrease in renal function resulting in oliguria or anuria. Increased IAP may also lead to an increase in intracranial pressure. In spite of the potential for the negative effects of the laparoscopic approach, the majority of such procedures are done without complications and there is an increasing trend favoring this approach.

Appendectomy

Acute appendicitis can have a variable presentation, including right lower quadrant pain, nausea, vomiting, anorexia and fever. Vomiting, fever, and duration of illness influence the degree of dehydration and dictate fluid resuscitation. The preferred mode of induction of anesthesia is intravenous. Tracheal intubation allows for controlled ventilation and prevents aspiration of gastric contents. Patients who have laparoscopic surgeries have significant postoperative pain [35]. Traditionally, parenteral opioids supplemented with NSAIDs or acetaminophen have been used to manage postoperative pain. Regional techniques with the aid of ultrasound are increasingly being used. Regional approaches can include quadratus lumborum, paravertebral, trans*versus* abdominis and rectus sheath blocks or local injection at the port site(s) [36, 37] (Fig. **1**). The choice of which block to be employed depends on the preferences of both the anesthesiologist and the surgeon.

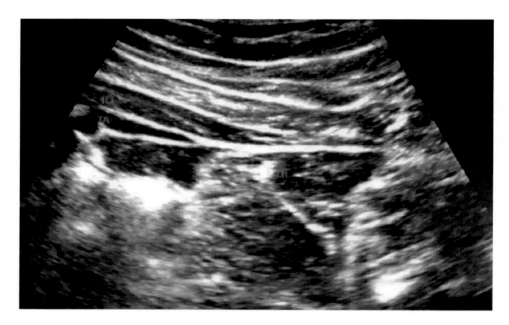

Fig. [1]. Ultrasound picture of abdominal anatomy: EO=External Oblique, IO=Internal Oblique, TA=Trans*versus* Abdominus, QL=Quadratus Lumborum (QL).

Pyloromyotomy

Pyloric stenosis is due to hypertrophy of the smooth muscle of the pylorus with an incidence of 0.9-5.1/1000 live births [38, 39]. It occurs 4-6 x more commonly in males than females and the most common age of presentation is between 1-3 months [39 - 41]. Classically, patients present with projectile vomiting of non-bilious stomach contents, loss of weight, or failure to gain weight. The classic electrolyte abnormalities are hypokalemic, hypochloremic, and metabolic alkalosis.

Pyloromyotomy is not an emergency and electrolyte abnormalities should be corrected such that serum chloride is greater than 100 mEq/L and HCO_3- is less than 30 mEq/L [38]. Metabolic alkalosis can cause respiratory depression and apnea. Preterm infants less than 60 weeks postmenstrual age are known to be at risk of postoperative apnea and apnea has also been reported in term infants after pyloromyotomy [42]. To decrease the risk of postoperative apnea, alkalosis must be corrected prior to surgery. All infants should be monitored after pyloromyotomy for 12- 24 hours. To minimize the risk of aspiration, gastric contents should be aspirated prior to induction of anesthesia. Induction can be achieved by IV or inhalation technique [43]. Neuromuscular relaxation with either succinylcholine or rocuronium can facilitate tracheal intubation. Because the infant airway is compressible and easily deformed, intubation may be more challenging with cricoid pressure [44]. Gentle bag mask ventilation is performed after induction to avoid hypoxemia and bradycardia. Volatile anesthetic combined with air and oxygen is preferred to N_2O because N_2O may expand the bowel gas and cause abdominal distension. Analgesia can be achieved by local infiltration of the port sites and acetaminophen. Rectus sheath blocks, transversus abdominis, and paravertebral blocks have been used successfully [45 - 47]. Considering the age (neonatal) and the small size of the incision necessary to perform the surgery, local anesthetic infiltration by the surgeon is commonly used.

Pyloromyotomy can be performed laparoscopically. Studies have shown a decreased length of hospital stay, less postoperative pain and shorter time to full feeds [38, 48 - 52].

Tonsillectomy and Adenoidectomy (T&A)

Indications for T&A are recurrent throat infections and obstructive sleep disordered breathing. Patients can present with multiple symptoms, including but not limited to learning disabilities, aggressive and impulsive behavior, sleepwalking, enuresis, snoring as well as obstructive sleep apnea (OSA). Preoperatively, it is important to assess for coexisting conditions. The procedure can be intracapsular or extracapsular. Intracapsular surgery is less painful but the tonsils may regrow and may even require a second tonsillectomy if symptoms persist. On the other hand, extracapsular surgery, also known as a 'total tonsillectomy' eliminates the possibility of tonsillar regrowth, but has more pain associated with it. Most tonsillectomies with or without adenoidectomy are performed on an outpatient basis. Young children (< 3 years old) and children with comorbid conditions such as severe OSA, craniofacial syndromes, obesity, cranial base disorders, trisomy 21, and storage disorders are at higher risk for postoperative respiratory complications. Such patients should be monitored overnight. For OSA, what constitutes 'severe' is variable from institution to institution. However, a guideline is provided by the American Academy of otolaryngologists, which defines severe OSA as "an apnea-hypopnea index greater than or equal to 10 obstructive events/hour, oxygen saturation less than 80% or both" [53]. Patients with OSA are known to have an increased sensitivity to opioid analgesics [54].

Patients for tonsil and adenoidectomy can be pre-medicated based on patient and family dynamics and presence of comorbidities. Anesthesia induction may cause pharyngeal obstruction secondary to loss of pharyngeal tone and may require a jaw thrust, oral or nasopharyngeal airway, and continuous positive airway pressure. Either an endotracheal or LMA may be used for the surgery depending on surgeon and anesthesia provider preference and comfort. The table is turned 90 degrees and a mouth gag is inserted by the surgeon, at which point tube dislodgement or compression can occur. Also, it is important to make sure the mouth gag does not pinch the lips. Again, surgeon preference dictates the use of local anesthesia within the tonsillar bed to decrease postoperative pain. The FiO_2 should be reduced to the lowest level possible in order to minimize the risk of airway fire. Analgesia can be provided with opioids (fentanyl, morphine) as well as nonopioid analgesics (acetaminophen, NSAIDS). NSAIDs decrease pain, postoperative opioid requirements, and nausea and vomiting. Some surgeons avoid NSAIDs due to concern for postoperative bleeding, but a Cochrane database has not found this association [55]. Dexamethasone (0.15 mg/Kg maximum 8-25 mg) helps to decrease edema as well as attenuates PONV. [53] Dexmedetomidine 1 mcg/Kg and Morphine 0.1 mg/KG have been shown to increase the time to first analgesia postoperatively and decrease the need for additional rescue analgesia in PACU. [56] A 5HT-3 antagonist can also be administered to decrease PONV. Extubation can be deep or awake. Deep extubation allows for quick turnover, no coughing or bucking, but the airway blood and secretions may lead to laryngospasm. Awake extubation has the benefit of airway patency, but the patient may cough and buck on the ETT. The patient can be placed on their side with the head lower than the body to facilitate drainage of blood and secretions from the mouth.

CONCLUSION

Although surgical emergencies are frequent in the pediatric population, the majority of surgical procedures are elective and can be performed as same day surgeries. Some of the more common pediatric surgeries such as strabismus correction, tonsillectomy and adenoidectomy, pyloromyotomy, appendectomy, circumcision, and hernia repair are discussed in this chapter. Thorough preoperative preparation is essential for a safe anesthetic administration and a good perioperative outcome. Even a non-pediatric anesthesiologist should be familiar with the issues relating to the anesthetic management of these children.

CONSENT FOR PUBLICATION

Not applicable.

CONFLICT OF INTEREST

The author declares no conflict of interest, financial or otherwise.

ACKNOWLEDGEMENTS

Declared none.

REFERENCES

[1]   Perry JN, Hooper VD, Masiongale J. Reduction of preoperative anxiety in pediatric surgery patients using age-appropriate teaching interventions. J Perianesth Nurs 2012; 27(2): 69-81.
[http://dx.doi.org/10.1016/j.jopan.2012.01.003] [PMID: 22443919]

[2]   Kain ZN. Postoperative maladaptive behavioral changes in children: incidence, risks factors and interventions. Acta Anaesthesiol Belg 2000; 51(4): 217-26.
[PMID: 11129622]

[3]   Kain ZN, Caldwell-Andrews AA, Maranets I, *et al.* Preoperative anxiety and emergence delirium and postoperative maladaptive behaviors. Anesth Analg 2004; 99(6): 1648-54. [table of contents.].
[http://dx.doi.org/10.1213/01.ANE.0000136471.36680.97] [PMID: 15562048]

[4]   Fortier MA, Kain ZN. Treating perioperative anxiety and pain in children: a tailored and innovative approach. Paediatr Anaesth 2015; 25(1): 27-35.
[http://dx.doi.org/10.1111/pan.12546] [PMID: 25266082]

[5]   Kain ZN, Mayes LC, O'Connor TZ, Cicchetti DV. Preoperative anxiety in children. Predictors and outcomes. Arch Pediatr Adolesc Med 1996; 150(12): 1238-45.
[http://dx.doi.org/10.1001/archpedi.1996.02170370016002] [PMID: 8953995]

[6]   Kain ZN, Caldwell-Andrews AA, Mayes LC, *et al.* Family-centered preparation for surgery improves perioperative outcomes in children: a randomized controlled trial. Anesthesiology 2007; 106(1): 65-74.
[http://dx.doi.org/10.1097/00000542-200701000-00013] [PMID: 17197846]

[7]   Yuen VM, Hui TW, Irwin MG, *et al.* A randomised comparison of two intranasal dexmedetomidine doses for premedication in children. Anaesthesia 2012; 67(11): 1210-6.
[http://dx.doi.org/10.1111/j.1365-2044.2012.07309.x] [PMID: 22950484]

[8]   Mace SE, Barata IA, Cravero JP, *et al.* Clinical policy: evidence-based approach to pharmacologic agents used in pediatric sedation and analgesia in the emergency department. Ann Emerg Med 2004; 44(4): 342-77.
[http://dx.doi.org/10.1016/j.annemergmed.2004.04.012] [PMID: 15459618]

[9]   Naaz S, Ozair E. Dexmedetomidine in current anaesthesia practice- a review. J Clin Diagn Res 2014; 8(10): GE01-4.
[http://dx.doi.org/10.7860/JCDR/2014/9624.4946] [PMID: 25478365]

[10]   Lexicomp Online. Lexicomp Online, Pediatric and Neonatal Lexi-Drugs Online. Hudson, Ohio: Wolters Kluwer Clinical Drug Information 2014.

[11]   Chhabra A, Pandey R, Khandelwal M, Subramaniam R, Gupta S. Anesthetic techniques and postoperative emesis in pediatric strabismus surgery. Reg Anesth Pain Med 2005; 30(1): 43-7.
[http://dx.doi.org/10.1016/j.rapm.2004.08.023] [PMID: 15690267]

[12]   Choi SR, Park SW, Lee JH, Lee SC, Chung CJ. Effect of different anesthetic agents on oculocardiac reflex in pediatric strabismus surgery. J Anesth 2009; 23(4): 489-93.
[http://dx.doi.org/10.1007/s00540-009-0801-0] [PMID: 19921355]

[13]   Oh AY, Kim JH, Hwang JW, Do SH, Jeon YT. Incidence of postoperative nausea and vomiting after paediatric strabismus surgery with sevoflurane or remifentanil-sevoflurane. Br J Anaesth 2010; 104(6): 756-60.
[http://dx.doi.org/10.1093/bja/aeq091] [PMID: 20418533]

[14]   Oh AY, Yun MJ, Kim HJ, Kim HS. Comparison of desflurane with sevoflurane for the incidence of

oculocardiac reflex in children undergoing strabismus surgery. Br J Anaesth 2007; 99(2): 262-5.
[http://dx.doi.org/10.1093/bja/aem145] [PMID: 17556352]

[15] Ebert TJ, Perez F, Uhrich TD, Deshur MA. Desflurane-mediated sympathetic activation occurs in humans despite preventing hypotension and baroreceptor unloading. Anesthesiology 1998; 88(5): 1227-32.
[http://dx.doi.org/10.1097/00000542-199805000-00013] [PMID: 9605682]

[16] Picker O, Schwarte LA, Schindler AW, Scheeren TW. Desflurane increases heart rate independent of sympathetic activity in dogs. Eur J Anaesthesiol 2003; 20(12): 945-51.
[http://dx.doi.org/10.1097/00003643-200312000-00002] [PMID: 14690095]

[17] Madan R, Bhatia A, Chakithandy S, et al. Prophylactic dexamethasone for postoperative nausea and vomiting in pediatric strabismus surgery: a dose ranging and safety evaluation study. Anesth Analg 2005; 100(6): 1622-6.
[http://dx.doi.org/10.1213/01.ANE.0000150977.14607.E1] [PMID: 15920184]

[18] Subramaniam B, Madan R, Sadhasivam S, et al. Dexamethasone is a cost-effective alternative to ondansetron in preventing PONV after paediatric strabismus repair. Br J Anaesth 2001; 86(1): 84-9.
[http://dx.doi.org/10.1093/bja/86.1.84] [PMID: 11575416]

[19] Brandt ML. Pediatric hernias. Surg Clin North Am 2008; 88(1): 27-43, vii-viii. [vii-viii.].
[http://dx.doi.org/10.1016/j.suc.2007.11.006] [PMID: 18267160]

[20] Chang SJ, Chen JY, Hsu CK, Chuang FC, Yang SS. The incidence of inguinal hernia and associated risk factors of incarceration in pediatric inguinal hernia: a nation-wide longitudinal population-based study. Hernia 2016; 20(4): 559-63.
[http://dx.doi.org/10.1007/s10029-015-1450-x] [PMID: 26621139]

[21] Chen YH, Wei CH, Wang KK. Children With Inguinal Hernia Repairs: Age and Gender Characteristics. Glob Pediatr Health. 2018.

[22] Davidson AJ, Morton NS, Arnup SJ, et al. Apnea after Awake Regional and General Anesthesia in Infants: The General Anesthesia Compared to Spinal Anesthesia Study--Comparing Apnea and Neurodevelopmental Outcomes, a Randomized Controlled Trial. Anesthesiology 2015; 123(1): 38-54.
[http://dx.doi.org/10.1097/ALN.0000000000000709] [PMID: 26001033]

[23] Frawley G, Bell G, Disma N, et al. Predictors of Failure of Awake Regional Anesthesia for Neonatal Hernia Repair: Data from the General Anesthesia Compared to Spinal Anesthesia Study--Comparing Apnea and Neurodevelopmental Outcomes. Anesthesiology 2015; 123(1): 55-65.
[http://dx.doi.org/10.1097/ALN.0000000000000708] [PMID: 26001028]

[24] Jackson OJ, Moglen LH. Umbilical hernia. A retrospective study. Calif Med 1970; 113(4): 8-11.
[PMID: 5479354]

[25] Burcharth J, Pedersen MS, Pommergaard HC, Bisgaard T, Pedersen CB, Rosenberg J. The prevalence of umbilical and epigastric hernia repair: a nationwide epidemiologic study. Hernia 2015; 19(5): 815-9.
[http://dx.doi.org/10.1007/s10029-015-1376-3] [PMID: 25840852]

[26] Relland LM, Tobias JD, Martin D, et al. Ultrasound-guided rectus sheath block, caudal analgesia, or surgical site infiltration for pediatric umbilical herniorrhaphy: a prospective, double-blinded, randomized comparison of three regional anesthetic techniques. J Pain Res 2017; 10: 2629-34.
[http://dx.doi.org/10.2147/JPR.S144259] [PMID: 29184439]

[27] Isaac LA, McEwen J, Hayes JA, Crawford MW. A pilot study of the rectus sheath block for pain control after umbilical hernia repair. Paediatr Anaesth 2006; 16(4): 406-9.
[http://dx.doi.org/10.1111/j.1460-9592.2005.01785.x] [PMID: 16618294]

[28] Mattei P. Minimally invasive surgery in the diagnosis and treatment of abdominal pain in children. Curr Opin Pediatr 2007; 19(3): 338-43.
[http://dx.doi.org/10.1097/MOP.0b013e32810c8eaf] [PMID: 17505197]

[29]   Phillips S, Walton JM, Chin I, Farrokhyar F, Fitzgerald P, Cameron B. Ten-year experience with pediatric laparoscopic appendectomy--are we getting better? J Pediatr Surg 2005; 40(5): 842-5.
[http://dx.doi.org/10.1016/j.jpedsurg.2005.01.054] [PMID: 15937827]

[30]   Sauerland S, Jaschinski T, Neugebauer EA. Laparoscopic *versus* open surgery for suspected appendicitis. Cochrane Database Syst Rev 2010; (10): CD001546
[http://dx.doi.org/10.1002/14651858.CD001546.pub3] [PMID: 20927725]

[31]   Markar SR, Blackburn S, Cobb R, *et al*. Laparoscopic *versus* open appendectomy for complicated and uncomplicated appendicitis in children. J Gastrointest Surg 2012; 16(10): 1993-2004.
[http://dx.doi.org/10.1007/s11605-012-1962-y] [PMID: 22810297]

[32]   Aziz O, Athanasiou T, Tekkis PP, *et al*. Laparoscopic *versus* open appendectomy in children: a meta-analysis. Ann Surg 2006; 243(1): 17-27.
[http://dx.doi.org/10.1097/01.sla.0000193602.74417.14] [PMID: 16371732]

[33]   De Waal EE, Kalkman CJ. Haemodynamic changes during low-pressure carbon dioxide pneumoperitoneum in young children. Paediatr Anaesth 2003; 13(1): 18-25.
[http://dx.doi.org/10.1046/j.1460-9592.2003.00973.x] [PMID: 12535034]

[34]   Pennant JH. Anesthesia for laparoscopy in the pediatric patient. Anesthesiol Clin North America 2001; 19(1): 69-88.
[http://dx.doi.org/10.1016/S0889-8537(05)70212-1] [PMID: 11244921]

[35]   Tomecka MJ, Bortsov AV, Miller NR, *et al*. Substantial postoperative pain is common among children undergoing laparoscopic appendectomy. Paediatr Anaesth 2012; 22(2): 130-5.
[http://dx.doi.org/10.1111/j.1460-9592.2011.03711.x] [PMID: 21958060]

[36]   Splinter WM, Thomson ME. Somatic paravertebral block decreases opioid requirements in children undergoing appendectomy. Canadian journal of anaesthesia = Journal canadien d'anesthesie 2010; 57(3): 206-10.
[http://dx.doi.org/10.1007/s12630-009-9239-y]

[37]   Carney J, Finnerty O, Rauf J, Curley G, McDonnell JG, Laffey JG. Ipsilateral trans*versus* abdominis plane block provides effective analgesia after appendectomy in children: a randomized controlled trial. Anesth Analg 2010; 111(4): 998-1003.
[http://dx.doi.org/10.1213/ANE.0b013e3181ee7bba] [PMID: 20802056]

[38]   Kamata M, Cartabuke RS, Tobias JD. Perioperative care of infants with pyloric stenosis. Paediatr Anaesth 2015; 25(12): 1193-206.
[http://dx.doi.org/10.1111/pan.12792] [PMID: 26490352]

[39]   To T, Wajja A, Wales PW, Langer JC. Population demographic indicators associated with incidence of pyloric stenosis. Arch Pediatr Adolesc Med 2005; 159(6): 520-5.
[http://dx.doi.org/10.1001/archpedi.159.6.520] [PMID: 15939849]

[40]   MacMahon B. The continuing enigma of pyloric stenosis of infancy: a review. Epidemiology 2006; 17(2): 195-201.
[http://dx.doi.org/10.1097/01.ede.0000192032.83843.c9] [PMID: 16477261]

[41]   Aboagye J, Goldstein SD, Salazar JH, *et al*. Age at presentation of common pediatric surgical conditions: Reexamining dogma. J Pediatr Surg 2014; 49(6): 995-9.
[http://dx.doi.org/10.1016/j.jpedsurg.2014.01.039] [PMID: 24888850]

[42]   Andropoulos DB, Heard MB, Johnson KL, Clarke JT, Rowe RW. Postanesthetic apnea in full-term infants after pyloromyotomy. Anesthesiology 1994; 80(1): 216-9.
[http://dx.doi.org/10.1097/00000542-199401000-00031] [PMID: 8291713]

[43]   Scrimgeour GE, Leather NW, Perry RS, Pappachan JV, Baldock AJ. Gas induction for pyloromyotomy. Paediatr Anaesth 2015; 25(7): 677-80.
[http://dx.doi.org/10.1111/pan.12633] [PMID: 25704405]

[44]   Walker RW, Ravi R, Haylett K. Effect of cricoid force on airway calibre in children: a bronchoscopic assessment. Br J Anaesth 2010; 104(1): 71-4.
[http://dx.doi.org/10.1093/bja/aep337] [PMID: 19942611]

[45]   Breschan C, Jost R, Stettner H, *et al.* Ultrasound-guided rectus sheath block for pyloromyotomy in infants: a retrospective analysis of a case series. Paediatr Anaesth 2013; 23(12): 1199-204.
[http://dx.doi.org/10.1111/pan.12267] [PMID: 24112798]

[46]   Kumar A, Wilson GA, Engelhardt TE. Ultrasound guided rectus sheath blockade compared to peri-operative local anesthetic infiltration in infants undergoing supraumbilical pyloromyotomy. Saudi J Anaesth 2014; 8(2): 229-32.
[http://dx.doi.org/10.4103/1658-354X.130725] [PMID: 24843338]

[47]   Mata-Gómez J, Guerrero-Domínguez R, García-Santigosa M, Ontanilla A. Ultrasound-guided paravertebral block for pyloromyotomy in 3 neonates with congenital hypertrophic pyloric stenosis. Braz J Anesthesiol 2015; 65(4): 302-5.
[http://dx.doi.org/10.1016/j.bjane.2014.03.012] [PMID: 26123148]

[48]   St Peter SD, Holcomb GW III, Calkins CM, *et al.* Open *versus* laparoscopic pyloromyotomy for pyloric stenosis: a prospective, randomized trial. Ann Surg 2006; 244(3): 363-70.
[http://dx.doi.org/10.1097/01.sla.0000234647.03466.27] [PMID: 16926562]

[49]   Craig R, Deeley A. Anaesthesia for pyloromyotomy. BJA Educ 2018; 18(6): 173-7.
[http://dx.doi.org/10.1016/j.bjae.2018.03.001] [PMID: 33456829]

[50]   Lansdale N, Al-Khafaji N, Green P, Kenny SE. Population-level surgical outcomes for infantile hypertrophic pyloric stenosis. J Pediatr Surg 2018; 53(3): 540-4.
[http://dx.doi.org/10.1016/j.jpedsurg.2017.05.018] [PMID: 28576429]

[51]   Kethman WC, Harris AHS, Hawn MT, Wall JK. Trends and surgical outcomes of laparoscopic *versus* open pyloromyotomy. Surg Endosc 2018; 32(7): 3380-5.
[http://dx.doi.org/10.1007/s00464-018-6060-0] [PMID: 29340829]

[52]   Lemoine C, Paris C, Morris M, Vali K, Beaunoyer M, Aspirot A. Open transumbilical pyloromyotomy: is it more painful than the laparoscopic approach? J Pediatr Surg 2011; 46(5): 870-3.
[http://dx.doi.org/10.1016/j.jpedsurg.2011.02.019] [PMID: 21616243]

[53]   Mitchell RB, Archer SM, Ishman SL, *et al.* Clinical Practice Guideline: Tonsillectomy in Children (Update). Otolaryngol Head Neck Surg 2019; 160(1_suppl) (Suppl.): S1-S42.
[http://dx.doi.org/10.1177/0194599818801757] [PMID: 30798778]

[54]   Brown KA, Laferrière A, Moss IR. Recurrent hypoxemia in young children with obstructive sleep apnea is associated with reduced opioid requirement for analgesia. Anesthesiology 2004; 100(4): 806-10.
[http://dx.doi.org/10.1097/00000542-200404000-00009] [PMID: 15087614]

[55]   Cardwell M, Siviter G, Smith A. Non-steroidal anti-inflammatory drugs and perioperative bleeding in paediatric tonsillectomy. Cochrane Database Syst Rev 2005; (2): CD003591
[PMID: 15846670]

[56]   Olutoye OA, Glover CD, Diefenderfer JW, *et al.* The effect of intraoperative dexmedetomidine on postoperative analgesia and sedation in pediatric patients undergoing tonsillectomy and adenoidectomy. Anesth Analg 2010; 111(2): 490-5.
[http://dx.doi.org/10.1213/ANE.0b013e3181e33429] [PMID: 20610555]

SUBJECT INDEX

A

Abdominal trauma 202, 229
Abnormalities 53, 93, 135, 143, 248
  cardiac 53, 143
  craniofacial 135
  syndromic 248
Abnormal pulmonary function tests 131
ACE inhibitors 53
Acetaminophen toxicity 41
Acetylcholinesterase 33, 34, 223
  inhibitors 33, 34, 223
Acid 40, 52, 56, 260
  arachidonic 40
  ethacrynic 56
  glycyrrhizic 52
  lactic 260
Acidosis 7, 33, 46, 47, 53, 131, 132, 133, 156,
  162, 260, 296, 303
  concomitant 46
  hypochloremic 260
  lactic 47
Acids, amino 10
Adenoidectomy 134, 166, 322, 323, 324, 333,
  362, 369, 370
ADH 49, 50, 55
  production 50
  secretion 49, 55
Age, postmenstrual 368
Agents 39, 40, 42, 53, 150, 152, 218, 219,
  226, 228, 264, 278, 294, 296, 322, 328,
  352
  anticholinergic 42
  anti-cytokine 296
  antiepileptic 150
  anti-inflammatory 40
  hypnotic 264
  prebiotic 296
  sedative-hypnotic 39
  vasodilating 352
Air 64, 66, 72, 75, 83, 84, 124, 197, 217, 229,
  263, 297, 369

aspiration 83
  gastric 72
Airway 3, 167, 184, 190, 195, 199, 262, 268,
  331, 349, 354, 355, 356
  abnormalities 199, 349
  assessment 268
  compromise 262, 356
  devices 184, 331, 349, 354, 355
  emergency 262
  resistance 3
  secretions 167, 190
  techniques 184, 195
  trauma 195
Alcohol dehydrogenase 21
Algorithm 171, 172, 205, 213, 331
  laryngospasm treatment 331
Allergic reactions 107, 221, 222, 246
  systemic 246
Amide hydrolysis 39
Aminoglycosides 33
Amnesia 28, 82, 117, 223
  temporary anterograde 117
Analgesia 29, 31, 35, 37, 41, 43, 82, 118, 123,
  307, 309, 366, 369, 370
  opioid 366
  spinal 35
Analgesic properties 31, 231
Anemia 9, 97, 109, 115, 130, 132, 170, 274,
  294, 327
  sickle cell 115
  in premature infants 130
Anesthesia 108, 114, 170, 348, 365
  cardiac 114
  genetic 108
  spinal 170, 365
Anesthesia 8, 157, 163, 238, 239, 350, 369
  care 238, 350
  gas 163
  history 157
  induction 8, 369
  -related cardiac arrest 239

Bharathi Gourkanti, Irwin Gratz, Grace Dippo, Nathalie Peiris and Dinesh K. Choudhry (Eds.)
All rights reserved-© 2022 Bentham Science Publishers

Made in the USA
Las Vegas, NV
11 May 2024

89790607R10240